Women, Children and Addiction

This proposed book draws on the expertise of 35 experts in the field of Addiction Medicine to provide the reader with a current and comprehensive view of addiction as related to women, pregnancy, newborns, infants and children. The volume begins by placing current attitudes towards addicted women in a historical context, and continues with contributions on the relationship of gender to substance abuse research, addiction as a general health issue in women, and ethical dilemmas faced when approaching drug use during pregnancy.

The volume discusses high-risk pregnancies and HIV infection related to maternal drug abuse. It details specific pharmacotherapy such as methadone and buprenorphine, and assesses society's punitive view toward illicit drug-using women. Finally, the book describes outcomes of newborns, infants and children born following intrauterine drug exposure.

Health providers in many related disciplines, specialists in Addiction Medicine, social workers and ethicists are among those who will gain insight into the complex interdisciplinary matrix of abuse in women, its unique relationship to pregnancy, and its impact on drug-exposed children.

This book was published as a special issue in the *Journal of Addictive Diseases.*

Loretta P. Finnegan is President of Finnegan Consulting which addresses education, research, and treatment in issues relating to women's health and perinatal addiction. She is a retired Professor of Pediatrics, Psychiatry and Human Behavior, Thomas Jefferson University, Philadelphia, PA and Former Senior Advisor on Women's Issues, National Institute on Drug Abuse. NIH, DHHS, Bethesda, Maryland. Dr. Finnegan is recognized nationally and internationally as an expert in these fields and credited with the development of an assessment tool for neonatal opioid abstinence which is used widely in neonatal intensive care units in this country and abroad. Dr. Finnegan developed a landmark program which provided comprehensive services for drug dependent women and their children. She has authored or co-authored 170 articles and book chapters and lectured throughout the United States and in many international settings to disseminate her clinical and research knowledge in women's health and perinatal addiction.

Stephen R. Kandall is the former Chief of Neonatology at Beth Israel Medical Center in New York and Professor of Pediatrics at the Albert Einstein College of Medicine. He has published over 70 articles and book chapters on perinatal addiction, authored a history of women and addiction in the United States, *Substance and Shadow* (Harvard University Press, 1996), lectured widely nationally and internationally, and served on a number of national panels related to perinatal addiction. He currently serves on the Board of the North Carolina March of Dimes and a number of state legislative committees in North Carolina.

Women, Children and Addiction

Edited by

Loretta P. Finnegan and Stephen R. Kandall

Routledge
Taylor & Francis Group
LONDON AND NEW YORK

First published 2011
by Routledge
2 Park Square, Milton Park, Abingdon, Oxon, OX14 4RN

Simultaneously published in the USA and Canada
by Routledge
605 Third Avenue, New York, NY 10017

Routledge is an imprint of the Taylor & Francis Group, an informa business

This book is a reproduction of the *Journal of Addictive Diseases*, vol. 29, issue 2. The Publisher requests to those authors who may be citing this book to state, also, the bibliographical details of the special issue on which the book was based.

Typeset in Times by Taylor & Francis Books

British Library Cataloguing in Publication Data
A catalogue record for this book is available from the British Library

ISBN 13: 978-0-415-60103-0 (hbk)

Disclaimer
The publisher would like to make readers aware that the chapters in this book are referred to as articles as they had been in the special issue. The publisher accepts responsibility for any inconsistencies that may have arisen in the course of preparing this volume for print.

Contents

Notes on Contributors vii

1. **Introduction to Women, Children and Addiction**
Loretta P. Finnegan 1

2. **Women and Drug Addiction: A Historical Perspective**
Stephen R. Kandall 5

3. **Women and Addiction: The Importance of Gender Issues in Substance Abuse Research**
Ellen Tuchman 15

4. **Substance Use and Women's Health**
Abigail Kay, *Trusandra E. Taylor*, *Andrea G. Barthwell*, *Jana Wichelecki*, and *Vera Leopold* 27

5. **Ethical Issues and Addiction**
Binta Lambert, *Melissa Scheiner*, and *Deborah Campbell* 52

6. **Addiction in Pregnancy**
Joan Keegan, *Mehdi Parva*, *Mark Finnegan*, *Andrew Gerson*, and *Michael Belden* 63

7. **Human Immunodeficiency Virus Risk Behavior Among Female Substance Abusers**
Susan E. Ramsey, *Kathryn M. Bell*, and *Patricia A. Engler* 80

8. **Pharmacotherapy in the Treatment of Addiction: Methadone**
Mary Jeanne Kreek, *Lisa Borg*, *Elizabeth Ducat*, and *Brenda Ray* 88

9. **Gender Issues in the Pharmacotherapy of Opioid-Addicted Women: Buprenorphine**
Annemarie Unger, *Erika Jung*, *Bernadette Winklbaur*, and *Gabriele Fischer* 105

10. **Punishing Pregnant Drug-Using Women: Defying Law, Medicine, and Common Sense**
Jeanne Flavin and *Lynn M. Paltrow* 119

11. **Prenatal Drug Exposure: Infant and Toddler Outcomes**
Emmalee S. Bandstra, *Connie E. Morrow*, *Elana Mansoor*, and *Veronica H. Accornero* 133

12. **Children of Addicted Women**
Barry M. Lester and *Linda L. Lagasse* 147

Index 165

Notes on Contributors

Emmalee S. Bandstra, **Connie E. Morrow**, **Elana Mansoor**, and **Veronica H. Accornero** are affiliated with the University of Miami Miller School of Medicine, Department of Pediatrics, Miami, FL.

Andrea G. Barthwell is affiliated with EMGlobal, LLC, Arlington, VA.

Loretta P. Finnegan is affiliated with Finnegan Consulting, LLC, Avalon, New Jersey.

Jeanne Flavin is affiliated with the Department of Sociology and Anthropology, Fordham University, Bronx, NY.

Andrew Gerson and **Michael Belden** are affiliated with Thomas Jefferson University, Philadelphia, PA.

Stephen R. Kandall is Retired Professor of Pediatrics, Albert Einstein College of Medicine, Bronx, NY.

Abigail Kay is affiliated with the Department of Psychiatry and Human Behavior–Division of Substance Abuse, Medical Director N.A.R.P., Thomas Jefferson University Hospital, Philadelphia, PA.

Joan Keegan, **Mehdi Parva**, **Mark Finnegan**, and **Andrew Gerson** are affiliated with the Lankenau Hospital, Wynnewood, PA.

Mary Jeanne Kreek, **Lisa Borg**, **Elizabeth Ducat**, and **Brenda Ray** are affiliated with the Laboratory of the Biology of Addictive Diseases, The Rockefeller University, New York, NY.

Binta Lambert, **Melissa Scheiner**, and **Deborah Campbell** are affiliated with Albert Einstein College of Medicine, Bronx, NY.

Barry M. Lester and **Linda L. Lagasse** are affiliated with Brown Center for the Study of Children at Risk, The Warren Alpert Medical School of Brown University, Women and Infants Hospital of Rhode Island, Providence, RI.

Lynn M. Paltrow is affiliated with National Advocates for Pregnant Women, New York, NY.

Susan E. Ramsey, **Kathryn M. Bell**, and **Patricia A. Engler** are affiliated with The Warren Alpert Medical School of Brown University, Providence, RI.

Trusandra E. Taylor is affiliated with JEVS Human Services, Philadelphia, PA.

Ellen Tuchman is affiliated with the Silver School of Social Work, New York University, New York, NY.

Annemarie Unger, **Erika Jung**, **Bernadette Winklbaur**, and **Gabriele Fischer** are affiliated with Medical University of Vienna, Department of Psychiatry and Psychotherapy, Vienna, Austria.

Jana Wichelecki and **Vera Leopold** are affiliated with Human Resources Development Institute, Inc., Chicago, IL.

Introduction to Women, Children and Addiction

Loretta P. Finnegan, MD, LLD (Hon), ScD (Hon)

Addiction in women is a major public health problem. Approximately 90% of women using drugs are of reproductive age.[1] Societal moral attitudes have stigmatized and dehumanized women who are drug-dependent, particularly those who become pregnant.[2] As a result, barriers exist for women who are addicted to drugs when they attempt to obtain optimal and appropriate medical and obstetrical care, as well as gender-specific services for their addiction. These barriers apply to women of all races and socioeconomic status. The best public health result can be obtained once these barriers have been removed, allowing women to find appropriate services in supportive, multidimensional treatment facilities for themselves and their children.[3] Much has been learned over the past several decades from research in the field of drug dependence, but continued attention to evidence-based studies is essential to provide the best possible care for women who are addicted, to determine the intricacies of neonatal abstinence syndrome, and to assess the overall immediate and long-term effects of in utero drug exposure. To delineate the multi-factorial aspects of addiction in women and the effects of in utero exposure, it will take many more dedicated researchers and a large funding commitment by government agencies and private foundations.

This supplement will address the major effects of addiction in women and the impact of in utero exposure on their infants and children. Commencing with the history of addiction in women, documents show that female addiction is not a new phenomenon in America, but rather has existed for more than 150 years and was "the result of inappropriate overmedication practices by physicians and pharmacists, media manipulation, or the woman's own attempts to cope with social or occupational barriers preventing equality and self-fulfillment."[2] One could look at current societal mores and practices and see that history truly repeats itself.

Epidemiological and clinical research has indicated that predictors for and progression to drug abuse and dependence are often gender-specific or gender-sensitive. Differences between men and women have been identified in evidence-based studies examining the epidemiology of drug abuse, biological and subjective responses to drugs, patterns of use, progression from use to dependence, gender differences in medical consequences of drug addiction, concomitant psychiatric disorders with drug use, victimization and violence against women, midlife and older women, specific barriers to entry, retention, and completion of treatment.[4,5] In contrast to men, women have a higher vulnerability to the adverse consequences of addiction, show a more rapid progression to entry into treatment despite fewer years of active illicit drug abuse; however, they are underrepresented in addiction treatment.[6]

Significant to women addicted to alcohol, nicotine, opioids or stimulants is the tremendous effect on their health. The medical literature clearly indicates that women progress more rapidly than men into addiction to alcohol and other drugs with the development of serious health consequences. Numerous medical complications occur as a result of addiction in women, including hepatitis, cirrhosis, cardiovascular disease, diabetes mellitus, osteoporosis, lung, breast and endometrial cancer, chronic obstructive pulmonary disease, infections, neurological dysfunctions, and HIV/AIDS.[3]

Drug use during pregnancy is a major risk factor for maternal morbidity and neonatal complications. To normalize the pregnancy and protect the unborn fetus, considerable challenges exist with regard to identification, assessment, and treatment of woman who addicted while pregnant. The numerous medical and psychosocial complications listed above are compounded during pregnancy with the risk of preterm birth, intrauterine growth restriction, and placental accidents. Infants born to women who are addicted have a higher incidence of morbidity and mortality as a result of prematurity, infection, neonatal abstinence syndrome, and the development of potentially lethal fetal anomalies due to some exposures (i.e., alcohol). Unfortunately, drug abuse treatment providers frequently do not have the facilities or the obstetrical staff available to provide the specialized services that the woman who are addicted while pregnant requires. Pregnancy is an opportune time for women and treatment staff to encourage the woman to seek recovery from an addictive lifestyle.[7] Both the health care and lay communities need to advocate for the ethical, moral, and just treatment of pregnant women who are addicted and their children.

Women who are addicted contribute to the incidence of HIV infection as a result of their risky behaviors as a result of their injection practices and because of increased engagement in high-risk sexual behaviors. During pregnancy, HIV infection confers the added risk of perinatal transmission, and this transmission accounts for nearly all new HIV infections in children.[8] Screening, risk reduction interventions, and treatment of the mother and infant represent the current approach to HIV-infected dyads. More specific risk reduction interventions for women are greatly needed.

Medication-assisted treatment has been instituted and used over the past 40 years. Numerous studies have reported on the efficacy, drug-drug interaction, side effects, and dosing issues regarding methadone. Basic clinical research addressing the molecular neurobiological aspects of opiate addiction, as well as human molecular genetic studies by Kreek et al.[9] and Kreek,[10] have found few differences between males and females. Although women have a different opioid binding capacity than men that will influence dosing regimens in opioid pharmacotherapy,[11] both pregnant and non-pregnant women have been successfully treated with methadone.

In recent years in the United States, buprenorphine has been approved for use in medication-assisted treatment in men and non-pregnant women. Buprenorphine has been shown to be well tolerated, and due to its partial agonist properties appears to be a safe therapeutic agent, especially because severe side effects such as respiratory depression develop only with severe over-dosing. It is clinically and scientifically desirable to have treatment options when selecting medication-assisted treatment for opioid dependent individuals.[12,13]

Although there has been considerable controversy concerning the use of methadone in pregnancy, it remains both the medication of choice and the standard treatment in the United States. Many studies suggesting that lower methadone doses in pregnancy decrease the incidence and severity of neonatal abstinence have been criticized due to poor research designs and confounding variables. More recent studies have demonstrated that dose is probably not related to the incidence or severity of neonatal methadone abstinence.[14] During pregnancy, significantly more benefits have been identified than risks when methadone and comprehensive services are provided. The main risk is the incidence of neonatal abstinence in 60% of the neonates exposed, equal to that of heroin but with less overall morbidity for the infant.[15]Some studies show that neonatal abstinence in infants exposed to buprenorphine may be less severe than that seen with methadone.[16] Numerous studies in the United States and in Europe have shown the usefulness of buprenorphine in pregnant women; however, we await results from the international MOTHER Study to further support its efficacy and safety in the perinatal period.[17]

Of great concern to many in the medical and legal professions is the practice of punishing or prosecuting pregnant women using drugs in several areas of the United States. The plight of the pregnant women who are drug dependent can best be stated by Flavin and Paltrow within their section of the current supplement:

> The arrests, detentions, prosecutions and other legal actions taken against drug-dependent pregnant women distract attention from significant social problems such as our lack of universal health care, the dearth of policies to support pregnant and parenting women, the absence of social supports for children, and the overall failure of the drug war. The attempts to "protect the fetus" undertaken through the criminal justice system (as well as in family and drug courts) actually undermine maternal and fetal health and discourage attempts to identify and implement effective strategies for addressing the needs of pregnant drug using women and their families.

Some of the flawed premises on which these arrests, detentions, and prosecutions are based are exposed in their section; the issues viewed through legal, moral, and ethical lenses broaden this volume's perspective.

One of the areas in the field of addiction that may evoke a great deal of emotion, controversy, and even anger is the relationship of prenatal drug exposure to the outcome of exposed infants and children. Numerous studies of animals and humans have reported the potential adverse effects on infants and children; however, many have not considered the confounding effects of multiple drugs (licit and illicit) as well as the environment to which the child is exposed. It is acknowledged that some drugs, such as alcohol, are teratogenic; however, the negative impact that nicotine may have on the developing fetus and the child are frequently discounted by the lay public.

After careful research designs were implemented, illicit drugs that had been considered seriously harmful to the offspring are now considered to have only subtle effects. Cocaine and opioids have the potential to affect growth at birth and in the toddler years. In contrast to opioids, which have a high incidence of neonatal abstinence and infant neurobehavioral deficits, prenatal cocaine exposure appears to be associated with subtle decrements in neurobehavioral, cognitive, and language function.[18–20]

In older children, numerous studies have cited the effects of prenatal cocaine exposure to include behavior problems and attention, language, and cognition deficits. Follow-up studies of children exposed to opioid (mostly methadone exposed), many that dealt with small numbers of participants, have been unable to adequately control for separate potentially confounding variables. In older children, studies report school behavior problems, disruptive behavior, and a diagnosis of ADHD.[21] Generally, no differences in children exposed to opioid have been noted on cognitive tests in contrast to comparison groups. However, one important issue in the long-term follow-up of these children is that they grow up in high risk environments. Similar learning and behavior problems have been reported in school-age children not only exposed to drugs in utero,[22] but also those living with drug-dependent parents who didn't have intrauterine exposure.[23,24] A key issue to consider in reporting the outcomes of infants and children is that the children and their families, as well as society in general, would be well served by providing appropriate prevention and intervention services to address the unique needs of drug-abusing pregnant and postpartum women and the developing fetus. These models of treatment have been described in the literature and many currently exist throughout major cities in the United States and abroad.[25] Unfortunately, not enough comprehensive services exist to meet the current needs of the vast population of women and children suffering from the disease of addiction.

This compilation of articles on women and children and addiction will provide the reader with up-to-date information prepared by clinicians and scientists who have had extensive clinical experiences and who have done some of the seminal research in this field. The areas covered include historical accounts, the importance of gender, health of the women including HIV risk behaviors and incidence, ethical issues, pregnancy, medication-assisted treatment with methadone and buprenorphine, society's need to punish women who are addicted and pregnant, and infant and toddler outcomes should provide the reader with an excellent background to deal with the effects of addiction on women and children. Finally, we must strive for excellence in research and in the clinical care of women and children afflicted by addiction. Government agencies and private foundations must recognize their responsibility to provide adequate funding to provide the appropriate and unique services and the needed research for women who are dependent on drugs and their children. Only if this responsibility is taken seriously will this country be able to cope with the pathophysiological and behavioral effects seen in women and children as a result of addiction.

REFERENCES

1. Kuczkowski K. The effects of drug abuse on pregnancy. Current Opinion in Obstetrics and Gynecology 2007; 19:578–85.

2. Kandall SR. Substance and shadow: women and addiction in the United States. Cambridge, MA: Harvard University Press, 1996.

3. Finnegan LP, Hagan T, Kaltenbach K. Opioid dependence: scientific foundations for clinical practice, pregnancy and substance abuse: perspectives and directions. Proceedings of the New York Academy of Medicine 1991; 67:223–39.

4. Wetherington CL. Sex-gender differences in drug abuse: a shift in the burden of proof? Exp and Clin Psychopharmacol 2007; 15:411–7.

5. Brady KT, Randall CL. Gender differences in substance use disorders. Psychiatr Clin North Am 1999; 22:241–52.

6. Hernandez-Avila C, Rounsaville B, Kranzler H. Opioid-, cannabis- and alcohol-dependent women show more rapid progression to substance abuse treatment. Drug and Alcohol Dependence 2004; 74:265–72.

7. Hagan TA, Finnegan LP, Nelson-Zlupko L. Impediments to comprehensive treatment models for substance-dependent women: treatment and research questions. Journal of Psychoactive Drugs 1994; 26:163–71.

8. Centers for Disease Control. HIV/AIDS surveillance report. [8]. 1996.

9. Kreek MJ, Bart G, Lilly C, LaForge KS, Nielsen DA. Pharmacogenetics and human molecular genetics of opiate and cocaine addictions and their treatments. Pharmacol Rev 2005; 57:1–26.

10. Kreek MJ. The role of qualitative and quantitative analysis of drugs and their metabolites in maternal-neonatal studies. In: National Institute on Drug Abuse Symposium on Comprehensive Health Care for Addicted Families and Their Children, Washington, DC: Services Research Report (USGPO), #017-024-00598-3, 1977: 67–73.

11. Zubieta JK, Dannals RF, Frost JJ. Gender and age differences on human brain mu-opioid receptor binding measured by PET. Am J Psychiatry 1999; 156: 842–8.

12. Johnson RE, Eissenberg T, Stitzer ML, Strain EC, Liebson IA, Gibelow GE. Buprenorphine treatment of opioid dependence: clinical trial of daily versus alternate-day dosing. Drug Alcohol Depend 1995; 40:27–35.

13. Fischer G, Johnson RE, Eder H, et al. Treatment of opioid-dependent pregnant women with buprenorphine. Addiction 2000; 95:239–44.

14. Berghella V, Lim PJ, Hill MK, Cerpes J, Chennat J, Kaltenbach K. Maternal methadone dose and neonatal withdrawal. Am J Obstet Gynecol 2003; 189: 312–7.

15. Finnegan LP, Kaltenbach K. 1992, Neonatal abstinence syndrome. In: Hoeckelman RA, Nelson NM, eds. Primary pediatric care (2nd ed.). St. Louis: Mosby Year Book Inc., 1991: 1367–78.

16. Jones HE, Johnson RE, Jasinski DR, et al. Buprenorphine versus methadone in the treatment of pregnant opioid-dependent patients: effects on the neonatal abstinence syndrome. Drug and Alcohol Dependence 2005; 79:1–10.

17. Jones HE, Arria AM, Baewert A, Heil SH, Kaltenbach K, Martin PR, Coyle MG, Selby P, Stine SM. Evolution and innovation in the agonist treatment of opioid-dependent pregnant women: development of a multi-center randomized controlled clinical trial maintenance in the addictions. Journal of Opioid Management, in press.

18. Weiner SM, Finnegan LP. Drug withdrawal in the neonate. In: Carter B and Gardner S, eds. Handbook of neonatal intensive care (6th ed.). St. Louis: Mosby-Year Book, Inc., 2009.

19. Bandstra ES, Accornero VH. Infants of substance abusing mothers. In Fanaroff and Martin, eds. Neonatal-perinatal medicine: diseases of the fetus and infant (8th ed., vol. 1). Philadelphia: Elsevier Mosby, 2006:733–57.

20. Bauer CR, Shankaran S, Bada H, et al. The maternal lifestyle study (MLS): drug exposure during pregnancy and short-term maternal outcomes. Am J Obstet Gynecol 2002; 186:487–95.

21. Hans SL. Prenatal drug exposure: behavioral functioning in late childhood and adolescence. NIDA Res Monogr 1996; 164:261–76.

22. Olofsson M, Buckley W, Andersen GE, Friis-Hansen B. Investigation of 89 children born by drug-dependent mothers. II. Follow-up 1-10 years after birth. Acta Paediatr Scand 1983; 72:407–10.

23. Hejanic B, Barredo V, Hejanic M, Tomelleri C. Children of heroin addicts. The International Journal of the Addictions 1979; 14:919–31.

24. Nichtem S. The children of drug users. Journal of the American Academy of Child Psychiatry 1973; 12:24–31.

25. Finnegan LP. ed. Treatment services for substance abusing women. National Institute on Drug Abuse Research Monograph Series. Washington, DC: U.S. Government Printing Office, 1997.

Women and Drug Addiction: A Historical Perspective

Stephen R. Kandall, MD

ABSTRACT. The history of women and addiction in America extends back more than 150 years. Although the true epidemiology of women and addiction has always been difficult to determine, the spectrum of female addicts extends well beyond those women who make sensationalistic headlines by "abandoning" or "battering" their children. Historically, female addiction has been largely the result of inappropriate overmedication practices by physicians and pharmacists, media manipulation, or individuals own attempts to cope with social or occupational barriers preventing equality and self-fulfillment. From the mid-nineteenth century, uneasy tolerance, social ostracism, vilification, persecution, and legal prosecution have grudgingly, but not completely, given way to more humane treatment opportunities in the setting of more enlightened comprehensive care.

INTRODUCTION

Although the crescendo of media coverage surrounding heroin-related crime in the 1960s and 1970s followed by the sensationalistic treatment of the "crack epidemic" may have suggested that America was fighting its first "war on drugs," the problem of uncontrolled and illicit use of addicting drugs has existed in America for more than 150 years.[1]

Legal use of opiates, such as reliance on gum opium by colonial militias, dates back to the Revolutionary War. However, drug use in America was first acknowledged to be a "problem" in the mid-nineteenth century. During that period, increased use of narcotics could be attributed primarily to the fact that physicians had a limited ability to treat patients pharmacologically, resorting to opiates as a mainstay of their pharmaceutical armamentarium. Opiates were used to treat a wide variety of conditions, such as hiccoughs, neuralgias, alcoholism, chronic respiratory disorders, malaria, syphilis, rheumatism, insomnia, anxiety, and fatigue.[2] Because opiates reduce intestinal motility, they were widely prescribed during cholera outbreaks in 1832–1833 and 1848–1854 and dysentery in 1847–1851. During the Civil War, approximately ten million opium pills and 2.8 million ounces of opium tinctures and powders were distributed to Union forces alone; many wounded veterans became dependent on opiates to soothe painful and inadequately treated wounds.[3]

In addition to medicinal use, recreational opium use found its way to America in the mid-nineteenth century. The Opium Wars of 1839–1842 and 1856–1860, launched by Great Britain to force China to accept opium into their country to offset a trade imbalance created by the British thirst for Chinese tea, opened the world market to China. In addition, large numbers of Chinese workers immigrated to America to help its westward expansion. Difficult working conditions drove those immigrants to opium dens for gambling, prostitution, and drugs; during this period an estimated 20% to 25% of Chinese workers in America smoked opium.[4] Although contacts between Chinese and Whites were initially limited, transfer of opium from Chinese to Whites began to occur after 1870, primarily through underworld contacts. All of these factors contributed to the seven-fold increase in opiate use in the general population from less than 1 per 1,000 in 1842 to approximately 5 per 1,000 in the 1890s.[5]

The end of the nineteenth century also saw a dramatic increase in cocaine use. Although a raw, impure form of cocaine had been chewed in Peru and Bolivia for more than 5,000 years, its origins in America can be traced to the late 1870s, when cocaine found wide acceptance as a topical anesthetic, especially in ophthalmic surgery, and even wider (and often inappropriate) medical application as a stimulant, in treatment of "wasting diseases," dyspepsia, typhoid fever, kidney disease, hay fever, colds, and sinus conditions.[6] After the 1880s, E. R. Squibb and Company, McKesson and Robbins, and Parke-Davis all marketed cocaine to meet the growing demand in America. In addition, cocaine-laced products were widely available in a vast array of "commercial folk medicines," home remedies, and tonics. In addition to the growing problem of opiates and cocaine, the use of ether, chloroform, and chloral hydrate were all considered fashionable during the end of the nineteenth century.[7]

Although modern culture has tended to view addiction as a "men's issue," the use and abuse of addicting substances by women is inextricably woven into this history and dates back to the earliest days of this country. Through the mid- to late nineteenth century, drug use increased more rapidly by women than men; by the end of the nineteenth century, approximately two-thirds to three-quarters of the opium addicts, as well as significant numbers of users of cocaine, chloroform, and cannabis, were women.[8-10]

The most important reason for the increase in opiate consumption among mid- to late nineteenth-century women, as with men, was the prescribing and dispensing of legal opiates by physicians and pharmacists. Victorian women were considered less capable of managing painful disorders and thus more in need of medication. R.V. Pierce, who built a huge business based on opiate-laden medications, advised that when woman, "the last and crowning handiwork of God . . . is disturbed by disease, when the nicely-adjusted balance of her complex nature deviates from its true and intended poise . . . its importance should elicit . . . the scientific administration of the choicest, rarest, and purest medicinal elements in the whole range of nature" (p. 684).[11]

The most common conditions for which women were medicated with opiates were "female problems."[12,13] In 1879, Dr. T. Gaillard Thomas, President of the American Gynecological Society, wrote: "For the relief of pain, the treatment is all summed up in one word, and that is *opium*. This divine drug overshadows all other anodynes. . . .you can easily educate her to become an *opium-eater*" (p. 316).[14] R. V. Pierce offered pages of testimonials from satisfied women who had used his patent medications for conditions such as "falling of the womb" (p. 733), "paralysis and uterine disease" (p. 737), " indigestion, constipation, and uterine disease"(p. 737), "female weakness" (p. 739), "severe flowing" (p. 741), "vaginitis" (p. 744), and "suppressed menstruation and nervous disability" (p. 746).[15] As late as 1913, women who suffered from painful menstruation were counseled that "paregoric, laudanum, etc. is a specific" (p. 724).[16]

Women were also widely treated for "neurasthenia," or "nervous weakness,' a vague disorder which encompassed an enormous spectrum of real and imagined symptoms, including tenderness of the scalp, spine and body; vague pains and "flying neuralgias"; flushing and fidgitiness; variability of pulse and palpitations; strength giving out or legs giving way; sensitivity to hot or cold water; sensitivity to weather changes; ticklishness; insomnia; nervous dyspepsia; partial memory failure; sexual exhaustion; depression and morbid fears; headache; pain and heaviness; floating specks before the eyes; noises in the ears; and chills and hot flashes.[17,18] As an 1886 medical textbook explained: "To women of the higher classes, ennuyée and tormented with neuralgias or the vague pains of hysteria and hypochondriasis, opium brings tranquility and self-forgetfulness" (p. 649).[19]

In addition to opiates, cocaine was also used to treat women for neurasthenia. In his *History of Coca,* W. Golden Mortimer, acknowledging that sufferers of this condition were more often women, noted that among physicians "fully one-half of those who went into detail advocated the use of Coca . . . " (p. 390) as the most beneficial treatment.[20] Cocaine was also used extensively to treat a range of gynecological complaints, including painful intercourse, cervical endometritis, urethral irritation, dysmenorrhea, and cervical lacerations following childbirth.

In addition to medical uses, cocaine was used recreationally by women of all social classes. Along with well-documented reports of use by women of privileged classes, reports can be found of "cocaine debauchery," raids on cocaine joints frequented by "lower classes of fallen women" and "lower class prostitutes, black as well as white" (pp. 464–5).[21]

Hypnotics, such as ether, chloroform, and chloral hydrate were also widely prescribed for women. Chloroform, first used as an anesthetic in the 1840s, came into wider use in treating nervous headaches and "trifling ailments."[22] Similar to opiates and cocaine, chloroform was marketed in many patent remedies such as Shilo's Consumptive Cure, King's New Discovery, and Edison's Polyform, as well as liniments. By the 1850s, chloroform had already found use as a non-medicinal agent. An undercover female reporter for the *New York Herald* wrote in 1894 that a doctor advised her "there was probably no form of disease where the gas had been so beneficial as in nervous troubles of all descriptions" (p. 681). In 1901, *The Boston Globe* reported that upper-class women were flocking to "oxygen parties," at which they inhaled a nitrous oxide mixture to liven up the festivities.[23] Finally, chloral hydrate could be easily purchased and by 1872, a physician noted that the drug enjoyed wide use among "school teachers, bookkeepers [and] invalid women made weaker by family cares" (p. 525). In addition, he found that "in obstetric practice, many physicians have used chloral hydrate with the happiest effect" (p. 525).[24]

During the mid- to late nineteenth century, words of caution regarding the dangers of drug use were issued by responsible physicians, and drug use was frowned on by many. However, the relatively benign approach that society as a whole took regarding drug use in women was predicated largely on the prevailing stereotype of the woman who used drugs. Although, in reality, the spectrum of female drug use was broad and spanned all socioeconomic strata of society, women who used drugs tended to be portrayed as genteel, southern, White, upper-middle class women, whose addiction "problems" tended to be family-centered rather than posing a danger to society. Such prototypes made their loosely fictionalized appearances in characters such as Helen Matthews in Maria Weed's 1895 novel, *A Voice in the Wilderness*, and better known figures such as Lily Bart, the chloral hydrate addict in Edith Wharton's 1905 novel, *The House of Mirth*, and later opium addicts such as Mary Tyrone in Eugene O'Neill's *Long Day's Journey into Night* and Mrs. Henry Lafayette Dubose in Harper Lee's *To Kill a Mockingbird.*

Although drug use by women was readily acknowledged to be widespread, the fact that the majority of them had become addicted through the misuse and overuse of legal but addicting substances suggested that they posed no immediate threat to society and, as such, did not incite sentiment for anti-drug legislation. The fact that anti-drug legislation in America experienced an upsurge between 1876 and 1920 is explained by dramatic changes in the sociodemographics of drug use in this country. As drug use patterns changed predominantly from female to male, White to minority, southern rural to northern urban, and wealthy to poor (in other words, from mainstream to deviant) it became easier to mobilize America in a campaign to eradicate drug use. Following passage of the first anti-opium legislation in San Francisco in 1875, which was intended to keep Whites from frequenting Chinese opium dens, similar laws were passed in Virginia City, Nevada, in 1876 and in New York State in 1882. National anti-drug legislation was unsuccessfully introduced in Congress in 1880 and 1884, but by 1912 every state except Delaware and many American cities had passed ordinances against opiates, cocaine, or both. In 1906, Congress passed the Pure Food and Drug Act, which exerted a measure of control over the production and sale of patent medicines. In 1914, Congress passed the Harrison Anti-Narcotic Act, which, although subject to interpretation, led to a hard-line anti-drug approach by the U.S. government following two 1919 Supreme Court decisions. In *U.S. v. Doremus,* the Supreme Court ruled that the Harrison Act was constitutional, and in *Webb et al. v. U.S.*, the Supreme Court ruled that physicians could not prescribe narcotics solely for addiction maintenance. These legislative and legal actions ushered in the repressive approach to drug control that has characterized the country's stance toward drug use for approximately 100 years.

As suggested, much of the early anti-drug legislation passed in the United States was intended to counter the growing social and economic threats posed by emerging minorities such as Asian immigrants or African Americans. To advance this initiative, women began to be portrayed as helpless targets of drug-crazed, sexually predatory minority men. The sensationalistic Hearst-dominated lay press frequently ran stories about women lured into prostitution through Chinese opium dens or the White slave trade. San Francisco authorities feared that "many women and young girls ... were being introduced to visit the dens, where they were being ruined morally and otherwise" (p. 1).[25] Hamilton Wright, one of the architects of our formative drug policy, was extremely concerned about opium and "the large numbers of women who have become involved and were living as common-law wives or cohabitating with Chinese in the Chinatowns of our various cities" (p. 44).[26] In response to the increasing use of cocaine by southern African American men, testimony was offered before the U.S. House of Representatives in 1910 that its use was involved in "a great many of the southern rape cases" (p. 93).[27] In the 1930s, Harry Anslinger, head of the Federal Bureau of Narcotics, advanced his anti-marijuana agenda with the warning that "it would be well for law-enforcement officers everywhere to search for marijuana behind cases of criminal and sex assault."[28]

Once drug use was essentially criminalized after the Harrison Act and the two 1919 Supreme Court decisions, addicted women were forced to support their drug habits as best they could. Women of the "smart chic set" could maintain their drug habits in private clinics or with the help of personal physicians. Sanitaria, however, which had been in existence since the late nineteenth century, numbering about 100 by 1910, had largely closed following exposure of their unsuccessful results by physicians and the press. Most famous of these sanitaria were the John Harvey Kellogg clinic in Battle Creek, Michigan, and the national chain of Keeley Institutes, which by 1892-1893 were treating approximately 15,000 addicts and were not finally closed until 1920.

Although some women found help, many more without means were forced into the shadowy margins of society, using prostitution and crime to support their drug habits. When it was realized that a large number of addicts had been suddenly forced on to the streets without any organized treatment, a primitive network of 44 clinics hurriedly sprung up around the country to bolster the few scattered clinics that had been started as early as 1912 in Jacksonville, Florida.[29] During the last 6 months of 1919, the New York City clinic treated 1,532 women, approximately one-quarter of the total of registered addicts. In many other clinics throughout the country, women constituted 25% to 35% of the patients.[30] Drug clinics reduced crime in their cities and, despite wide variability in their quality, offered women the chance to cope with their addiction in a medically supervised manner. However, because these clinics ran counter to the repressive anti-drug approach being promoted by the federal government, they never found favor with the Narcotics Unit of the Treasury Department, and the last clinic in Shreveport, Louisiana, was closed in March 1925.

Not all women using drugs were poor or wanted treatment. Society women, movie stars, and the "idle rich" dabbled with cocaine, marijuana, and opium smoking during the 1920s and 1930s. Hollywood found that drug use combined with sexuality made for big business.

Beginning in 1894 with a 30-second kinetograph entitled "Chinese Opium Den," which was made for Thomas Edison, Hollywood produced more than 200 films dealing with drug themes, many portraying women as the vulnerable targets of drug-involved men.[31] Top stars such as Norma Shearer, Pola Negri, and W.C. Fields starred in these movies, while other stars such as Mabel Normand and Tallulah Bankhead developed off-screen cocaine habits, often leading to lurid scandals.

Jazz age music also gave expression to the interaction of drug use and female sexuality.[32] Duke Ellington's "Hophead" and Louis Armstrong's "Muggles," about marijuana, Leadbelly's refrain about cocaine, "Ho, ho, baby, take a whiff on me," Cab Calloway's "Minnie the Moocher," "Kicking the Gong Around," and "Reefer Man," as well as other songs such as "Sweet Marijuana Brown," "If You're a Viper," and "The Girl in the Velvet Band" all spoke to the permeation of drug use into that segment of society. In the case of "Cocaine Lil," a popular cult figure of the 1920s who lived in "Cocaine Town upon Cocaine Hill," her drug use proved fatal: "She died as she lived-sniffing cocaine."

Somewhat later, through the 1940s and 1950s, treatment options for women addicted to drugs remained limited. Between 1941 and 1965, approximately 15,000 female patients, constituting 18% of all admissions, were treated at the Lexington, Kentucky Federal Farm, ostensibly a centralized drug treatment facility but in reality akin to a prison run by the Public Health Service under the vigilant supervision of the Justice Department and the Federal Bureau of Narcotics.[33] Living conditions were primitive and depressing[34] and were compared to those described in *The Snake Pit*, Mary Jane Ward's expose of conditions in asylums treating mental disorders. Not surprisingly, relapse rates were high among women discharged from Lexington, and many became "winders," patients who spent much of their lives in and out of treatment seeking elusive cures for their addictions.

Treatment options did begin to expand in the 1960s. Detoxification, which had the longest history, remained a therapeutic option but showed limited success. Women were among early enrollees in therapeutic communities, which began in 1958 with Synanon in Ocean Park, California, followed by other programs such as Daytop, Odyssey House, and Phoenix House. Religion-based alternatives, outpatient non-maintenance treatment, inpatient chemical dependency treatment, and correctional treatment programs all offered drug treatment to women in limited ways but most were based on models more suited to treatment of male addicts. In many of these male-dominated "therapeutic" settings, women often had to contend with gender-based insensitivity, hostility, voyeurism, and even outright sexual abuse.

The most important therapeutic option for women was the development of methadone maintenance. During the early 1960s, Drs. Vincent Dole, Marie Nyswander and Mary Jeanne Kreek, working at the Rockefeller Institute in New York, pioneered the use of methadone, a synthetic opiate they found could block the euphoriant effects of heroin and the addict's craving for that drug. Although the original methadone trials excluded women, a small group of female addicts soon entered treatment and appeared to derive significant benefit from maintenance replacement therapy. Between 1969 and 1973, as methadone maintenance gained wider acceptance, women comprised 10,000 of the 40,000 patients in federally funded treatment programs. This percentage remained relatively stable over the next 20 to 30 years; in every year from 1992 to 2005, women comprised approximately 35% of the 100,000 to 125,000 patients treated in publicly funded methadone maintenance programs.

As increased awareness of drug addiction was beginning to benefit women, newer forms of addiction offset some of that progress. Psychoactive drug use mushroomed during the 1950s and early 1960s. Disproportionately affecting women, prescriptions, often inappropriately prescribed, were written for minor tranquilizers, hypnotics, stimulants, sedatives, major tranquilizers, and antidepressants. By the late 1960s, women comprised two-thirds of all psychoactive prescription drug users.[35] Some claimed that sexism played a major role in shaping physicians' attitudes toward their female patients. Much like chloral hydrate and bromides prescribed a century earlier, these new psychotropic agents were offered to middle-aged, middle-class women for anxiety, mild depression, and a general sense of dissatisfaction that had no known organic basis.

Throughout the 1970s, women remained the major users of prescription drugs. The National Institute on Drug Abuse reported early in the decade that between one and two million women experienced some degree of addiction to prescription drugs. In addition, the National Institute on Drug Abuse (NIDA) noted that 60% of all drug-related hospital emergency room visits involved women; two-thirds of those visits were the result of suicide attempts and one-third were due to drug dependency or adverse drug reactions.[36] Even as late as the 1990s, despite the widely-known dangers of such drugs, 3.7 million women were reportedly taking prescription drugs non-medically.[37]

Momentum in the push to provide treatment options for addicted women was provided by the Women's Movement in the 1970s, which created an atmosphere in which a more enlightened discussion of women and drugs could flourish. NIDA opened in 1974 with a forward-looking approach to female addictions; by 1975, NIDA had launched several innovative comprehensive drug treatment demonstration grants in six cities, using pregnancy as the entry point. Thus, programs such as the Family Center Program in Philadelphia, the Pregnant Addicts and Addicted Mothers Program in New York, and the Hutzel Hospital program in Detroit pioneered efforts to provide women using drugs with a network of comprehensive and interrelated services to meet their varied needs. Whereas in the past treatment for addicted women had been clumsily grafted onto models more suitable for males, by the early 1970s the idea of "comprehensive care" for pregnant drug-users was taking shape. For the first time, although in a limited number of programs, women could receive their medical, obstetric, and drug treatment care in a single facility. This concept has been subsequently expanded and it is now recognized that truly "comprehensive" care should include: a continuum of addiction services (residential, outpatient, and home-based); counseling on other issues such as sexual abuse and domestic violence; services for children (day care, play therapy, child developmental monitoring, and parental training); concrete services such as housing, food and transportation; comprehensive health care (family planning, prenatal care, and HIV and STD prevention and treatment); educational training such as job training and high school equivalency; appropriate staffing (female, supportive, non-confrontational, and culturally and racially sensitive); legal and advocacy services; and aftercare (12-step, transitional housing, and individual counseling).[38]

By the end of the 1970s, the "treatment glass" for women could be viewed as half-full or half-empty. On the positive side, an enlightened attitude had taken hold and more women were finding their way into drug treatment. However, on the negative side the need for services continued to overwhelm available treatment slots, too many programs did not accept women, many programs were still providing inadequate gender-based services, and women were having difficulty reaching levels of administrative responsibility within programs. A 1979 nationwide survey found that only 25 programs described themselves as specifically geared to female addicts.[39] Even in those programs, more than half of the women did not receive gynecologic care, three-fourths did not receive contraceptive counseling, and non-minority women received the majority of available treatment.

Despite the fact that slow but perceptible progress in treating women addicted to drugs was being made through the 1970s and into the 1980s, a venomous attack on these women began in the mid-1980s. Anger against these women, stereotypically cast as poor, urban, minority women, fit well with the Reagan administration's plan to limit women's reproductive options, reduce social welfare spending, and socially marginalize the "welfare queens who were bankrupting the country." A continuing tough "zero tolerance" anti-drug policy led to the Comprehensive Crime Control Act of 1984, the Anti-Drug Abuse Act of 1986, and the Anti-Drug Abuse Amendment of 1988. Although funding for interdiction and policing increased between 1981 and 1985, the budgetary allotment for drug prevention, education, and treatment decreased by approximately 65 million dollars.

Anger against women using drugs, typified by their prosecution (see related article by Flavin and Paltrow in this edition) could be explained by several interrelated factors. The first was the increasing number of babies exposed to drugs being delivered in the United States due to the persistence of heroin use and the increasing use of cocaine. Data from individual cities, primarily in the northeast, such as New York, Boston, Philadelphia, and Providence, confirmed this increase in drug-related births. Nationally, these figures varied considerably, but exploitation of the highest figure, 375,000 babies annually or 11% of newborn babies,[40] fit the agendas of activists on both sides of the political spectrum: those who wished to demonize women using drugs and those who wished to maximize the problem to secure additional funding for drug treatment programs.

Second, with the heightened attention paid to newborns exposed to drug, women were also chastised, prosecuted, and incarcerated for their deficiencies as "child rearers." With little sympathy for women who felt forced to avoid the healthcare system for fear of anger, resentment, discrimination, removal of their children, and even prosecution, the media and public tended to condemn these women as unfit mothers who lacked a maternal instinct and cared little about their children. As a result, the number of reports of child abuse and neglect tripled when both parents were drug users, which led to a nationwide increase in foster care placements. In 1994, the New York State Council on Children reported that the parents of 75% of the children in foster care were substance abusers.[41] Nationally, the number of children in foster care increased from 280,000 to 360,000 between 1986 and 1989, and increased again to 500,000 by 1997.[42]

A third factor contributing to the anger and resentment toward women using substances was the increase in medical problems seen in babies following prenatal drug exposure. Congenital syphilis, which had all but disappeared, reappeared and increased in numbers in the mid-late 1980s. Even more devastating was the increase in HIV infection among women using drugs and their offspring (see article by Ramsey, Bell, and Engler in this edition). By 1984, 50% to 60% of street addicts were HIV-positive; by 1993, 40,000 (12% of the 330,000 known AIDS cases in the United States) were women. Despite this, it was not until 1993 that the Office of Research on Women's Health acknowledged that women were being systematically excluded from trials of useful and potentially life-saving drugs. This issue took on critical significance in 1994 when it was shown that zidovudine (AZT) treatment during pregnancy and continued treatment of the infant after birth could reduce the rate of perinatal HIV transmission by two-thirds.[43]

Other pediatric medical issues contributing to the national anger against women using drugs were the increase in drug-related infant mortality, as well as low birth weight and its associated costs. For example, in New York City drug-related pregnancies were associated with a quadrupling of low birth weight infants between 1985 and 1987.[44] This coincided with pressure being brought by the government and managed care organizations to reduce health care costs. The Inspector General's Office of the Health and Human Services Department estimated that the birth of 100,000 babies exposed to cocaine would cost the nation $20 billion dollars annually.[45] It would hardly be unreasonable for society to conclude that valuable healthcare dollars were being siphoned from "legitimate" medical needs to fund the care of "innocent" babies born to "unfeeling" and "uncaring" mothers who used drugs.

A fourth factor contributing to national resentment toward women who used drugs was the increased presence of such women in the criminal justice system. Increased incarceration rates for women both fueled anger about the associated monetary costs and provided confirmation for the common belief that addiction was a "moral failing" rather than a sociological-medical problem. As previously noted, women who used drugs were more visible in the criminal justice system after passage of the Harrison Act in 1914. By the 1960s and 1970s, narcotics violations among women increased from just over 1% of total arrests to more than 6%.[46] Even more striking was the increase in narcotics-related juvenile arrests from less than 7 per 100,000 people to more than 150 per 100,000 people.[47] As a byproduct of the recent "war on drugs," the number of women arrested for drug-related offenses increased by 89% between 1982 and 1991. A national survey found that one of three female inmates was serving a drug-related sentence in 1991 compared to one of eight in 1986.[48] By the late 1990s, the rate of incarceration for women had followed a steeper trajectory than for men among the nearly 300,000 drug offenders in our nation's prisons. Incarceration appeared to be more punitive than rehabilitative since drug treatment services have always been grossly inadequate; a national survey in 1990 found that only approximately 11% of incarcerated female addicts received drug treatment.[49]

Over time, society's view of women who use drugs has varied according to the cultural norms of the period and how mainstream America has chosen to define the "drug problem." Throughout the past 150 years, women who use drugs and those who are addicted have been subjected to a range of indignities, from benign neglect in the mid- to late nineteenth century to a progressive pattern of repression, victimization, persecution and prosecution in the twentieth century. As a group, these women have been pushed to the shadowy margins of society, usually ostracized and frequently hated. This marginalization, aided by propagation of the myth that drug users are "them" and not "us," and that the stereotypical female addict is a poor, minority, urban "crack mother" has done little to foster a dialogue as how best to help them. Sensationalistic press coverage, dating back to the Hearst portrayals in the early twentieth century, sells newspapers and television advertising spots but does little to untangle the many roots of addiction.

The need to help women who are struggling with addiction has taken on added urgency. In the nineteenth century, many women trapped in their personal prisons of addiction lived in secure, intact families and had no need to resort to crime to support their habits. Passage of the Harrison Act in 1914 and the Webb and Doremus Supreme Court decisions of 1919 set the stage for an increase in female drug-related poverty and crime, as well as disintegrating family structure. Addicted women have faced increased risk from "hard drugs," as well as acquisition of potentially life-threatening diseases from "crack houses" and "shooting galleries." To make matters worse, these dangers are being faced in a society that has become more socially, politically and fiscally conservative, and thus less willing to allocate dollars that might benefit marginal, non-voting members of society. Candidates for national political office in the 1990s and into this new century, as well as our new president, have not been willing to present any innovative approach to societal drug issues.

Although answers to the problem of women and addiction remain elusive, it is clear that although providing services may not always work, certainly not providing services will never work. Unfortunately, history provides few answers as to what really works. Past attempts at treatment for women, whether by private physicians, in sanitaria, in short-lived drug clinics from 1912-1925, or later at the Lexington facility, were limited in scope, lacked firm scientific foundation, and were never properly assessed.

Even today, effective therapeutic interventions such as methadone maintenance are misunderstood and maligned. Overwhelming evidence exists that methadone maintenance offers significant benefit to those women addicted to opiates seeking to restructure their lives. As one San Francisco addict said in Marsha Rosenbaum's important studies, "with methadone, you don't have to go out and use other dugs. You have a choice" (p. 4).[50] Women who give up heroin in favor of methadone treatment engage in less illegal behavior, decrease their rates of needle use and HIV acquisition, experience an improvement in general health and nutrition, receive more consistent prenatal care, show better obstetrical outcomes, and are better prepared for parenting. However, the stigma remains that methadone is "just another addiction," akin to substituting whiskey for gin.

Several major themes recur as we look back over the 150-year history women and addiction in America. First, the spectrum and extent of female drug use has always been wider than acknowledged. Second, the excessive and often inappropriate medication of women by physicians and pharmacists, compounded by women's self-medication, has been a significant component of the problem. Third, the unique role of women as child-bearers and child-rearers has rendered them vulnerable to social ostracism, vilification, and prosecution. Fourth, the association of female sexuality and drug use has been persistent. Last, addicted women have largely remained on the shadowy margins of society, receiving little help until the 1970s, bound in a common circumstance often socially and politically ignored, at an inestimable human cost.

REFERENCES

1. Kandall SR. Substance and shadow: women and addiction in the United States. Cambridge, MA: Harvard University Press, 1996.

2. Kandall SR. Substance and shadow: women and addiction in the United States. Cambridge, MA: Harvard University Press, 1996: 20–1.

3. Courtwright D. Opiate addiction as a consequence of the civil war. Civil War History 1978; 24:101–11.

4. Hirata LC. Chinese immigrant women in nineteenth-century America. In: Berkin CR and Norton MB, ed. Women in America: a history. Boston: Houghton Mifflin, 1979:232.

5. Kandall SR. Substance and shadow: women and addiction in the United States. Cambridge, MA: Harvard University Press, 1996:10–4.

6. Kandall SR. Substance and shadow: women and addiction in the United States. Cambridge, MA: Harvard University Press, 1996:32–36.

7. Kandall SR. Substance and shadow: women and addiction in the United States, Cambridge, MA: Harvard University Press, 1996:36–37.

8. Marshall O. The opium habit in Michigan. Michigan State Board of Health Annual Report 1878; 6:63–73.

9. Earle CW. The opium habit: a statistical and clinical lecture. Chicago Medical Review 1880; 2:442–6.

10. Nolan DW. The opium habit. Catholic World 1881; 33:827–35.

11. Pierce RV. The people's common sense medical advisor in plain English. Buffalo: World's Dispensary, 1895:684.

12. Marshall O. The opium habit in Michigan. Michigan State Board of Health Annual Report 1878; 6:63–73.

13. Mattison JB. Opium habituation. Medical Record 1879; 16:332–333.

14. Thomas TG. Clinical lecture on diseases of women. Medical Record 1879; 16:316.

15. Pierce RV. The people's common sense medical advisor in plain English. Buffalo: World's Dispensary, 1895:727–71.

16. Wholey CC. Psychopathologic phases observable in individuals using narcotic drugs in excess. Pennsylvania Med J 1913; 16:724.

17. Beard GM. Certain symptoms of nervous exhaustion. Virginia Med Monthly. Repr in New York Academy of Medicine pamphlet No. 1280.

18. Mortimer WG. History of Coca. Repr San Francisco: And/Or Press, 1901.

19. Wilson JC. The opium habit and kindred affections. In: Pepper W, ed. System of practical medicine. Philadelphia: Lea Brothers, 1886:649.

20. Mortimer WG. History of Coca. Repr San Francisco: And/Or Press, 1901:390–1.

21. Waterhouse ER. Cocaine debauchery. Eclectic Medical J 1886; 56:464–5.

22. The choloroform habit as described by one of its victims. Detroit Lancet 1884; 8:254.

23. Silver G, ed. The dope chronicles (1850–1950). San Francisco: Harper and Row, 1979:681.

24. Etheridge JH. Lectures on chloral hydrate. Chicago Med J 1872; 29:525.

25. Kane HH. Opium smoking in America and China. New York: GP Putnam's Sons, 1882:1.

26. Wright H. Report on international opium, opium problem. 61st Cong., 2d sess., February 21, 1910. S. Doc. 377:44.

27. Morgan HW. Drugs in America: a social history, 1800–1980. Syracuse: Syracuse University Press, 1981: 93.

28. Anslinger H. Marijuana: assassin of youth. American Magazine 1937.

29. Kandall SR. Substance and shadow: women and addiction in the United States. Cambridge, MA: Harvard University Press, 1996: 84–93.

30. Kandall SR. Substance and shadow: women and addiction in the United States. Cambridge, MA: Harvard University Press, 1996:87.

31. Starks M. Cocaine fiends and reefer madness: an illustrated history of drugs in the movies. New York: Cornwall Books, 1982.

32. Kandall SR. Substance and shadow: women and addiction in the United States. Cambridge, MA: Harvard University Press, 1996:107–108.

33. Kandall SR. Substance and shadow: women and addiction in the United States. Cambridge, MA: Harvard University Press, 1996:131–138.

34. Hughes HM. The fantastic lodge. Boston: Houghton Mifflin, 1961.

35. Balter MB, Levine J. The nature and extent of psychotropic drug usage in the United States. Psychopharmacology Bulletin 5, No. 4, 1969:3–13.

36. Women and prescription drugs. NIDA Capsule, April 1978.

37. Women and drug abuse. NIDA Capsule, June 1994.

38. Finnegan LP, Connaughton JF, Emich JP, et al. Comprehensive care of the pregnant addict and its effect on maternal and infant outcome. Contemp Drug Probl 1972; 1:795–809.

39. Beschner GM, Thompson P. Women and drug abuse treatment: needs and services. Washington, DC: U.S. Department of Health and Human Services, National Institute on Drug Abuse. DHHS Pub. No. (ADM) 81–1057, 1981.

40. Chasnoff IJ. Drug use and women: establishing a standard of care. Annals of the NY Academy of Sciences 1990; 562: 208–10.

41. Charting new directions; planning substance abuse treatment services in New York City. New York City: Health Systems Agency of New York City, Inc., 1994.

42. Kilborn PT. Priority on safety keeping more children in foster care. New York Times April 20, 1997: A1.

43. Connor EM, Sperling RS, Gelber R et al: Reduction of maternal infant transmission of human immunodeficiency virus type 1 with zidovudine treatment. New Engl J Med 1994; 331:1173–1180.

44. Maternal drug abuse-New York City. City health information. New York City Department of Health 1989; vol. 8, no. 8.

45. Wagner L. Cost of maternal drug abuse drawing notice. Modern Healthcare; March 26, 1990:21.

46. Silverman IJ. Women, crime and drugs. J Drug Issues 1982; 12:167–83.

47. Silverman IJ. Women, crime and drugs. J Drug Issues 1982; 12:46.

48. Snell TJ. Women in prison: survey of state prison inmates. Bureau of Justice Statistics special report. Washington DC: US Department of Justice. Doc NCJ-145321, 1994.

49. Wellisch JM, Anglin MD, Prendergast ML. Numbers and characteristics of drug-using women in the criminal justice system: implications for treatment. J Drug Issues 1993; 23:7–30.

50. Wenger LD, Rosenbaum M. Drug treatment on demand-not. J Psychoactive Drugs 1994; 26:4.

Women and Addiction: The Importance of Gender Issues in Substance Abuse Research

Ellen Tuchman, PhD

ABSTRACT. Substance use was considered to be primarily a male problem, and many substance abuse studies are conducted with a predominance of male participants. However, recent substance abuse research indicates significant gender differences in the substance-related epidemiology, social factors and characteristics, biological responses, progressions to dependence, medical consequences, co-occurring psychiatric disorders, and barriers to treatment entry, retention, and completion. The epidemiology of women's drug use presents challenges separate from those raised by men's drug use. A convergence of evidence suggests that women with substance use disorders are more likely than men to face multiple barriers affecting access and entry to substance abuse treatment. Gender-specific medical problems as a result of the interplay of gender-specific drug use patterns and sex-related risk behaviors create an environment in which women are more vulnerable than men to human immunodeficiency virus. Individual characteristics and treatment approaches can differentially affect outcomes by gender. All of these differences have important clinical, treatment, and research implications.

INTRODUCTION

Historically, in substance abuse research, as in other fields of public health research, participants have largely been male. Emerging evidence in the past few years, however, is clearly establishing the importance of studying issues specific to women and studying male-female differences in all areas of substance abuse research. Studying outcomes separately in males and females expands our knowledge regarding women and drug abuse to include all areas of drug abuse and not just issues specific to women.[1] Accumulating epidemiological and clinical research indicates that the predictors for and progression to drug abuse and dependence are often gender-specific or are gender-sensitive.

Reasons for gender differences in drug abuse are not yet clear but could have important implications for the development of substance abuse treatment interventions and programs. The recent prevalence rates indicate that the number of female drug abusers is increasing, and the number of clinical studies in which sex and gender differences in drug abuse are investigated is steadily increasing.[2] Evidence presented in this article shows that there are noteworthy differences between men and women in the epidemiology of substance abuse, biological and subjective responses to drugs, patterns of use, progression from use to dependence, gender differences in medical consequences, co-occurring psychiatric disorders and substance abuse, women's history of victimization and violence, midlife and older women, specific barriers to treatment entry, retention, and completion for women.

EPIDEMIOLOGIC DATA

Epidemiologic data on substance abuse can provide an important basis for understanding the implications of drug abuse for women. Differences in patterns between women's and men's drug abuse are revealed through epidemiological data. The National Survey on Drug Use and Health is a yearly survey conducted through the Substance Abuse and Mental Health Services Office of Applied Studies. The most recent data report that an estimated 20.4 million people are currently using illicit drugs. Additionally, the number of people with substance dependence is 22.6 million in 2006.[3] Adult men are more likely than adult women to be current illicit substance abusers (10.5% vs. 6.2%, except prescription medications), alcohol users (65.9% vs. 57.9%), and tobacco users (36.4% vs. 23.3%).[3] However, men and women had similar rates of past month use of stimulants (0.5% for both), Ecstasy (0.2% for both), sedatives (0.1 and 0.2%, respectively), OxyContin (0.1% for both), LSD (0.1 and less than 0.1%, respectively), and PCP (less than 0.1% for both).

Among pregnant women aged 15 to 44 years, an estimated 11.8% reported current alcohol use, 2.9% reported binge drinking, and 0.7% reported heavy drinking. These rates were significantly lower than the rates for nonpregnant women in the same age group (53.0%, 23.6%, and 5.4%, respectively).[3]

Among those ages 50 years and older, men remain more likely than women to be dependent or abuse drugs (4.9 vs. 1.5%).[3] Alcoholism and prescription drug abuse are the top two chemical dependency issues for older women.[4] *Under the Rug: Substance Abuse and the Mature Woman* is a survey of primary care physicians and an analysis of prescriptions of psychoactive drugs for women older than 50 years (National Center on Addiction and Substance Abuse, 1998). Findings include the following: 1.8 million older women abuse or are addicted to alcohol, 2.8 million abuse or are addicted to psychoactive prescription drugs, and 4.4 million smoke cigarettes.[4] Of the 1.8 million mature women who need treatment for alcohol abuse and addiction, only 0.6%, or 11,000 women, are receiving it. Even when physicians refer midlife and older adult patients to substance abuse counseling or treatment, one-fifth say their referrals were denied because a managed care organization or insurance company would not cover the costs. In addition, the study also found that women older than 59 years are susceptible to abuse and addiction of alcohol and psychoactive prescription drugs because they get addicted faster and when using smaller amounts than any other group.

DEMOGRAPHIC AND CLINICAL CHARACTERISTICS OF WOMEN

Several demographic and clinical factors that differentiate women from men with regard to substance use have been identified. Women are more likely than men to come from families where one or more members are also addicted to drugs or alcohol,[5,6] attribute the cause of substance abuse to genetic predisposition, family history, or environmental stress,[7] and attribute their drinking to a traumatic event or stressor.[8]

Additional research indicates that women who are addicted have a history of over-responsibility in their families of origin and reportedly have experienced more disruption in their families than their male counterparts.[5] Women are also more likely than men to be in relationships with drug-abusing partners or spouses who are drug abusers[5–10] and to identify relationship problems as a cause for their substance abuse.[7] In addition to interpersonal stressors, women are more likely to experience affective disorders, whereas men who are addicted are more likely to engage in sociopathic or criminal behavior. Although many women support their habits through prostitution or petty larceny, men are more likely to rely on robbery, con games, and burglary to support their substance abuse.[7]

Several differences between older male and female alcohol abusers have been reported.

Women are more likely than men to be widowed or divorced, to have had a problem drinking spouse, to have experienced depression, and to report more negative effects of alcohol.[11] Older women have later onset of alcohol problems,[12,13] more vulnerability to addiction stigma, greater use of prescribed psychoactive medications,[14] and are more likely to abuse multiple substances.[5,7,10] Women are more likely to combine their prescription drug abuse with marijuana, cocaine, or other drugs.[6,10] Investigators also find that women may view substance abuse more negatively and that the social stigma attached to the substance dependence may act as a deterrent for women, leading them to obtaining their drugs from legitimate sources such as physicians.[5,7,10] These factors may have implications for understanding the effects of gender and widowhood on the development of late-onset problem drinking.

It is well documented that women face greater medical exposure to psychotropic drugs than men, but little research examines whether women also have increased use of prescription drugs with abuse potential.[15] Data about women's abuse of or dependence on prescription medications are virtually nonexistent. This is significant considering that women, particularly midlife and older women, are the largest consumers of prescription painkillers, antidepressants, and benzodiazepines. Clinical evidence reported in the literature suggests that prescription drugs, especially benzodiazepines, sedatives, and hypnotics, are frequently prescribed for and abused by older women. Older women are prescribed benzodiazepines more than any other age group.[16] Age-related changes in drug metabolism, interactions with other prescriptions, and over-the-counter drugs and alcohol contribute to greater risks for cognitive impairment, dementia, and falls.[16]

Women incarcerated for drug-related offenses represent one of the fastest growing populations in jails and prisons. Women confined in prison increased from 7.8% in 1974 to 10.3% in 2001, and more than half of the incarcerated women surveyed by the Bureau of Justice Statistics reported that they committed their offenses under the influence of drugs or alcohol.[17]

GENDER DIFFERENCES IN BIOLOGICAL RESPONSE

Research suggests that men and women differ in their biological and subjective responses to abused drugs. Women initiate cocaine use sooner, take less time to become addicted to cocaine,[18] and report less euphoria and dysphoria compared to men.[19] Women and men given equal doses of cocaine experience the same cardiovascular response despite the fact that blood concentrations of cocaine did not rise as high in women as in men. In studies involving long-term cocaine users, women and men showed similar impairment in tests of concentration, memory, and academic achievement following sustained abstinence, even though women in the study had substantially greater exposure to cocaine.[20] Women cocaine users also were less likely than men to exhibit abnormalities of blood flow in the brain's frontal lobes. These findings suggest a sex-related mechanism that may protect women from some of the damage cocaine inflicts on the brain.[20]

Biological indicators point toward clear differences between men and women in the metabolism[21] and other physiological effects of alcohol.[22] Women become intoxicated after drinking smaller quantities of alcohol than men and achieve higher blood alcohol concentrations.[23] Retrospective reports from alcoholics reveal that women consume lesser amounts and are less likely than men to drink daily or to engage in binge patterns of alcohol use.[24] This may be related to the fact that women have less total body water than men of comparable size, meaning that they achieve higher blood-alcohol concentrations than men after drinking equivalent amounts of alcohol.

Important gender differences also exist in the physiologic effects of nicotine. Women and men are equally likely to become addicted to nicotine, yet women typically smoke cigarettes with lower nicotine content than those smoked by men, smoke fewer cigarettes per day, and inhale less deeply than men.[20] Females report positive mood increases to a greater extent after nicotine smoking and show a great decline in positive mood during smoking abstinence that men.[25]

PROGRESSION TO DEPENDENCE

Research is beginning to show that the progression, or developmental stages, of drug involvement is not identical for men and women. In the progression from legal drug use to illicit drug use, for example, cigarette smoking plays a relatively larger role for women than for men, and alcohol use plays a relatively larger role for men than for women.

Studies of self-quitters find that women are less likely to quit initially[26] or to remain abstinent at follow-up.[27,28] Perkins' review of cessation trials with nicotine replacements reports on 9 of 10 studies that provided sex-specific outcome results and found poorer absolute abstinence rates in women, although one study found equal outcomes at a later follow-up.[25] Possible explanations for this sex difference have been suggested, such as women's greater concern about weight gain, greater difficulty with negative mood (and higher prevalence of affective disorders), greater need for social support to quit smoking, and the effects of cigarette advertising targeted at women.[29,30]

The progression to dependence, particularly alcohol-use disorder, also seems to be different for women than for men. The interval between the age of first drinking and treatment-seeking tends to be shorter for women than for men.[31] In addition, women progress between landmarks associated with the developmental course of alcoholism (e.g., regular drinking or loss of control) sooner than men.[32] These findings have led to the theory that "telescoping" may occur in women. This theory posits that there may be a shorter timeframe for the development of medical consequences and behavioral and psychological factors characteristic of an alcohol dependence disorder.

With regard to initiation into illicit drugs, data suggest that women are more likely to begin or maintain cocaine use to develop more intimate relationships, while men are more likely to use the drug with male friends and in relation to the drug trade. Kosten et al. found that female cocaine abusers had more severe cocaine use and significantly shorter periods of time of cocaine abstinence compared to when they abstained from using cocaine, and male cocaine abusers were more likely to abuse alcohol to intoxication. However, female cocaine abusers used opiates longer, which is another example of their more severe drug use problem.[18]

Westmeyer and Boedicker compared men and women as to patterns of tobacco, caffeine, alcohol, cannabis, opiate, sedative, cocaine, inhalant, amphetamine, hallucinogen, and phencyclidine (PCP) use and found that women used each drug, except cocaine, for a shorter time period compared to men. However, rates of dependence were similar between women and men, suggesting that women take less time to progress to dependence than men.[33]

GENDER DIFFERENCES IN MEDICAL CONSEQUENCES

Women who abuse drugs have been found to get sicker more quickly and suffer higher rates of liver problems, hypertension, anemia, and gastrointestinal disorders than male drug users. Women also experience gender-specific medical problems as a result of their addiction, such as a higher risk for infertility, vaginal infections, repeat miscarriages, and premature delivery.[5,6]

Despite lower levels of alcohol intake and shorter periods of drinking, women suffer more severe medial consequences than men, including liver cirrhosis.[34] Postmenopausal women who drink moderate to heavy amounts of alcohol also have other health problems, including breast cancer. They are at higher risk for breast cancer and heart disease even if the amount they drink is less than that of their male counterparts.[35–37] Women who chronically abuse alcohol have death rates 50% to 100% higher than men who have the same alcohol use patterns.[38]

Some research suggests that the impact of a given amount of smoking on lung cancer risk may be greater among women than men, and that exposure to environmental tobacco smoke may be associated with increased risk for breast cancer.[39] Particularly alarming is that women may be at even greater risk than men for smoking-related diseases, including lung cancer[40,41] and myocardial infarction.[42] Men have higher prevalence rates of chronic obstructive pulmonary disease than women, which has been attributed tothe historically higher rates of cigarette smoking in men. However, the increased rates of cigarette smoking in women within the past several decades have been associated with steadily increasingrates of chronic obstructive pulmonary disease in women.[43]

The interplay of gender-specific drug use patterns and sex-related risk behaviors creates an environment in which women are more vulnerable than men to infection with the human immunodeficiency virus (HIV).[44,45] Women using intravenous drugs are at higher risk than men for acquiring HIV.[46] Women are more likely than men to inject drugs, use drugs with many partners, share paraphernalia with an injection partner, exchange sex for money or drugs, and have difficulty negotiating condom use with their sex partners.[44] Women account for 26% of all reported adult AIDS cases in the United States, which represents a doubling over the past decade. High-risk heterosexual contact was the source of 80% of newly diagnosed infections. However, an estimated one in five new HIV diagnoses for women are related to injection drug use.[46]

CO-OCCURRING PSYCHIATRIC DISORDERS AND SUBSTANCE ABUSE

It is well established that women with substance abuse disorders present for treatment with significant psychiatric co-morbidity. Women show higher rates of certain co-occurring psychiatric disorders compared to men, such as major depression, social phobia, post-traumatic stress disorders, and eating disorders.[47–54]Gender differences in depression are generally thought to be related to the interaction of biological and psychosocial factors. Higher rates of depression occur among women who are poor, less educated, welfare-dependent, and unemployed.[54] Although depression is common among women with drug abuse problems, it often goes undetected in this population.

Gender differences in the relationships between depressive symptoms and drinking behavior have been reported in problem drinkers, indicating that depression can play a dual role, at least for women.[55] More specifically, if men and women are motivated to stop drinking, depression can trigger a change in the beginning of treatment of both genders. However, following treatment, depression seems to be associated with relapse, primarily in women.

Studies of comorbid psychiatric disorders in opiate[56] and cocaine[57] abusers have shown higher percentages of affective and anxiety disorders in women than in men. In a recent study of treatment-seeking opiate abusers, lifetime psychiatric comorbidity was more than twice as common in women compared with men.[56]

Women dependent on methamphetamine are more likely to report depression, suicidal ideation, and a need for psychiatric assistance than men. Increased risk for depressive symptoms was observed for both women and men reporting methamphetamine dependence compared to those not reporting dependence. Furthermore, women, but not men, reporting methamphetamine dependence were more likely than those not reporting methamphetamine dependence to report suicidal ideation and a need for psychiatric care.[58]

HISTORY OF VICTIMIZATION AND VIOLENCE

Another area of particular importance for women is substance abuse and victimization and violence. Prevalence rates of intimate partner violence among women in drug treatment have been found to range between 25% and 57%.[59] These rates of intimate partner violence are substantially higher than the range of 1.5% to 16% prevalence rates found in epidemiological surveys of community-based samples of non-drug using women.[60,61] Furthermore, a growing body of evidence suggests that interpersonal stress and relationship conflicts are major triggers for relapse among women in drug treatment and that intimate partner violence may result in continued drug use and relapse.[62]

MIDLIFE AND OLDER WOMEN

Because of the projected growth of the midlife and older adult population in the coming decades, the treatment of substance abuse problems among midlife and older women is of increasing interest. With the aging of the drug using population, a majority of women in substance abuse treatment are perimenopausal or menopausal.[63] Risk factors for a more complicated menopausal transition (e.g., alcohol, smoking and illicit substance use, medical comorbidities, HIV/AIDS and hepatitis, premorbid and current psychological distress, few social and economic resources, and negative life events) are fairly widespread in substance abusing women.[64] The rate of HIV infection in midlife women, 15% of all cases among women older than 50 (a number that has doubled in the past 12 years), is attributable to the risk behaviors associated with their drug use or sexual practices with heterosexual partners.[65]

No longer concerned with pregnancy prevention, postmenopausal women may not continue barrier methods of contraception, which may include diaphragms, condoms, and cervical caps, and face increased risk of sexually transmitted diseases, including HIV from male sex partners who have a current or past drug history.[66] Furthermore, many of the symptoms associated with menopause (hot and cold flashes, sweats, fatigue, loss of libido, menstrual irregularity, and sleep disturbances) are similar to those associated with substance abuse, especially opiate withdrawal and methadone treatment with improper doses.[63] Those women who are sensitive to these symptoms and experience increased levels of physical discomfort, insomnia, irritability, anxiety, and depression may be at a high risk for relapse to drug use and HIV sexual risk behaviors.

SPECIFIC BARRIERS TO TREATMENT ENTRY FOR WOMEN

Women are underrepresented in substance abuse treatment programs. In 2002, 30% of the admissions to substance abuse treatment programs were women, but the ratio of women to men with dependence on illicit drugs is larger.[4] Research indicates that women seek treatment for substance abuse less often than men.[67,68] The low rates of substance abuse treatment entry among women may reflect the specific barriers they face. Barriers for young women that have been documented in the past two decades include pregnancy, lack of services for pregnant women, fear of losing custody when the baby is born, or fear of prosecution, voyeurism, and sexual harassment.[69–73] Perhaps the most substantial obstacle for these young women is available, affordable childcare.[74,75] Few treatment programs provide on-site childcare or provide assistance with making child care arrangements. Even when women are able to make alternative arrangements, they are likely to face resistance or hostility from family members.[5]

Women seeking treatment have been found to have more substance-related problems, and those problems tend to be more severe than those of men entering treatment.[76,77] For instance, women are more likely to encounter difficulty with transportation to treatment sites,[71] inadequate health insurance, poverty,[75] dealing with a relationship with a drug-abusing partner,[5–7,9,10,74] and being less likely than their male counterparts to have someone actively supporting them in treatment.

Wechsberg et al. found that women entering substance abuse treatment were younger, had lower education and employment levels, were more concerned about child-related issues, were less likely to be married, had more health and mental health problems, had greater exposure to physical and sexual abuse, and had greater concerns about issues related to children compared with men.[78] Women enter treatment with problems related to health, higher HIV/AIDS risk, and family and employment situations[79,80]

Treatment entry for men seems to be facilitated by social institutions such as employers or the criminal justice system, whereas for women treatment entry more often results from social work referral, suggesting that contact with social agencies eases women's entry into treatment.[81]

TREATMENT RETENTION AND COMPLETION

Controversy exists as to whether research varies as to whether greater treatment retention is achieved for women or men. Some studies have positive findings for women. For instance, women remain in treatment longer[82] and were less likely to drop out or not complete treatment compared with men.[83] Other studies have negative findings. For example, women were more likely than men to drop out of substance abuse treatment,[76] women attend fewer treatment sessions than men, [84] and women with substance use disorders differ significantly from men with substance use disorders in terms of the risk factors for, and natural history of, substance use problems, reasons for relapse, presenting problems, and motivations for treatment.[85–89] However, no gender differences in treatment retention or length of stay were shown in three studies.[90–92]

Sayre et al. examined factors affecting treatment attrition in individuals seeking treatment for cocaine dependence. Sixty-five percent dropped out before completing all 20 therapy sessions. Treatment dropouts were more likely to be women, to be separated from their spouses, to have poorer family/social functioning, and to have fewer years of education. Individuals with higher education levels and those with poorer psychiatric functioning tended to remain in treatment longer.[93] Treatment program characteristics may be associated with retention and completion rates among women. These findings have direct implications for identifying individuals at higher risk for attrition from outpatient substance abuse programs.

Women report that services such as health care, domestic violence counseling, transportation, and child care, along with relationships with individual counselors, are the primary reasons they remain in treatment.[94,95] Women's failure rates in treatment programs have been attributed in part to the fact that traditional programs are designed by and for men and that their approaches have been informed by research conducted on the male substance-abusing population.[5,9,75] Previous research indicates that male clients are more likely to evidence greater denial of their drug problem. As such, traditional treatment programs are centered on aggressively confronting the addict about his abuse and resulting consequences. Relapse is often met with a punitive response instead of an exploration of possible environmental factors that may have contributed to recurring drug use. In contrast, women are more likely to experience higher levels of guilt and shame in acknowledging their substance abuse. Therefore, confrontational approaches, which serve to enhance guilt and shame, have been found to be ineffective with female clients.[5,75]

Nearly all prison-based substance abuse treatment programs have also been designed with male prisoners in mind, and little research is available describing the effectiveness of interventions developed for substance abusing female prisoners. Two studies examined county jail inmates in a 6-week residential substance abuse treatment program and federal prisoners who participated in a 9- or 12-month residential substance abuse treatment program, respectively.[96,97] Both studies reported gender differences: female prisoners had more serious patterns of drug use, were more likely to have grown up in homes where drug use was present, were more likely to have experienced physical and sexual abuse as children, and were more likely to have mental and physical health problems compared to male prisoners.[96,97] If treatment services in criminal justice settings are not expanded to address the needs of female substance abusers, large numbers of these individuals will continue to be involved in drug-related crime and will return to the criminal justice system.

Whether women should be in women-specific versus mixed-gender groups is an issue of debate.[98,99] An evaluation of women-only versus mixed-gender addiction groups found that women identified several issues that they would discuss only in women's groups, including guilt regarding being an inadequate mother.[5] Another study found superior outcomes for women treated in specialized women's programs versus mixed-gender programs[100] while other studies found no differences.[101,102]

A meta-analysis examining effectiveness of single-gender substance abuse treatment for women concluded that single-gender treatment was effective, but that its strongest impact was on pregnancy outcomes. Psychological well-being, attitudes and beliefs, and HIV risk reduction were also substantially improved by treatment but psychiatric outcomes improved only modestly. Treatment resulted in only small improvements in alcohol use, other drug use, and reduced criminal activity.[24] However, few studies in this meta-analysis compared gender-sensitive or gender-specific treatment to mixed-gender programs, making conclusions tentative, suggesting the need for additional research on women's outcomes.

Several studies have suggested that gender differences in interaction styles and men's traditional societal dominance may negatively affect women in mixed-gender group treatment.[103–105] As a result, it is generally asserted that substance abuse treatment for women, particularly pregnant women and women with dependent children, must differentially address these complex psychosocial issues.[106–109] As such, treatment programming designed specifically for women is needed to address not only women's substance abuse related problems, but also their special needs and barriers to treatment.

FUTURE RESEARCH DIRECTIONS

Evidence indicates there are significant gender differences in the epidemiology of substance use disorders, social factors and characteristics, biological responses, patterns of use, progressions to dependence, health consequences, co-occurring psychiatric disorders, and factors related to treatment entry, retention, and completion.

The epidemiology of women's drug use presents challenges separate from those raised by men's drug use. High-risk subpopulations of women (homeless, mentally ill, HIV positive, violence victims, incarcerated, and midlife and aging) necessitate more intensive and specialized services.

Progression, or developmental stages, of drug involvement is not identical for men and women. If the phenomenon of telescoping is, in fact, common to most drugs of abuse, further research is needed. Areas for exploration include pathophysiology to determine whether biological or hormonal differences in response to drugs, societal differences regarding entry into treatment, or gender differences in seeking medical treatment explain the shorter time course for women than men. It may also imply that women have a smaller window of opportunity for intervention before the disease progresses, which has implications on programming and treatment protocols.

Gender-specific medical problems as a result of the interplay of gender-specific drug use patterns and sex-related risk behaviors create an environment in which midlife and older women are more vulnerable than men to HIV. There is a need to develop, engage, and test effective treatments for women across the life cycle with substance use disorders, particularly midlife and older women.

There is a dearth of research related to the effectiveness of treatment interventions designed specifically for women who abuse substances. Although many service providers acknowledge and address gender differences among clients in substance abuse treatment, these differences and the programming that addresses them have not been adequately studied. Because women remain under-represented in substance abuse treatment programs, new studies on treatment effectiveness are needed to assess gender differences in response to different treatment strategies. In addition, there is a need to develop and examine gender-specific assessment scales and treatment protocols to optimize treatment effectiveness. Future research should be theoretically based and methodologically sound to advance the evidence base of substance abuse treatment for women.

At the national, state, and local levels, policymakers and service providers need new knowledge to understand how male and female clients differ in terms of sociodemographics, substance use characteristics, treatment entry, retention, and completion. Future research examining the factors that underlie gender differences may allow for the development of safe and effective gender-specific interventions for drug abuse.

The research evidence makes it clear that there are significant gender differences in drug abuse and that more research is necessary. The translation of these research findings to the treatment community to improve treatment outcomes for both sexes will be an exciting challenge for the field. Increased and improved policies, services, and new research will continue to improve the lives of women substance abusers.

REFERENCES

1. Wetherington CL. Sex-gender differences in drug abuse: a shift in the burden of proof? Exp Clin Psychopharmacol 2007; 15:411–7.

2. Brady KT, Randall CL. Gender differences in substance use disorders. Psychiatr Clin North Am 1999; 22:241–52.

3. Substance Abuse and Mental Health Services Administration. Results from the 2006 National Survey on Drug Use and Health: national findings. Rockville, MD: Office of Applied Studies; 2007. NSDUH Series H-32, DHHS Publication, No. SMA 07–4293.

4. Brady T M, Ashley OS, eds. Women in substance abuse treatment: results from the Alcohol and Drug Services Study (ADSS). Rockville, MD: Substance Abuse and Mental Health Services Administration, Office of Applied Studies; 2005. DHHS Publication, No. SMA 04-3968, Analytic Series A-26.

5. Nelson-Zlupko L, Kauffman E, Dore MM. Gender differences in drug addiction and treatment: implications for social work intervention with substance-abusing women. Soc Work 1995; 40:45–54.

6. US Department of Health and Human Services. Treatment Methods for Women. Rockville, MD: US Department of Health and Human Services, National Institutes of Health, National Institute on Drug Abuse, 2003.

7. Kauffman SE, Silver P, Poulin J. Gender differences in attitudes toward alcohol, tobacco, and other drugs. Soc Work 1997; 42:231–41.

8. Lex BW. Gender differences and substance abuse. Adv Subst Abuse 1991; 4:225–96.

9. Bloom B, Covington S. Gender-specific programming for female offenders: what is it and why is it important? Washington, DC: American Society of Criminology, 1998.

10. Manhal-Baugus M. The self-in-relation theory and women for sobriety: female-specific theory and mutual help group for chemically dependent women. J Addict Offender Counseling 1998; 18:78–85.

11. Gomberg ESL. Recent developments in alcoholism: gender issues. In: Galanter M, ed. Recent developments in alcoholism (vol. 11). New York: Plenum Press, 1993:95–107.

12. Graham K, Braun K. Concordance of use of alcohol and other substances among older adult couples. Addict Behav 1999; 24:839–56.

13. Brennan PL, Moos RH, Kim JY. Gender differences in the individual characteristics and life contexts of late-middle-aged and older problem drinkers. Addiction 1993; 88:781–90.

14. Gomberg ESL. Risk factors for drinking over a woman's life span. Alcohol Health Res World 1994; 18:220–7.

15. Simoni-Wastila L. The use of abusable prescription drugs: the role of gender. J Womens Health and Gender-based Med 2000; 9:289–97.

16. Colletti SD. Service providers and treatment access issues. In: Wetherington CL, Roman AB, eds. Drug addiction research and the health of women. Rockville, MD: National Institute on Drug Abuse, 1998:236-244. NIH Publication, No. 98–4290.

17. US Department of Justice. Fact Sheet: Drug-Related Crime. Washington, DC: Office of Justice Programs, Bureau of Justice Statistics, 1994. Publication No. NCJ–149286.

18. Kosten TR, Kosten TA, McDougle CJ, et al. Gender differences in response to intranasal cocaine administration to humans. Biol Psychiatry 1996; 39:147–8.

19. Lucas LR, Angulo JA, Le Moal M, McEwen BS, Piazza PV. Neurochemical characterization of individual vulnerability to addictive drugs in rats. Eur J Neurosci 1998; 10:3153–63.

20. National Institute of Drug Abuse. Gender differences in drug abuse risks and treatment. NIDA Notes 2000; 15(4):1–4.

21. Dawson DA, Archer L. Gender differences in alcohol consumption: effects of measurement. Br J Addict 1992; 87:119–23.

22. Thomasson HR. Gender differences in alcohol metabolism: physiological responses to ethanol. Recent Dev Alcohol 1995; 12:163–79.

23. Mumenthaler MS, Taylor JL, O'Hara R, Yesavage, JA. Gender differences in moderate drinking effects. Alcohol Res Health 1999; 23:55–64.

24. Orwin RG, Francisco L, Bernichon T. Effectiveness of women's substance abuse treatment programs: a meta-analysis. Arlington, VA: Substance Abuse and Mental Health Services Administration (SAMHSA), Center for Substance Abuse Treatment, 2001. NEDS Contract, No. 270-97–7016.

25. Perkins KA. Sex differences in nicotine versus non-nicotine reinforcement as determinants of tobacco smoking. Exp Clin Psychopharmacol 1996; 4: 166–77.

26. Killen JD, Fortmann SP. Craving is associated with smoking relapse: findings from three prospective studies. Exp Clin Psychopharmacol 1997; 5:137–42.

27. Killen JD, Fortmann SP. Role of nicotine dependence in smoking relapse: results from a prospective study using population-based recruitment methodology. Int J Behav Med 1994; 1:320–34.

28. Kabat GC, Wnyder EL. Determinants of quitting smoking. Am J Public Health 1987; 77:1301–5.

29. Ockene JK. Smoking among women across the lifespan: prevalence, interventions, and implications for cessation research. Ann Behav Med 1993; 15: 135–48.

30. Pierce JP, Lee L, Gilpin EA. Smoking initiation by adolescent girls, 1944 through 1988: an association with targeted advertising. JAMA 1994; 271:608–11.

31. Piazza NJ, Vrbka JL, Yeager RD. Telescoping of alcoholism in women alcoholics. Int J Addict 1989; 24:19–28.

32. Randall CL, Roberts JS, DelBoca FK, Carroll KM, Connors GC, Mattson ME. Telescoping of landmark events associated with drinking: a gender comparison. J Stud Alcohol 1999; 60:252–60.

33. Westermeyer J, Boedicker AE. Course, severity, and treatment of substance abuse among women versus men. Am J Drug Alcohol. 2000; 26(4):523–35.

34. Jarque-López A, Gonzalez-Reimers E, Rodriguez F. Prevalence and mortality of heavy drinkers in a general medical hospital unit. Alcohol Alcohol 2001; 36:335–8.

35. Urbano-Marquez A, Estruch R, Fernández-Solá J, Nicolás JM, Paré JC, Rubin E. The greater risk of cardiomathopathy and myopathy in women compared with men. JAMA 1995; 274:149–54.

36. Smith-Warner SA, Spiegelman D, Yaun SS, van den Brandt PA, Folsom AR, Goldbohm RA, Graham S, Holmberg L, Howe GR, Marshall JR, Miller AB, Potter JD, Speizer FE, Willett WC, Wolk A, Hunter DJ. Alcohol and breast cancer: a pooled analysis of cohort studies. JAMA 1998; 279:535–40.

37. Zhang Y, Kreger BE, Dorgan JF, Splansky GL, Cupples LA, Ellison RC. Alcohol consumptions and risk of breast cancer: The Framingham Study revisited. Am J Epidemiol 1999; 149:93–101.

38. Wilsnack SC, Bechman LJ, eds. Alcohol problems in women: antecedents, consequences, and intervention. New York: Guilford Press, 1984.

39. US Department of Health and Human Services. Women and smoking: a report of the surgeon general–2001. Washington, DC: Government Printing Office, 2001:343–67.

40. Kure EH, Ryberg D, Hewer A, Phillips DH, Skaug V, Baera R, Haugen A. Mutations in lung tumors: relationship to gender and lung DNA adduct levels. Carcinogenesis 1996; 17:2201–5.

41. Zang EA, Wynder EL. Differences in lung cancer risk between men and women: examination of the evidence. J Natl Cancer Inst 1996; 88:183–92.

42. Prescott E, Osler M, Hein HO, Borch-Johnsen K, Lange P, Schnohr P, Vestbo J. Gender and smoking-related risk of lung cancer. Epidemiology 1998; 9:79–83.

43. Silverman EK, Chapman HA, Drazen JM, Weiss ST, Rosner B, Campbell EJ, O'Donnell WJ, Reilly JJ, Ginns L, Mentzer S, Wain J, Speizer FE. Gender-related differences in severe, early-onset chronic obstructive pulmonary disease. Am J Respir Crit Care Med 2000; 162:2152–8.

44. Stevens SJ, Tortu S, Coyle SL. Women drug users and HIV prevention: overview of findings and research needs. In: Stevens SJ, Tortu S, Coyle SL, eds. Women, drug use, and HIV prevention. Binghamton, NY: The Hawthorne Medical Press, 1998:19–47.

45. Weeks MR, Singer M, Himmelgreen DA, Richmond P, Grier M, Radda K. Drug use patterns in substance abusing women: gender and ethnic differences in an AIDS prevention program. In: Stevens SJ, Wexler HK, eds. Women and substance abuse. Binghamton, NY: The Hawthorne Medical Press, 1998:35–61.

46. Center for Disease Control and Prevention. HIV/AIDS Surveillance Report, 2005 (vol. 17, Rev ed). Atlanta: US Department of Health and Human Services, 2007:1-46. Accessed December 9, 2007.

47. Denier CA, Thevos AK, Latham PK, Randall CL. Psychosocial and psychopathology differences in hospitalized male and female cocaine abusers: a retrospective chart review. Addict Behav 1991; 16:489–96.

48. Fornari VM, Kent J, Kabo L, Goodman B. Anorexia nervosa: "thirty something." J Subst Abuse Treat 1994: 11:45–54.

49. Grella CE, Anglin D, Annon JJ. HIV risk behaviors among women in methadone maintenance treatment. Subst Use Misuse 1996; 31:277–301.

50. Grella CE. Services for perinatal women with substance abuse and mental health disorders: the unmet need. J Psychoactive Drugs 1997; 29:67–78.

51. Merikangas KR, Stevens DE, Fenton B, Stolar MS, O'Malley S, Woods SW, Risch N. Co-morbidity and familial aggregation of alcoholism and anxiety disorders. Psychol Med 1998; 28:773–88.

52. Najavits LM, Weiss RD, Shaw SR. The link between substance abuse and posttraumatic stress disorder in women. Am J Addict 1997; 6:273–83.

53. Sonne SC, Back SE, Zuniga CD, Randall CL, Brady KT. Gender differences in individuals with comorbid alcohol dependence and posttraumatic stress disorder. Am J Addict 2003; 12:412–3.

54. Westermeyer J, Kopka S, Nugent S. Course and severity of substance abuse among patients with comorbid major depression. Am J Addict 1996; 6:284–92.

55. Schutte KK, Seable JH, Moos RH. Gender differences in the relations between depressive symptoms and drinking behavior among problem drinkers: a three-wave study. J Consult Clin Psychol 1997; 65:392–404.

56. Brooner RK, King VL, Kidorf M, Schmidt CW Jr, Bigelow GE. Psychiatric and substance comorbidity among treatment-seeking opioid abusers. Arch Gen Psychiatry 1997; 54:71–80.

57. Rounsaville BJ, Anton SF, Carroll K, Budde D, Prusoff BA, Gawin F. Psychiatric diagnoses of treatment-seeking cocaine abusers. Arch Gen Psychiatry 1991; 48:43–51.

58. Kalechstein AD, Newton TF, Longshore D, Anglin MD, van Gorp WG, Gawin FH. Psychiatric comorbidity of methamphetamine dependence in a forensic sample. J Neuropsychiatry Clin Neurosci 2000; 12:480–4.

59. El-Bassel N, Gilbert L, Shilling R, Wada T. Drug abuse and partner violence among women in methadone treatment. J Fam Violence 2000; 15:209–28.

60. Caetano R, Nelson S, Cunradi C. Intimate partner violence: dependence symptoms and social consequences from drinking among White, Black and Hispanic couples in the United States. Am J Addict 2001; 10:60–9.

61. Tjaden P, Thoennes N. Prevalence, incidence, and consequences of violence against women: findings from the national violence against women survey. Washington, DC: Department of Justice, National Institute of Justice, 1998:3–18.

62. Gilbert L, El-Bassel N, Rajah V, Foleno A, Frye E. Linking drug-related activities with experiences of partner violence: a focus group study of women in methadone treatment. Violence Vict 2001; 16:517–36.

63. Tuchman E. Methadone and menopause: midlife women in drug treatment. J Soc Work Pract Addict 2003; 3:43–56.

64. Tuchman E. Exploring the prevalence of menopause symptoms in midlife women in methadone maintenance treatment. Soc Work Health Care 2007; 45:43–62.

65. Zablotsky D, Kennedy M. Risk factors and HIV transmission to midlife and older women: knowledge, options, and the initiation of safer sexual practices. J Acquir Immune Defic Syndr 2003; 33:S122–30.

66. Levy JA, Ory MG, Crystal S. HIV/AIDS interventions for midlife and older adults: current status and challenges. JAIDS 2003; 33(2):S59–S67.

67. Shober R, Annis HM. Barriers to help-seeking for change in drinking: a gender-focused review of the literature. Addict Behav 1996; 21:81–92.

68. Weisner C, Schmidt L. Gender disparities in treatment for alcohol problems. JAMA 1992; 268: 1872–6.

69. Paltrow LM. Punishing women for their behavior during pregnancy: an approach that undermines the health of women and children. In: Wetherington CL, Roman AB, eds. Drug addiction research and the health of women. Rockville, MD: National Institute on Drug Abuse, 1998:467-502. NIH Publication, No. 98–4290.

70. Pelissier B, Jones N. A review of gender differences among substance abusers. Crime Delinquency 2005; 51:343–72.

71. Ayyagari S, Boles S, Johnson P, Kleber H. Difficulties in recruiting pregnant substance abusing women into treatment: problems encountered during the cocaine alternative treatment study. Assoc Health Serv Res 1999; 16:80–1.

72. DeAngelis T. Better research, more help needed for pregnant addicts. APA Monitor 1993; 24(9):7–8.

73. Finkelstein N. Treatment issues for alcohol and drug dependent pregnant and parenting women. Health Soc Work 1994; 19:7–15.

74. Bride BE. Single-gender treatment of substance abuse: effect on treatment retention and completion. Soc Work Res 2001; 25:223–32.

75. Hodgins DC, Ed-Guebaly N, Addington J. Treatment of substance abusers: single or mixed gender programs? Addiction 1997; 92:805–12.

76. Arfken CL, Klein C, diMenza S, Shuster CR. Gender differences in problem severity at assessment and treatment retention. J Subst Abuse Treat 2001; 20:53–7.

77. Farid B, Clarke ME. Characteristics of attenders to community based alcohol treatment centre with special reference to sex difference. Drug Alcohol Depend 1992; 30:33–6.

78. Wechsberg WM, Craddock SG, Hubbard RL. How are women who enter substance abuse treatment different than men? A gender comparison from the Drug Abuse Treatment Outcome Study (DATOS). Drugs Soc 1998; 13:97–115.

79. Halikas JA, Crosby RD, Pearson VL, Nugent SM, Carlson GA. Psychiatric comorbidity in treatment-seeking cocaine abusers. Am J Addict 1994; 3:25–35.

80. Marsh JC, Miller NA. Female clients in substance abuse treatment. Int J Addict 1985; 20:995–1019.

81. Grella CE, Joshi V. Gender differences in drug treatment careers among clients in the National Drug Abuse Treatment Outcome Study. Am J Drug Alcohol Abuse 1999; 25:385–406.

82. Chou CP, Hser YI, Anglin MD. Interaction effects of client and treatment program characteristics on retention: an exploratory analysis using hierarchical linear models. Subst Use Misuse 1998; 33:2281–301.

83. Hser YI, Polinsky ML, Maglione M, Anglin MD. Matching clients' needs with drug treatment services. J Subst Abuse Treat 1999; 16:299–305.

84. McCaul ME, Svikis DS, Moore RD. Predictors of outpatient treatment retention:patient versus substance use characteristics. J Subst Abuse 2001; 62: 255–70.

85. Davis S. Drug treatment decisions of chemically-dependent women. Int J Addict 1994; 29:1287–304.

86. Hughes P, Coletti S, Neri R, Urmann C, Stahl S, Sicillian D, Anthony J. Retaining cocaine-abusing women in a therapeutic community: the effect of a child live-in program. Am J Public Health 1995; 85:1149–52.

87. Pelissier BMM, Camp SD, Gaes GG, Saylor WG, Rhodes W. Gender differences in outcomes from prison-based residential treatment. J Subst Abuse Treat 2003; 24: 149–60.

88. Saunders JB, Aasland OG, Babor TF, de la Fuente JR, Grant M. Development of the Alcohol Use Disorders Identification Test (AUDIT): WHO collaborative project on Early Detection of Persons with Harmful Alcohol Consumption-II. Addiction 1993; 88:791–804.

89. Green CA, Polen MR, Dickinson DM, Lynch FL, Bennett MD. Gender differences in predictors of initiation, retention, and completion in an HMO-based substance abuse treatment program. J Subst Abuse Treat 2002; 23:285–95.

90. Kosten TA, Gawin FH, Kosten TR, Rounsaville BJ. Gender differences in cocaine use and treatment response. J Subst Abuse Treat 1993; 10:63–6.

91. Mertens JR, Weisner CM. Predictors of substance abuse treatment retention among women and men in an HMO. Alcohol Clin Exp Res 2000; 24:1525–33.

92. Veach LJ, Remley TP, Kippers SM, Sorg JD. Retention predictors related to intensive outpatient programs for substance use disorders. Am J Drug Alc Abuse 2000; 26:417–28.

93. Sayre SL, Schmitz JM, Stotts AL, Averill PM, Rhoades HM, Grabowski JJ. Determining predictors of attrition in an outpatient substance abuse program. Am J Drug Alcohol Abuse 2002; 28:55–72.

94. Nelson-Zlupko L, Dore MM, Kauffman E, Kaltenbach K. Women in recovery: their perceptions of treatment effectiveness. J Subst Abuse Treat 1996; 13:51–9.

95. Strauss SM, Falkin GP. The relationship between the quality of drug user treatment and program completion: understanding the perceptions of women in a prison-based program. Subst Use Misuse 2000; 35:2127–59.

96. Peters RH, Strozier AL, Murrin MR, Kearns WD. Treatment of substance-abusing jail inmates: examination of gender differences. J Subst Abuse Treat 1997; 14:339–49.

97. Langan NP, Pelissier BMM. Gender differences among prisoners in drug treatment. Journal of Substance Abuse 2001; 13:291–301.

98. McCrady BS, Raytek H. Women and substance abuse: treatment modalities and outcomes. In: Gomberg ESL, Nirenberg TD, eds. Women and substance abuse. Norwood, NJ: Ablex, 1993:314–338.

99. Vannicelli M. Barriers to treatment of alcoholic women. Subst Alcohol Actions/Misuse 1984; 5: 29–37.

100. Dalhgren L, Willander A. Are special treatment facilities for female alcoholics needed? A controlled two-year follow-up study from a specialized female unit (EWA) versus a mixed male/female treatment facility. Alcohol Clin Exp Res 1989; 13:499–504.

101. Copeland J, Hall W, Didcott P, Biggs V. A comparison of a specialist women's alcohol and other drug treatment service with two traditional mixed-sex services: client characteristics and treatment outcome. Drug Alcohol Depend 1993; 2:81–92.

102. Dodge K, Potocky-Tripodi M. The effectiveness of three inpatient intervention strategies for chemically dependent women. Res Soc Work Pract 2001; 11:24–39.

103. LaFave LM, Echols LD. An argument for choice: an alternative women's treatment program. J Subst Abuse Treat 1999; 16:345–352.

104. Schliebner CT. Gender-sensitive therapy: an alternative for women in substance abuse treatment. J Subst Abuse Treat 1994; 11:511–5.

105. Wilke D. Women and alcoholism: how a male-as-norm bias affects research, assessment, and treatment. Health Soc Work 1994; 19:29–35.

106. Jansson LM, Svikis D, Lee J, Paluzzi P, Rutigliano P, Hackerman F. Pregnancy and addiction: a comprehensive care model. J Subst Abuse Treat 1996; 13:321–9.

107. Knight DK, Hood PE, Logan SM, Chatham LR. Residential treatment for women with dependent children: one agency's approach. J Psychoactive Drugs 1999; 31: 339–51.

108. Substance Abuse and Mental Health Services Administration (SAMHSA). 45 CFR 96: Rules and Regulations. Available at: www.treatment.org/legis/45CFR961.html. Accessed December 1, 2007.

109. Volpicelli J, Markman I, Monterosso J, Filing J, O'Brien C. Psychosocially enhanced treatment for cocaine-dependent mothers: evidence of efficacy. J Subst Abuse Treat 2000; 18:41–9.

Substance Use and Women's Health

Abigail Kay, MD, MA
Trusandra E. Taylor, MD, FASAM, MPH
Andrea G. Barthwell, MD, FASAM
Jana Wichelecki
Vera Leopold

ABSTRACT. Scientific findings show that substance abuse in women yields a higher risk of a variety of health problems than substance abuse in men. Research suggests that women experience addiction telescoping when they abuse alcohol, tobacco, specific stimulants, and possibly opioids. Medical side effects also develop more rapidly in women than men when they abuse many substances. Cancer and cardiac complications, specifically, pose a significant threat for women who abuse almost all types of substances. However, the physical consequences are not the only ones women suffer when they engage in substance abuse. Research on substance abuse in women ties opioids to mood and anxiety disorders, heroin to neurological deficiencies, cocaine to immune system suppression, and alcohol to intimate partner abuse. Additionally, female substance abusers, on average, have a lower level of education and lower rates of employment. In light of these gender-specific concerns, physicians should give particular consideration to detecting substance abuse in women.

INTRODUCTION

Substance use among women is a widespread and costly problem that can lead to a variety of medical complications. In 2006, 571,748 women in the United States were admitted into substance abuse treatment programs that receive public funding,[1] a number significantly higher than the number of new breast cancer cases (182,460) for that same year. Additionally, on an annual basis, $180.9 billion is spent in the United States on the associated costs of substance abuse overall.[2] Given the fact that substance abuse contributes to many of the leading threats to women's health, it is essential to understand the relationships between the abuse of different substances and

This manuscript received administrative and logistical support from Human Resources Development Institute, Inc. (HRDI). The authors thank Ryan Williams for his assistance in the preparation of the paper and Joe Macare for his editorial input.

the incidence of medical problems in the female population.

WOMEN'S HEALTH RESEARCH

Comprehensive research data on the physiological effects of addiction in women has been difficult to obtain prior to the past decade. The recent attention given to and the improved understanding of women's health was precipitated by the larger women's social movement beginning in the 1960s, which focused on addressing the social exclusion of women (e.g., from traditionally male-dominated careers).[3] This push for inclusion was exemplified in the biomedical field in grass-roots publications such as *Our Bodies, Ourselves*.[4] This work, released in 1973, encouraged women to seek information about their health directly instead of relying on what the publication called "paternalistic" male medical doctors.[4]

The National Institutes of Health (NIH) is the primary federal agency responsible for funding medical research, with a budget of approximately $30 billion annually.[5] It was not until 1994, however, that the NIH officially established guidelines requiring that women be included in federally funded health studies. At that time, the federal government officially created the NIH Office of Research on Women's Health and specifically requested the inclusion of women into federal research because of concerns that women were underrepresented in medical studies.[6]

Research into the effects of alcohol and smoking on women's health is more available than research into the effects of opioids and stimulants on women's health. Researchers have only recently undertaken studies on the effects of these latter substances on women's health. This delay is due to the aforementioned under-representation of women in biomedical research, along with concerns over fetal health and the subsequent legal implications[3] of exposing women who may become pregnant to highly addictive stimulants shown to cause premature birth,[7] lower birth weight,[8] and slow language development.[9,10]

FEMALE-SPECIFIC CHARACTERISTICS OF SUBSTANCE ABUSE

Research shows that substance use disorders take a different course in women than in men. Women generally begin using substances later than do men.[11,12] Studies on female substance abuse treatment clients have found that they have lower education levels than male clients, lower rates of employment, and lower average age at admission into treatment.[13,14] In a study of Los Angeles substance abuse treatment clients, Hser et al. found that 39% of female clients had less than a high school education, compared with 19% among males.[14] Additionally, substance-dependent females are more likely than substance-dependent males to have spouses or partners who are also substance dependent.

Additionally, women who are addicted to substances are more likely than men to have psychiatric disorders. A study of individuals with opioid abuse disorders found that female users were twice as likely as male users to have a mood or anxiety disorder. Female users are also more likely to have psychiatric disorders that predate their substance use disorders.[15,16]

Telescoping

The telescoping of alcohol addiction has been well established in women—that is, the medical literature confirms that women progress more quickly than men into addiction to alcohol and development of the physiological consequences of alcohol abuse.[17,18] For example, there is considerable evidence that women move quickly from first use to addiction.[19–21] In an analysis of retrospective reports of over 2,000 substance abuse treatment facility clients, Johnson et al. found a faster progression in women from initiation of regular alcohol use to problem use than in men.[21]

A number of studies have also found that medical problems associated with alcohol use progress more swiftly in women.[22–24] Female alcoholics have 50 to 100% higher rates of premature death than do male alcoholics. Also, more female alcoholics die from circulatory disorders and cirrhosis of the liver than male alcoholics.[25]

Additionally, research has demonstrated that even with shorter durations of heavy drinking than their male counterparts, women have comparable incidence rates of diseases associated with alcoholism (ulcer disease, gastrointestinal hemorrhage, fatty liver, hypertension, obesity, anemia, malnutrition).[24]

Emerging research suggests that this telescoping phenomenon may also occur in women using other substances, such as tobacco, opioids, and stimulants.

Screening for Substance Use Disorders

Though substance use leads to many social and medical consequences, few seek treatment for substance use disorders. In 2002, the Substance Abuse Mental Health Services Administration (SAMHSA)'s National Survey on Drug Use and Health found that while 26.3 million people had diagnosable chemical abuse disorders, only about 6% of these individuals believed that they should seek treatment.[26] People with substance use disorders may visit a physician to seek treatment for other medical issues, and physicians must use these opportunities to screen patients; users often present with medical ailments that are related to, and may even be caused by, the substance use disorder itself.

While screening tools can be adapted to be gender-specific, it is key that physicians themselves understand the differences in the course of addiction for women, as identifying and treating substance use can mitigate or prevent many health problems in women, as described below. Medical professionals can thereby help to significantly reduce suffering and health care costs—for both the patient and society as a whole—by addressing an underlying source of medical distress. Through a review of current and past literature, this article will lay out the possible physiological consequences of substance use in women, focusing specifically on the use of alcohol, tobacco, opioids, and stimulants.

Alcohol

In women who use alcohol, telescoping—the rapid onset of addiction and of the physiological consequences of alcohol abuse—is a result of the way that women's bodies process alcohol. Though this process is not completely understood, it is theorized that the lower average amount of body water in women leads to higher blood alcohol concentrations, even when they consume the same amount of alcohol as men.[27,28] Another possible contributing factor to women's increased susceptibility to alcohol is the fact that women's digestive systems may contain less alcohol dehydrogenase, an enzyme that helps to metabolize alcohol, resulting in reduced metabolizing of alcohol and more alcohol absorption.[29]

Although previous research shows that women tend to begin using substances at later ages than do men,[11,12] more recent research suggests that women are beginning to use alcohol at younger ages.[30,31] Binge drinking among 19- to 22-year-old women has increased from 28% to 34% between 1995 and 2007.[31] In addition, although men and boys generally have higher rates of alcohol use than women and girls, the gender gap in binge drinking among teenagers has narrowed over the years. One indication of this change is the percentage-point difference between rates of binge drinking among male and female 12th graders. The difference between the prevalence of 12th-grade boys consuming five or more drinks in a row and the prevalence of 12th-grade girls engaging in the same activity has decreased from 23 points in 1975 to 7 points in 2006.[31]

The increased alcohol intake among young adult women is of particular concern in light of the medical complications that alcohol causes, and the more rapid onset of these complications that women face. It is essential, therefore, that physicians screen for alcohol use among these populations.

CONDITIONS ASSOCIATED WITH ALCOHOL USE

Liver Disease

Excessive alcohol consumption may lead to a spectrum of liver diseases, including fatty liver, alcoholic hepatitis, and cirrhosis.[32] In the United States between 1999 and 2005, deaths resulting from alcoholic liver syndromes among women increased by 15%.[33] Various studies have found that the female liver is more susceptible to alcohol than the male liver.[34,35] Although cirrhosis mortality rates are twice as high among men compared with women,[36] women develop cirrhosis faster than do men.[37] Becker et al. studied alcohol consumption and alcohol-related liver disease in a group of more than 13,200 men and women over a 12-year period. The researchers found that the level of alcohol consumption above which women increased their relative risk of developing liver disease (seven to 13 drinks per week) was about half of that for men (14 to 27 drinks per week). In addition, at any level of alcohol intake, women had a significantly higher risk of developing liver disease than did men.[38]

Cardiovascular Disease

In 2006, cardiovascular disease affected 35% of women in the United States.[39] Evidence suggests that, in general, light drinking may be associated with lower risk of cardiovascular complications, whereas heavy drinking is associated with higher risk.[40,41] In a review of key animal and human studies, Saremi and Arora found that while there is evidence that moderate alcohol consumption (especially the consumption of red wine) may have a protective effect on cardiovascular health, consumption of three or more drinks a day was associated with hypertriglyceridemia, cardiomyopathy, hypertension, and stroke.[41]

Researchers have also found that both abstaining from alcohol and heavy alcohol consumption increase risk of cardiovascular disease among women. Ikehara et al. surveyed nearly 35,000 men and 49,000 women about lifestyle, medical history, and alcohol. On follow-up 14 years later, they found that more than 1,600 participants had died of stroke and more than 700 had died of heart disease. The researchers also found distinct trends for women versus men.[42] Men who drank greater than or equal to 69 grams of alcohol per day experienced increased risk of coronary heart disease. Meanwhile, women experienced increased risk of mortality from coronary heart disease if they consumed between 23 and 45.9 grams of alcohol per day. This risk was more than tripled in women who drank 46 grams or more of alcohol per day.[42]

This study confirmed that women's risk of cardiovascular disease is increased with use of lower amounts of alcohol than for men. The threshold for increased risk of coronary heart disease among men was found to be 69 grams of alcohol per day, an amount that is three times higher than the 23-gram threshold for increased coronary heart disease risk among the women in this study.[42] Additionally, although light drinking was associated with a reduced risk of mortality from coronary heart disease for both men and women, the amount of alcohol consumption that provided a protective effect for women was significantly less than the amount that had the same effect for men. For men, intake of up to 68.9 grams of alcohol per day was associated with lower risk of coronary heart disease. In contrast, for women, drinking only up to 22.9 grams of alcohol per day had this protective effect.[42]

Despite findings that light drinking reduces risk of cardiovascular disease in men and women, the American Heart Association (AHA) does not recommend drinking alcohol to protect against heart disease because alcohol may have overall negative consequences on health. Instead, the AHA recommends consulting a doctor about lowering cholesterol and blood pressure, along with making healthy lifestyle choices, such as eating a balanced diet, exercising regularly, and controlling weight, to protect against heart disease.[43]

Endocrine Diseases

Medical research shows that alcohol consumption causes disturbances in endocrine system functioning. Health care providers should be aware of the fact that alcohol consumption can lead to elevated levels of cortisol, which is related to hypertension, impaired immune function, and metabolism disturbances.[44–46] Evidence suggests that alcohol consumption affects the hypothalamic-pituitary-adrenal axis, increasing cortisol levels.[47] In one study, Badrick et al. found that in both men and women alcohol affected hypothalamic-pituitary-adrenal function. In women, heavy drinkers experienced greater cortisol awakening response (a marker of cortisol secretion) than did moderate drinkers.[47]

Obesity

Excess weight gain and obesity are increasing at an alarming rate among Americans of all ages and both genders. In 2005, 60.5% of women were overweight or obese;[48] rates were highest among non-Hispanic black women (79.9%) and Hispanic women (68.4%).[49] These observations present a significant public health challenge because being overweight or obese increases the chances of developing heart disease, hypertension, type 2 diabetes mellitus, respiratory problems, and certain types of cancers, in both men and women.

Heavy alcohol consumption is linked to disturbances in body weight and nutrition. An 8-year prospective study using multivariate analysis found a non-linear relationship between alcohol consumption and weight gain exceeding five kilograms.[50] Heavy drinking, defined as consumption of alcohol exceeding 30 grams per day, was associated with a slight increase in weight gain among all women. Among women younger than 35 years, heavy drinking was more strongly associated with weight gain. In fact, the risk of weight gain among this group was approximately 68% higher than non-drinkers. Additionally, among African American women, even light drinking was associated with an increased risk of weight gain compared with non-drinkers.[50]

Alcohol consumption may also be associated with abdominal obesity. Schröder et al. found that among men and women consumption of three or more drinks per day was associated with increased abdominal obesity.[51] Abdominal obesity should be of particular concern to health care providers because it is a risk factor for type 2 diabetes mellitus.[52]

Diabetes Mellitus

In the United States, 9.5 million women have been diagnosed with diabetes mellitus,[48] a leading cause of death and disability. An additional 2.5 million women are believed to have undiagnosed diabetes mellitus, whereas another 23 million have been diagnosed with prediabetes mellitus.[48] Diabetes mellitus is more common in women than in men, and is especially prevalent among non-Hispanic black women. In 2005, diabetes mellitus occurred in 106.8 per 1,000 people in this population compared with 69.1 per 1,000 in non-Hispanic White women.[49]

Current research suggests that both abstaining from alcohol and consuming large amounts of alcohol increase risk, whereas light-to-moderate consumption may decrease risk.[53] In a systematic review of literature published between 1963 and August 2003, Howard et al. concluded that, compared with abstaining from alcohol, moderate consumption (defined as one to three drinks per day) was associated with a 33% to 56% lower incidence of diabetes mellitus. Meanwhile, heavy consumption of alcohol (more than three drinks per day) was associated with up to a 43% increase in diabetes mellitus incidence.[53]

Few studies look at this phenomenon specifically in women. In a 20-year twin cohort study that also investigated alcohol use and diabetes mellitus in women, Carlsson et al. found that lean-to-normal weight women who consumed large amounts of alcohol, characterized by prolonged consumption and binge drinking, had an increased incidence of type 2 diabetes mellitus.[54] Hu et al. confirmed the finding that low-to-moderate alcohol consumption among women reduces diabetes mellitus risk.[55]

Although some studies suggest that alcohol may have a protective effect against type 2 diabetes mellitus or its complications,[56,55] the American Diabetes Association does not recommend use of alcohol to protect against diabetes mellitus. In fact, for people with diabetes mellitus, drinking alcohol can cause hypoglycemia. The American Diabetes Association recommends that people with diabetes mellitus must exercise more caution if consuming alcohol.[57]

Osteoporosis

Eight million women in the United States are affected by osteoporosis, comprising 80% of all osteoporosis cases.[58] It is well accepted that use of alcohol is a risk factor for osteoporosis.[60,59] Felson et al. followed participants for 35 years, collecting data on health and alcohol consumption. They found that heavy consumption, defined as seven ounces or more of alcohol per week, caused an increase in risk of hip fracture, especially for women. Women's risk increased by 54%, whereas the risk for men increased by 26%.[59] In a more recent analysis of data from three studies, comprising a total of nearly 6,000 men and 11,000 women, Kanis et al. found that found that participants who drank moderate or large amounts of alcohol had increased risk of fracture, osteoporotic fracture, and hip fracture.[60]

Recent research has suggested that light drinking may have a protective effect for women. In a study of twins, Williams et al. found that moderate alcohol consumption did not lead to lower bone density, and in fact may be beneficial.[61] In a study of women aged 65 years and older, Diaz et al. found that risk of vertebral deformity was reduced significantly in participants who consumed alcohol more than five days per week, especially compared with those who consumed alcohol less than once per week.[62]

Despite these findings, the National Osteoporosis Foundation does not recommend consuming alcohol as a preventive measure in its prevention materials for patients. The National Osteoporosis Foundation does, however, acknowledge that heavy drinking increases risk for osteoporosis and recommends no more than two drinks per day.[63]

Lung Cancer

Lung cancer affects 219,000 women in the United States.[64] In a review of literature published between 1966 and 2000, Bandera et al. found that although research is not conclusive, there is some evidence that alcohol, particularly beer, may be associated with lung cancer.[65] In one study, Pollack et al. found that participants who consumed more than 40 ounces of alcohol per month had almost twice the incidence of lung cancer of those who did not drink alcohol.[66] In another study, Djouseé et al. found that consumption of two drinks per day approximately doubled the incidence of lung cancer, controlling for age, smoking history and gender.[67]

Breast Cancer

In 2005, approximately 2.5 million women had breast cancer,[64] whereas more than 40,000 women died as a result of breast cancer that year.[68] Studies have consistently shown that alcohol consumption can increase risk for breast cancer.[69–74] One study found that regardless of the specific alcoholic beverage consumed (wine, beer, or liquor), breast cancer rates increase with alcohol consumption. The increased risk of developing breast cancer from consuming three or more drinks per day is roughly comparable to that associated with smoking one pack of cigarettes per day.[75,76] Various studies have confirmed elevated risk, up to 60% higher for heavy drinkers than for non-drinkers (1.19 to 1.6 relative risk). Definitions of heavy drinking varied among these studies, some of which considered 15 grams or more per day to be heavy while others considered 30 grams or more per day to be heavy.[69–72]

Other studies, however, have found that even light drinking may increase women's risk for breast cancer. In a study of 490,000 males and females with a nine-year follow up, Thun et al. found that mortality from breast cancer was 30% higher among women who consumed at least one drink daily compared with non-drinkers (relative risk, 1.3).[73] More recently, Allen et al. followed 1.28 million middle-aged women for an average of 7 years, and found that for each 10-gram increase of alcohol per day, risk of breast cancer increased by 12%.[77]

Evidence suggests that drinking at later ages also contributes to breast cancer risk in women. Longnecker et al. looked at the influence of age on the relationship between breast cancer and alcohol consumption. Study participants were women with an average age of 58.7 years, who either had breast cancer (6,600) or did not (9,100). These researchers confirmed a linear relationship between alcohol consumption and breast cancer risk. Women who reported moderate consumption (12 to 18 grams or about one drink per day) had a relative risk of 1.39, compared with a non-drinker, whereas women who reported heavy consumption (33 to 45 grams or about three drinks per day) had a relative risk of 2.3. They also found, however, that breast cancer risk was not affected by alcohol consumption before the age of 30 years.[78] In a similar study, Swanson et al. confirmed this finding and also found that heavy drinking during the 5-year period leading up to breast cancer diagnosis increased relative risk by 70%.[79]

Because alcohol consumption, perhaps even light consumption, increases women's risk of breast cancer, reduction of this risk factor is essential. Physicians should emphasize this to female patients and be sure to assess alcohol use in women, including those who have been diagnosed with breast cancer.

Genital/Urinary Cancer

Endometrial cancer is the most common cancer of the female reproductive tract.[80] An estimated 554,000 women had endometrial cancer as of 2005.[64] Although research is still inconclusive, some studies have found an association between alcohol consumption and endometrial cancer. In a hospital-based study of more than 700 endometrial cancer patients and 2,100 controls, Parazzini et al. found that as alcohol consumption increased, so did risk of endometrial cancer.[81] Although these findings do not establish a cause-effect relationship, they are consistent with the finding that alcohol use may spur an increase in blood estrogen levels in postmenopausal women.[82]

Other Cancers

Studies have linked alcohol consumption to other cancers as well. In 2009, Allen et al. completed the Million Women Study, in which approximately 1.28 million middle-aged women were surveyed and followed over an average of 7 years. During the follow-up period, more than 69,700 cancers occurred. Risk for other cancers increased with each 10-gram increase of alcohol per day. Cancer of the rectum increased 10%, cancer of the liver increased 24%, and cancer of the breast increased 12%. There was no significant difference in risk based on type of alcohol consumed.[77]

Allen et al. also found that a 10-gram increase of alcohol per day resulted in increases in risk of cancer of the upper aerodigestive tract (head and neck); cancer of the oral cavity and pharynx increased 29%; cancer of the esophagus increased 22%; and cancer of the larynx increased 44%. Alcohol-associated risk, however, was restricted to current smokers and did not apply to those who had never smoked or past-smokers.[77] Other studies[83,84] on the joint effects of smoking and alcohol consumption have found increased risk of cancer for both men and women. Castellsague et al. found an association between simultaneous alcohol drinking and tobacco smoking and esophageal cancer, although smoking alone or alcohol consumption alone did not correlate with esophageal cancer.[83]

Assessment

Given the evidence of alcohol's harmful effects on women's health, health care providers should address alcohol use among female patients. There are many scales for addressing alcohol use. It is useful to use questions that assess multiple domains because questions limited to quantity and frequency of alcohol use may not detect alcohol misuse or abuse.

Useful questionnaires include the CAGE (Cut down, Annoyed, Guilty, Eye-opener) questionnaire,[85] the Michigan Alcoholism Screening Test,[86] and the Self-Administered Screening Test.[87] Although these tests are useful, they have limited application to women in terms of quantity, frequency, and consequences, but they are better than no instrument. The TWEAK (Tolerance, Worry, Eye-Opener, Amnesia, Cut down), T-ACE (Tolerance, Annoyed, Cut-down, Eye-opener), and Alcohol Use Disorders Identification Test are more sensitive tools for evaluating women in general.[88]

Studies show that the CAGE questions, taught at most medical schools, are not as sensitive in picking up alcohol disorders in women. The MAST and SAST are lengthy, and responders may require clinical supervision.

In light of the telescoping problem, a physician should use these instruments with women who have vague complaints (anxiety, difficulty sleeping, weight loss, depression, fatigue), who are undergoing stressful life events,[89] who live with an alcohol- or drug-dependent partner, or who use alcohol as a medication.

Conclusion: Alcohol

The medical literature provides sufficient evidence as to the health consequences of alcohol use. As a result of the way the female body metabolizes alcohol, women experience these consequences more quickly than men. Evidence shows that alcohol consumption increases risk of several chronic or potentially fatal conditions, including liver disease, coronary heart disease, breast cancer, diabetes mellitus, and osteoporosis. In addition, evidence suggests that associations exist between alcohol use and other cancers, such as lung, liver, or rectal cancer. Given the myriad of negative health effects of alcohol consumption, physicians must prioritize addressing alcohol abuse with female patients.

TOBACCO

Tobacco use is known to be a major health hazard, contributing to a broad range of health conditions and disorders. Aside from the established direct causal link between cigarette smoking and lung cancer, tobacco use is also associated with an increased risk of other pulmonary diseases, cardiovascular diseases, and many types of cancers, including cancers of the breast, head and neck, esophagus, pancreas, intestinal tract, bladder, and reproductive system. Although a direct dose-dependent correlation has not been fully established in some cases for these other illnesses,[90] the literature strongly suggests that these associated risks are not only present but highly significant. Additionally, the telescoping effect described earlier may also occur with smoking in women, hastening many of the adverse health impacts of tobacco use.

Cigarette smoking annually causes an estimated 178,000 deaths of women in the United States.[91] The three leading smoking-related causes of death in women are lung cancer (45,000 lives per year), heart disease (40,000), and chronic lung disease (42,000).[91] Statistics show that women who smoke more than double their risk of developing coronary heart disease[92] and increase more than tenfold their likelihood of dying from chronic obstructive pulmonary disease.[93,94] The incidence of these smoking-related deaths and illnesses can only be expected to increase in the future because global rates of cigarette smoking in women are increasing, making tobacco use an issue of particular concern for women.

Conditions Associated with Tobacco Use

Pulmonary Diseases

Lung Cancer. The causal link between cigarette smoking and lung cancer has been well established, making tobacco use a major cause of death in both men and women. In the year 2000, an estimated 47% of lung cancer cases in women in the United States were deemed a consequence of tobacco smoking.[95] Moreover, approximately 80% of all lung cancer deaths in female smokers are attributable to smoking.[96] Since 1950, lung cancer deaths among women have increased by more than 600%.[93] By 1987, lung cancer had surpassed breast cancer as the leading cause of cancer-related deaths in U.S. women.[93,97] Studies also show that the incidence of lung cancer in women is steadily increasing worldwide, while lung cancer in men shows signs of stabilization.

Evidence suggests that tobacco use in women also has a telescoping effect with lung cancer. A study of lung cancer patients in Poland revealed that women developed lung cancer at younger ages than did men, despite consuming fewer cigarettes per day and smoking for a shorter duration.[98] The data suggests that women, therefore, have a greater susceptibility to the cancer-causing compounds in cigarette smoke due to a genetic predisposition. This theory is supported by the finding that the gene for the gastrin-releasing peptide receptor is located on the X chromosome. This receptor, when activated, has a demonstrated association with the proliferation of bronchial cells.[99]

Chronic Obstructive Pulmonary Disease. Chronic obstructive pulmonary disease (COPD) continues to be the fourth leading cause of death both worldwide[100] and in the United States.[101] Smoking, particularly heavy smoking, long-term use of tobacco, and smoking of high-tar cigarettes, is a risk factor that is strongly associated with the development of COPD. Figures suggest that 10% to 15% of all smokers, and up to 26% of heavy smokers, develop COPD.[102,103]

Since the 1970s, as the incidence of tobacco use in the United States has increased among women and slightly decreased in men, the percentage of total COPD deaths comprised by women has increased from 19% in 1970 to nearly 40% in 1993.[104] Female smokers may be at greater risk of COPD-related death than men because their pulmonary system may be more swiftly compromised by long-term smoking. In a study of the effect of smoking cessation on lung function over 5 years, women who continued smoking had a proportionately greater decline in lung functioning than men with similar rates of tobacco use.[105] Conversely, women in this study who quit smoking and remained tobacco-free showed greater early improvement in lung functioning than men who also quit.

Cardiovascular Disease

Tobacco smoking is generally considered the most important preventable cause of coronary heart disease for both genders.[106,107] Epidemiologic studies have strongly supported a greater incidence of cardiovascular disease, including fatal coronary artery disease and myocardial infarction, in both men and women who smoke.[108–110] This association appears to be true even when the tobacco is used in different forms; when compared with non-smokers, those using low-tar cigarettes and smokeless tobacco still exhibited an increased risk of cardiovascular events.[111,112] More research is needed on the components of cigarette smoke and the exact mechanisms causing this association.[90]

There have been few studies of factors that predict the occurrence and severity of coronary artery disease, specifically for women. Research has shown, though, the risk of future coronary events begins to decline within 1 to 2 years of the cessation.[113]An Australian study, however, found that the total amount of lifetime cigarette smoking, whether the habit was past or current, was the most relevant quantitative variable to independently predict and prevent premature coronary artery disease. Moreover, this study found that the total smoking dose was more predictive for coronary artery disease in women than in men.[114]

Research has also shown tobacco use to be a risk factor for sudden death with severe coronary disease in women. The mechanisms leading to sudden coronary death are not fully understood, but components of cigarette smoke are believed to erode coronary plaque, which is a collection of cholesterol, fats, and calcium inside blood vessels.[115] Plaque erosion can cause blockages in blood vessels, leading to a propensity for fatal clotting, especially in women.[116] Indeed, young female smokers without other relevant risk factors (such as high cholesterol or elevated body mass index) account for the majority of fatal acute coronary thrombosis cases caused by plaque erosion in women.[117] Tobacco smoking cessation would, therefore, appear to be the most significant lifestyle change needed in preventing these deaths of young women.[117]

Breast Cancer

As the worldwide leading cause of death from cancer in women (despite being surpassed by lung cancer in the United States),[118] breast cancer is clearly a key health concern for the female population. A direct relationship between cigarette smoking and breast cancer has not been clearly established because many epidemiologic studies have failed to find that tobacco use is a significant risk factor for the disease.[119] Other evidence, however, suggests that an association may exist; in four of eight case-control studies reviewed in Japan, moderate or strong associationsbetween smoking and breast cancer risk (odds ratio > 2.0) were observed.[120] This and other research supports the plausibility that tobacco smoking has a positive association with the incidence of breast cancer.[121]

Furthermore, experimental studies suggest that genotoxic agents in cigarette smoke are involved in causing breast cancer. In rodents, the genotoxic substances in tobacco smoke were found to be mammary carcinogens.[122] Certain women who smoke may be more susceptible to these carcinogens, depending on their phase of life and genetic characteristics. For example, sensitivity of the female breast to tobacco carcinogens is increased during adolescence and earlyadulthood, but decreases after first childbirth, when most breast tissue has terminally differentiated.[123]

An example of a specific genetic difference that may put some female smokers at greater breast cancer risk is the speed with which they metabolize a certain gene, NAT2, which encodes an enzyme to activate or deactivate drugs and carcinogens in the body. People fall into three categories: rapid, intermediate, and slow NAT2 acetylators.[124] A 1996 study showed that women who are genetically slow NAT2 acetylators (about 50% of the female population) have a significantly elevated risk of breast cancer from smoking. These results held up through 12 similar studies conducted over the next decade.[125,126] Although the relative risk is small ($\sim$1.5) for NAT2 slow acetylators, the sheer number of breast cancer cases worldwide means attention to these findings and further research into the association with smoking is merited.

Cancers of the Reproductive System

Cervical cancer and other cancers of the reproductive system are also important health concerns for women. Studies have suggested that tobacco use is associated with a higher incidence of both ovarian and cervical cancers. Cigarette smoking, however, also appears to interact with women's systems in unique ways, possibly reducing the risk of endometrial cancer and causing other estrogen-associated effects (please see "Other Female-Specific Consequences of Tobacco Use").

Cervical Cancer. In studies that controlled for the effect of human papillomavirus (HPV) infection (a recognized cause of the majority of cervical cancers) tobacco use increased the risk of cervical cancer among women who were already HPV-positive.[127]In cross-sectional studies, HPV cervical infectionhas not been found to be associated consistently with smoking.[128] Research that also investigated other environmental risk factors such as diet, oral contraceptive use, and sexual history while controlling for HPV infection found that smoking appears to be the most significant of these factors associated with cancer of the cervix.[129]

These cross-sectional studies conclude that: HPV infection cannot explain theassociation between cervical cancer and smoking; the effect of smoking is unlikely to represent only a surrogate markerof a woman's sexual behavior; and the association of tobaccosmoke with invasive cervical cancer, therefore,indicates a causal relationship.[128] An alarming prediction can be made based on these findings that the increasing rates of smoking in young women may lead to a much greater incidence of cervical cancer in coming years.

Ovarian Cancer. Compared with other cancers, comparatively little research has been done into the impact of tobacco use on the incidence of ovarian cancer. Some existing studies, however, do point to cigarette smoking as a risk factor for the disease because the incidence of ovarian cancer was found to be increased even for those women who smoked in the past, but later quit.[130] The findings of Green et al. were especially significant for the incidence of mucinous types of ovarian cancer.[130] Other research suggests that cigarette smoking may only play a role in these mucinous cancers but not in ovarian cancers of other cell types.[131] More research is needed to clarify this association.

Endometrial Cancer. Interestingly, some studies have found a connection between cigarette smoking and a decreased incidence of endometrial cancer.[132–134] The link appears to be most significant in postmenopausal women.[135,136] Given the myriad adverse and potentially fatal health impacts associated with cigarette smoking, this finding of one reduced risk is not of direct importance from a public health standpoint. It does, however, point to an opportunity to better understand and prevent endometrial cancer through more research into the mechanisms by which tobacco use reduces risk.[136]

Other Cancers

Women who smoke tobacco also put themselves at increased risk for other cancers, including cancers of the pancreas, bladder, gastrointestinal tract, head and neck, and esophagus.

Smoking has a significant association with pancreatic carcinoma[137] and bladder cancer,[138] and risks for both these diseases in women may be higher than in men with the same duration and amount of tobacco use. Additionally, a Norwegian study that tracked 26,000 men and women for nearly three decades found that there was a dose-response relationship between cigarette smoking and the risk of cancers of the urinary bladder and upper digestive tract, among other cancers already discussed.[139]

Tobacco use has been found to be a significant risk factor for head and neck cancers in women, including cancers of the oral cavity, pharynx, and larynx. The overall incidence of squamous (soft-tissue) cancers of the head and neck is approximately three times higher in men than in women. Female smokers, however, have been found in one study to have a higher hazard ratio for developing head and neck cancer when compared with men. Consequently, the authors of that study estimated that cigarette smoking accounts for 75% of head and neck cancer in women, compared with 45% of these same cancers in men.[140]

Esophageal cancer is one of the least studied cancers,[141,142] despite being the fifth most common cause of death from cancer in men and seventh most common in women worldwide.[118] Studies conducted on the influence of cigarette smoking, and other potential risk factors, on the incidence of esophageal cancer have found that tobacco use is a significant risk factor for the disease. The association was strongest for esophageal adenocarcinomas; smoking was shown to have a strong relationship with the eventual development of these cancers, even 20 years after quitting.[143] This relationship may be caused by the swallowing of carcinogenic material in condensed cigarette, cigar, and pipe smoke.[144]

Other Female-Specific Consequences of Tobacco Use

In addition to the increased risk of serious health threats caused by tobacco use in women, smoking has other pervasive effects on the female body. Through mechanisms not fully understood, cigarette smoking is believed to have an anti-estrogenic effect in women. Female smokers' resulting deficiency of estrogen could explain their reduced incidence of endometrial cancer.[145] A meta-analysis of 12 studies found that the lower hormonal level caused by smoking may also have an impact on fertility in women, leading to difficulty in getting pregnant and possibly even infertility.[146] Decreased estrogen levels associated with smoking may cause earlier menopause as well; a 1999 study showed that on average current smoking decreases the age of natural menopause by 2 years and past smoking by 1 year.[147]

Many studies have discovered that post-menopausal women who smoke have lower bone density than women who have never smoked.[148] A meta-analysis of 29 cross-sectional studies on smoking and bone density and 19 cohort and case-control studies on hip fractures and smoking found that the cumulative bone loss of smokers over many years is substantially higher than in non-smokers.[149] This finding indicates that women using tobacco after menopause are at increasingly greater risk of bone injury than non-smokers as they age. The authors of this meta-analysis estimated that smoking increases the risk of hip fracture by 17% at age 60, 41% at age 70, and 71% at 80 years of age.

Conclusion: Tobacco

The evidence in the literature leaves no doubt that tobacco use has severe and potentially fatal health consequences for women of all ages, from young adulthood through maturity and old age. Moreover, the same risks of cancers, cardiovascular ailments, and pulmonary diseases due to smoking that men experience may be exacerbated in women as a result of their genetic makeup and other physiological mechanisms yet to be revealed. Finally, given the increased risk of preterm delivery, stillbirth, low birth weight, and sudden infant death syndrome (SIDS) in babies born to mothers who smoked during pregnancy,[93] the harmful effects of smoking in women can even extend to impact the chances of survival and health of the next generation.

OPIOIDS

The incidence of opioid abuse, especially of opioid prescription medications, has been increasing at an alarming rate in the United States. Rates of prescription drug abuse are especially high among teens, young adults, and those older than 60.[150] Over the past decade, the number of people abusing prescription medications has more than doubled,[151] and the majority of this abuse believed to be of pain relievers. According to Substance Abuse and Mental Health Services Administration (SAMHSA) figures, in 2007 there were 2.1 million new users aged 12 or older of prescription pain relievers.[150]

Heroin use is also on the rise, possibly owing to its connection with the abuse of prescription opioids. This increase may be attributed to the growing number of teens trying prescription opioids such as OxyContin, which is similar to heroin in chemical composition and produces a similar high. OxyContin is a synthetic opioid that resembles morphine, the organic substance from which heroin is derived.[152,153] During 2007, 106,000 persons aged 12 or older used heroin for the first time.[150] Recent findings suggest that people who abuse opioid medications may be at risk of graduating to heroin. For example, in 2006 the number of opioid-related deaths (those comprised of prescription opioid and heroin overdoses) among young people in Massachusetts was five times greater than in 1997.[154]

Opioid use among women of all age groups appears to be increasing. Although levels of cocaine and alcohol abuse among adult women dropped an average of 10% between 1992 and 2006, addictions to opioids increased 260% in the same time frame.[1] Generally, rates of drug use are higher among men than women. However, according to SAMHSA girls aged 12 to 17 had higher rates of abuse of prescription pain relievers than did boys in the same age group (2.8% versus 2.5%).[150] Additionally, through a review of research published between 1990 and 2006, Simoni-Wastila and Yang concluded that up to 11% of older female adults may use prescription medications inappropriately.[155] This research points to opioid abuse as an issue of special and growing concern for women's health.

Evidence of Telescoping

Some studies on the patterns of telescoping that pertain to the course of opioid addiction in women have begun to emerge. Researchers have found evidence that women abusing opioids may progress more quickly to addiction.[20,156] In a study of 546 men and women addicted to heroin, Anglin et al. found that women were more likely than men to become addicted to heroin within 1 month of initial exposure.[156] This study also found that women escalated their use of heroin more rapidly, became addicted in a shorter period of time, and sought treatment earlier in the course of addiction than did men.[156]

Other research conducted more recently supports these findings. A 2004 study of 271 substance-dependent patients found that women entered treatment for heroin addiction sooner than men after initial exposure to the drug. These researchers also found that, although women had been addicted for less time than men, they reported equal levels of addiction severity.[20] Such findings on the strength and speed of addiction in women make it all the more essential for health professionals to prevent, discover, and treat opioid abuse in female patients.

Physiological Effects of Opioid Abuse

Although there is little research into the effects of opioid abuse on the health of women specifically, some researchers have found increased severity of general health problems in opioid-addicted women versus men. Hernandez-Avila et al. studied male and female substance-dependent patients, using the Addiction Severity Index (ASI) to assess the severity of addiction and related problems. This assessment consists of an hour-long interview during which subjects are asked about lifetime and recent severity of problems in several areas of functioning, including medical functioning. Hernandez-Avila et al. found that women addicted to opioids reported slightly more medical issues than did men addicted to opioids.[20] Arfken et al. also conducted a study of substance-dependent patients in which ASI scores were analyzed. Although these researchers did not categorize ASI results by substance of abuse, they found a general trend in which women reported more severe medical issues than did men.[157]

Although there is little female-specific research, the literature contains extensive evidence illuminating the medical consequences of opioid use. There is an accepted causal relationship between certain opioids and respiratory depression.[158–160] In a 1981 double-blind, placebo-controlled study, six healthy women were administered oral methadone and six were administered a placebo. In the methadone group, the women's ventilatory response to carbon dioxide, which initiates exhalation, was slowed significantly during and after the half-life of the methadone dose. The significance of this delay lead researchers to conclude that women suffered opioid-induced respiratory depression despite the higher levels of progesterone present during specific menstrual cycles normally regarded as having a regulatory effect on respiration.[158]

Methadone and oxycodone overdose has also been linked to specific and sometimes fatal cardiac events, such as myocardium or striated muscle damage and depressed heart rate, as measured by prolonged QTc intervals. In a 2009 Danish study, researchers examined 100 chronic nonmalignant pain patients being treated with methadone and oxycodone and found that higher doses led to equally long delays in QTc intervals and increases in torsade de pointes, an abnormally fast heart rhythm originating in one or more ventricles. In addition, in vitro testing revealed that most opioids can block cardiac potassium channels, possibly leading to other forms of arrhythmia.[161]

Furthermore, Toth and Varga found evidence for striated muscle damage in 78 opioid abuse-related deaths. The researchers found that microscopic examinations of individuals' heart muscles in autopsy revealed that all had suffered striated muscle or myocardium damage. The authors suggest that undiagnosed striated or myocardium damage may also sometimes be a cause of death in several cases.[162]

Additionally, research has found an association between opioid use and a higher incidence of several cancers. It has also been shown that opioids can lead to an increased chance of metastasis and a subsequent decreased survival rate among tumor-bearing animals. A 2008 hospital-based case-control study of 179 patients found that opium users were more likely to develop bladder cancer, a risk that increased six-fold when the user was also a heavy smoker.[163] These findings follow a 2004 study with similar results.[164]

A causal relationship has also been suggested between opioid exposure and esophageal squamous cell carcinoma[165] and laryngeal cancer.[166] Morphine sulfate, the main alkaloid in opium, has been shown to cause an alkylation increase in the esophagus, which can lead to overproduction of diethylnitrosamine and subsequent carcinogenesis, particularly in the esophagus and liver of animals.[167] Research suggests that opioid abuse may have a deleterious effect on the immune system,[168–170] and that it may increase the risk of bacterial and viral infection in animals.[171,172] More studies are needed to shed further light on the mechanisms of these health impacts, as well as the physiological effects of opioid abuse on specific populations such as women.

Neurological Consequences of Opioid Abuse

Opioid abuse can have several severe neurological consequences for both men and women. Heroin use in particular has been shown to have negative effects on brain function, impacting attention span, memory, and verbal fluency throughout the duration of addiction.[173,174] Trail-making tests, two-back and gambling tasks, and recognition memory tests have been used to show that heroin abusers and methadone-dependent patients alike suffer from deficits in psychomotor speed, working memory, decision making, and metamemory.[175–177] Studies have also found that heroin abusers exhibit impaired verbal function and visual-spatial analysis,[178] impulse control,[179] and mental planning.[180] Such effects on proper brain functioning may seriously impact an opioid-addicted individual's ability to function in society, care for his or her health, and successfully hold employment.

Although there is a lack of conclusive opioid research specific to female physiology, recent research has suggested that female heroin abusers may experience certain neurological deficits attributed to heroin abuse more acutely than men. In a study of 18 male and 19 female patients dependent on heroin at a detoxification clinic in China, patients were presented with a map on the floor of a room and asked to perform several tasks relevant to navigating the physical space, such as following arrows on the ground and walking to specific points marked by photographs in a particular order. In three out of the four tests, female study participants performed more poorly than both control subjects and male study participants.[181]

The female participants in this same study were also found to be deficient in their ability to perform left-oriented tasks. An earlier study suggested that the capacity to discriminate between left and right was especially impaired in women dependent on heroin, who performed more poorly than control women and men dependent on heroin on all tests. Men dependent on heroin only performed poorly on some of the tests.[182]

Conclusion: Opiates

The escalating rates of opioid abuse, as well as figures that suggest opioids have become the drug of choice for many women, make our understanding of addiction to these substances and its effects critical. Additional studies must be conducted regarding the detrimental health effects of opioid abuse, especially in light of the recently published research linking bladder cancer and other ailments to use of these drugs. Attention must be paid to the physiological and neurological conditions caused by opioid abuse that are specific to, or particularly prevalent among, female patients. Also, more research is clearly needed into female-specific characteristics of addiction to heroin and other opioids, especially prescription pain relievers.

STIMULANTS

In 2007, mor than 900,000 people aged 12 and older used cocaine for the first time.[150] The number of women seeking treatment for cocaine abuse has slightly decreased since 1992 from 102,076 admissions to 99,380 admissions in 2006. However, the overall percentage of women who use cocaine admitted into treatment facilities receiving public funding has increased from 37.8% to 39.7% over the same time frame.[1]

In addition to the danger of fatal overdose from cocaine abuse, behaviors and risks associated with use of the drug can also lead to premature death in both men and women. Marzuk et al. completed a review of data on New York City male and female residents who suffered fatal injury from 1990 to 1992 and found that more than 26% had used cocaine shortly before their deaths.[183] The researchers detected cocaine in the user's system in almost one of five fatal-injury cases, which included homicides, suicides, traffic accidents, falls, and other intentional and unintentional incidents. In fact, when compared with leading causes of death, including AIDS, cancer, and heart disease, fatal injuries following cocaine use were the most common cause of death for individuals aged 15 to 24 from all racial and ethnic groups and both genders in New York City, excluding White women.[183]

Evidence of Telescoping

Significant evidence exists of telescoping in women abusing cocaine.[184–186] The literature shows that women begin using cocaine earlier in their patterns of concurrent addictions, experience more severe health problems related to cocaine use,[187] and, therefore, seek treatment sooner than men. Women also move more quickly from their introduction to cocaine into abuse.[184,186,188]

In a study of individuals with polysubstance use issues who had been admitted into two Florida drug court programs, Haas et al. found that although women began using alcohol and marijuana later in life than men they progressed to using cocaine at an earlier point in the course of addiction. Additionally, in women there was a shorter duration between first cocaine use and cocaine abuse, and they reported more cocaine use-related problems.[186]

Physiological Effects

Sweeping physiological changes caused by prolonged abuse of stimulants, including alterations at the molecular, cellular, and tissue levels, can lead to mortality among chronic users. Research in this area is inconclusive and sparse, yet there is some evidence that these changes may affect women more severely than men. In their study of men abusing polysubstances and women in Florida drug court programs, Haas and Peters found that women reported more current health problems than did men.[186]

Potentially fatal myocardial alterations can occur following chronic cocaine use, including cardiac hypertrophy, myocardial fibrosis, and microangiopathy.[189] In a study of men and women addicted to crack cocaine, Evans et al. found that smoking cocaine produced more prolonged cardiovascular effects and higher cocaine plasma concentrations in women than in men.[190] Additionally, Dudish et al. found that women were more likely to report headaches and trips to the emergency room following crack cocaine use.[191]

Several studies have suggested that cocaine use may broadly suppress the immune system[192,193] and, as a result, may enhance the infectivity of HIV in users.[193] In a study of HIV-positive women, Cook et al. found that women who persistently used crack cocaine were three times more likely to die from AIDS. These women were also more likely to develop AIDS-defining illnesses and to have virologic and immunologic markers of HIV-1 disease progression.[194]

Although the link between cigarette smoking and lung cancer has been clearly established after decades of research, studies on the possible association between smoking of illicit drugs and lung cancer are still in their preliminary stages. A 1998 study, however, did suggest that cocaine and marijuana smoking has field cancerization effects on bronchial structures in the lung, potentially putting cocaine users at higher risk of developing lung cancer.[195] The field cancerization theory, first introduced by Slaughter et al., hypothesizes that genetic alterations can occur to whole areas of tissue, developing a "patch" of altered cells and explaining the development of multiple tumors and locally recurring cancers.[196,197] Little to no research has been done on the female-specific incidence of cancer in stimulant users.

Effects of Stimulant Use Specific to Female Physiology

Women's menstrual cycles affect how they experience the subjective effects of cocaine. In one study, women were shown to experience the mood-altering effects of cocaine more strongly during their follicular menstrual cycle (the earliest period of menstruation) when estrogen was high but progesterone was low. Later, in the luteal cycle, when progesterone was higher, the effects of the drug were not felt as strongly. Researchers believe that progesterone played a significant role in dampening the physical reaction to cocaine. The authors did not fully clarify the implications of their research, but these findings demonstrate a clear mechanism specific to women and should be further investigated.[198]

As in cocaine, there is evidence that women experience the euphoric and addictive effects of amphetamines more strongly in the early follicular stages of their menstrual cycle. Of additional concern was that women in one study also reported craving and enjoying the effects of amphetamines more during the early phases of menstruation, particularly in times of high estrogen.[199]

Psychological Effects

The use of stimulants may exacerbate psychological problems, such as depression, especially in women. Research has established an association between illicit drug use and higher concentrations of cortisol, which may lead to more depressive symptoms.[200] A 2005 study found that, among heroin and cocaine users, this association was more pronounced in women, and female users with elevated cortisol concentrations were significantly more depressed than all other participants in the study.[200] This mechanism is not yet fully understood because it is unknown whether high cortisol levels precede depression or are an associated effect. The "chicken and egg" relationship between depression and illicit drug use may make causative relationships difficult to uncover.

Conclusion: Stimulants

In future national surveys of individuals entering rehabilitation or clinical facilities, more data should be collected regarding the physical condition of subjects to better elucidate the associated health concerns and determine more accurately the cost to the national economy of drug addiction.

SOCIAL CONSEQUENCES

Intimate Partner Violence

In the United States, women experience 4.8 million instances of intimate partner-related physical assaults and rapes every year.[201] Additionally, during 2005, 1,181 women were murdered by an intimate partner.[202] Many studies have found an association between alcohol abuse and intimate partner violence.[203–207] Specifically, there is much evidence of an association between intimate partner violence and alcohol use by the perpetrator.[208,203]

Some studies have found a correlation between intimate partner violence and victims' alcohol use.[204,206,209] For example, Miller et al. surveyed alcoholic and non-alcoholic women and found that alcoholic women had higher levels of spouse-to-woman violence in their lives.[206] Additionally, in a study of female welfare recipients, Tolman and Rosen found that women who had experienced intimate partner violence had higher rates of alcohol dependence than did women who had not experienced intimate partner violence.[209] Additionally, an analysis of forensic data from intimate partner related homicides detected alcohol in 45% of victims and in 70% of suspects.[210] This finding does not suggest a causal relationship. Physicians should be aware of this association so that they can look for signs of possible intimate partner violence in women who abuse alcohol and identify signs of alcohol abuse in women who have experienced intimate partner violence.

HIV/AIDS and Other Sexually Transmitted Diseases

At the end of 2005, according to the World Health Organization, 17.5 million women worldwide were infected with HIV.[211] HIV disproportionately affects African-American and Hispanic women.[212] Together they represent less than 24% of all U.S. women, yet they account for more than 82% of AIDS cases in women.[213]

Problems of substance use in women are significantly correlated with high-risk behaviors involving injection drug use, unprotected sexual contact, and multiple sexual partners. Many studies have found a direct relationship between HIV seropositivity and the number of partners with whom injection equipment has been shared, frequency of injection, and frequency of needle sharing.[214–216] Studies have also found that female users have a greater risk of contracting sexually transmitted diseases than do male users. In a study of African American adolescents, Fullilove et al. found that female crack cocaine users were more likely to engage in high-risk activities than non-using females. For example, women who used crack cocaine were more likely to take part in high-risk sexual acts in exchange for money or drugs, and they were less likely to have used a condom during last sexual intercourse than their non-using counterparts.[217] Additionally, there is evidence that women who inject drugs or smoke crack cocaine have more sex partners than do their male counterparts, further placing them at risk of contracting STDs, including HIV.[218]

Research suggests that women who drink alcohol heavily may have a heightened risk of contracting sexually transmitted diseases, including HIV.[219,220] In a study of sexually transmitted disease clinic patients, Hutton et al. found that women who reported binge drinking were twice as likely to report having multiple sex partners and five times as likely to have gonorrhea than women who abstained from alcohol.[221] By screening for and addressing substance use disorders among women, physicians can help women to reduce their risk factors for HIV and other sexually transmitted diseases.

REFERENCES

1. U.S. Dept. of Health and Human Services, Substance Abuse and Mental Health Services Administration, Office of Applied Studies. TREATMENT EPISODE DATA SET (TEDS), 1992-2006 (Concatenated) [Computer file]. Prepared by Synectics, Incorporated. ICPSR02184-v8. Ann Arbor, MI: Inter-university Consortium for Political and Social Research [producer and distributor], 2006-12-08.

2. Executive Office of the President. Office of National Drug Control Policy. 2004, December. The economic costs of drug abuse in the United States 1992-2002. Available from: http://www.whitehousedrugpolicy.gov/publications/economic_costs/economic_costs.pdf. Accessed March 12, 2009.

3. Blehar MC. Women's mental health research: the emergence of a biomedical field. Annual Review of Clinical Psychology 2006; 2:135–60.

4. Norsigian J. Boston women's health book collective: our bodies, ourselves. Boston, MA: New England Free Press, 1973.

5. The Nation's Medical Research Agency. National Institutes of Health Web site. Available from: http://www.nih.gov/about/NIHoverview.html. Accessed March 12, 2009.

6. National Institutes of Health. NIH guidelines on the inclusion of women and minorities as subjects in clinical research. Bethesda, MD: NIH Guide, 1994: 23.

7. Frank DA, Jacobs RR, Beeghly M, Augustyn M, Bellinger D, Cabral H, Heeren T. Level of prenatal cocaine exposure and scores on the Bayley Scales of Infant Development: modifying effects of caregiver, early intervention, and birth weight pediatrics. Pediatrics 2002; 110:1143–52.

8. Lumeng JC, Cabral HJ, Gannon K, Heeren T, Frank DA. Pre-natal exposures to cocaine and alcohol and physical growth patterns to age 8 years. Neurotoxicol Teratol 2007; 29:446–57.

9. Morrow CE, Bandstra ES, Anthony JC, Ofir AY, Xue L, Reyes MB. Influence of prenatal cocaine exposure on early language development: longitudinal findings from four months to three years of age. J Dev Behav Pediatr 2003; 24:39–50.

10. Bandstra ES, Morrow CE, Vogel AL, Fifer RC, Ofir AY, Dausa AT, Xue L, Anthony JC. Longitudinal influence of prenatal cocaine exposure on child language functioning. Neurotoxicol Teratol 2002; 24:297–308.

11. Chou SP, Dawson DA. A study of the gender differences in morbidity among individuals diagnosed with alcohol abuse and/or dependence. J Subst Abuse 1994; 6:381–92.

12. Gomberg ES. Women and alcohol: use and abuse. J Nerv Ment Dis1993; 181:211–9.

13. Wong CJ, Badger GJ, Sigmon SC, Higgins ST. Examining possible gender differences among cocaine-dependent outpatients. Exp Clin Psychopharmacol 2002; 10:316–23.

14. Hser YI, Huang D, Teruya C, Anglin DM. Gender comparisons of drug abuse treatment outcomes and predictors. Drug Alcohol Depend 2003; 72:255–64.

15. Kessler RC, Crum RM, Warner LA, Nelson CB, Schulenberg J, Anthony JC. Lifetime co-occurrence of DSM-III-R alcohol abuse and dependence with other psychiatric disorders in the National Comorbidity Survey. Arch Gen Psychiatry 1997; 54:313–21.

16. Grella CE, Karno MP, Warda US, Niv N, Moore AA. Gender and comorbidity among individuals with opioid use disorders in the NESARC study. Addict Behav 2009; 34(6–7):498–504.

17. Orford J, Keddie A. Gender differences in the functions and effects of moderate and excessive drinking. Br J Clin Psychol 1985; 24:265–79.

18. Randall CL, Roberts JS, Del Boca FK, Carroll KM, Connors GJ, Mattson ME. Telescoping of landmark events associated with drinking: a gender comparison. J Stud Alcohol 1999; 60:252–60.

19. Diehl A, Croissant B, Batra A, Mundle G, Nakovics H, Mann K. Alcoholism in women: Is it different in onset and outcome compared to men? Eur Arch Psychiatry Clin Neurosci 2007; 257:344–51.

20. Hernandez-Avila CA, Rounsaville BJ, Kranzler HR. Opioid-, cannabis- and alcohol-dependent women show more rapid progression to substance abuse treatment. Drug Alcohol Depend 2004; 74:265–72.

21. Johnson PB, Richter L, Kleber HD, McLellan AT, Carise D. Telescoping of drinking-related behaviors: gender, racial. Subst Use Misuse 2005; 40:1139–51.

22. Mann K, Ackermann K, Croissant B, Mundle G, Nakovics H, Diehl A. Neuroimaging of gender differences in alcohol dependence: are women more vulnerable? Alcohol Clin Exp Res 2005; 29:896–901.

23. Halliday A, Bush B, Cleary P, Aronson M, Delbanco T. Alcohol abuse in women seeking gynecologic care. Obstet Gynecol 1986; 68:322.

24. Ashley MJ, Olin JS, le Riche WH, Kornaczewski A, Schmidt W, Rankin JG. Morbidity in alcoholics: Evidence for accelerated development of physical disease in women. Arch Intern Med 1977; 137:883–7.

25. Hill SY. Biological consequences of alcoholism and alcohol-related problems among women. In: Special Populations Issues. National Institute on Alcohol Abuse and Alcoholism. Alcohol and Health Monograph No. 4. DHHS Pub. No. (ADM)82-1193. Washington, DC: Superintendent of Documents, U.S. Government Printing Office, 1982: 43–73.

26. Coombs RH. Addiction counseling review: preparing for comprehensive, certification and licensing examinations. New York: Routledge, 2005.

27. Jones BM, Jones MK. Women and alcohol: intoxication, metabolism, and the menstrual cycle. In: Greenblatt M, Schuckit MA, eds. Alcohol problems in women and children. New York: Grne & Stratton, 1976: 103–136.

28. Van Thiel DH, Tarter RE, Rosenblum E, Gavaler JS. Ethanol, its metabolism and gonadal effects: does sex make a difference? Adv Alcohol Subst Abuse 1988; 3-4:131–69.

29. Frezza M, di Padova C, Pozzato G, Terpin M, Baraona E, Lieber CS. High blood alcohol levels in women: the role of decreased gastric alcohol dehydrogenase and first-pass metabolism. N Engl J Med 1990; 322:95–9.

30. Johnston LD, O'Malley PM, Bachman JG, Schulenberg JE. Monitoring the Future national survey results on drug use, 1975-2007. Volume I: Secondary school students (NIH Publication No. 08-6418A). Bethesda, MD: National Institute on Drug Abuse, 2008:707.

31. Johnston LD, O'Malley PM, Bachman JG, Schulenberg JE. Monitoring the Future national survey results on drug use, 1975-2007. Volume II: College students and adults ages 19-45 (NIH Publication No. 08-6418B). Bethesda, MD: National Institute on Drug Abuse, 2008:319.

32. Mann RE, Smart RG, Govoni R. The epidemiology of alcoholic liver disease. Alcohol Res Health 2003; 27:209–19.

33. Centers for Disease Control and Prevention, National Center for Health Statistics. Compressed Mortality File 1999-2005. CDC WONDER On-line Database, compiled from Compressed Mortality File 1999-2005 Series 20 No. 2K, 2008. Available at: http://wonder.cdc.gov/cmf-icd10.html. Accessed March 12, 2009.

34. Tuyns AJ, Péquignot G. Greater risk of ascitic cirrhosis in females in relation to alcohol consumption. Int J Epidemiol 1984; 13:53–7.

35. Colantoni A, Idilman R, De Maria N, La Paglia N, Belmonte J, Wezeman F, Emanuele N, Van Thiel DH, Kovacs EJ, Emanuele MA. Hepatic apoptosis and proliferation in male and female rats fed alcohol: role of cytokines. Alcohol Clin Exp Res 2003; 27:1184–9.

36. Yoon YH, Yi H, Grant BF, et al. Surveillance Report #57: liver cirrhosis mortality in the United States, 1970–98. Washington, DC: National Institute on Alcohol Abuse and Alcoholism, 2001.

37. Anderson P. Alcohol and risk of physical harm. In: Holder HD, Edwards G, eds. Alcohol and public policy: evidence and issues. Oxford: Oxford University Press, 1995: 82–113.

38. Becker U, Deis A, Sorensen TI, Gronbaek M, Borch-Johnsen K, Muller CF, Schnohr P, Jensen G. Prediction of risk of liver disease by alcohol intake, sex, and age: A prospective population study. Hepatology 1996; 23:1025–9.

39. American Heart Association. Heart Disease and Stroke Statistics-2009 Update. Statistics committee and stroke statistics subcommittee. Circulation. 2008 Dec 15.

40. Foerster M, Marques-Vidal P, Gmel G, Daeppen JB, Cornuz J, Hayoz D, Pécoud A, Mooser V, Waeber G, Vollenweider P, Paccaud F, Rodondi N. Alcohol drinking and cardiovascular risk in a population with high mean alcohol consumption. Am J Cardiol 2009; 103:361–8.

41. Saremi A, Arora R. The cardiovascular implications of alcohol and red wine. Am J Ther. 2008; 15:265–77.

42. Ikehara S, Iso H, Toyoshima H, Date C, Yamamoto A, Kikuchi S, Kondo T, Watanabe Y, Koizumi A, Wada Y, Inaba Y, Tamakoshi A. Alcohol consumption and mortality from stroke and coronary heart disease among Japanese men and women. Stroke 2008; 39: 2936–42.

43. American Heart Association. Alcohol, wine and cardiovascular disease. Available at: http://www.americanheart.org/presenter.jhtml?identifier=4422. Accessed March 12, 2009.

44. Plat L, Leproult R, L'Hermite-Baleriaux M, Fery F, Mockel J, Polonsky KS, Van Cauter E. Metabolic effects of short-term elevations of plasma cortisol are more pronounced in the evening than in the morning. J Clin Endocrinol Metab 1999; 84:3082–92.

45. Spiegel K, Leproult R, Van Cauter E. Impact of sleep debt on metabolic and endocrine function. Lancet 1999; 354:1435–9.

46. Whitworth JA, Williamson PM, Mangos G, Kelly JJ. Cardiovascular consequences of cortisol excess. Vasc Health Risk Manag 2005; 1:291–9.

47. Badrick E, Bobak M, Britton A, Kirschbaum C, Marmot M, Kumari M. The relationship between alcohol consumption and cortisol secretion in an aging cohort. J Clin Endocrinol Metab 2008; 93:750–7.

48. Lloyd-Jones D, Adams R, Carnethon M, De Simone G, Ferguson TB, Flegal K, Ford E, Furie K, Go A, Greenlund K, Haase N, Hailpern S, Ho M, Howard V, Kissela B, Kittner S, Lackland D, Lisabeth L, Marelli A, McDermott M, Meigs J, Mozaffarian D, Nichol G, O'Donnell C, Roger V, Rosamond W, Sacco R, Sorlie P, Stafford R, Steinberger J, Thom T, Wasserthiel-Smoller S, Wong N, Wylie-Rosett J, Hong Y. for the American Heart Association Statistics Committee and Stroke Statistics Subcommittee. Heart disease and stroke statistics—2009 Update: A report from the American Heart Association Statistics Committee and Stroke Statistics Subcommittee. Circulation 2009; 119:e21–181.

49. U.S. Department of Health and Human Services, Health Resources and Services Administration. Women's Health USA 2007. Rockville, Maryland: U.S. Department of Health and Human Services, 2007.

50. Wannamethee SG, Field AE, Colditz GA, Rimm EB. Alcohol intake and 8-year weight gain in women: a prospective study. Obes Res 2004; 12:1386–96.

51. Schröder H, Morales-Molina JA, Bermejo S, Barral D, Soler Mándoli E, Grau M, Guxens M, de Jaime Gil E, Domínguez Álvarez M, Marrugat J. Relationship of abdominal obesity with alcohol consumption at population scale. Eur J Nutr 2007; 46:369–76.

52. Hirani V, Zaninotto P, Primatesta P. Generalised and abdominal obesity and risk of diabetes, hypertension and hypertension: diabetes co-morbidity in England. Public Health Nutrition 2008; 11:521–7.

53. Howard AA, Arnsten JH, Gourevitch MN. Effect of alcohol consumption on diabetes mellitus: a systematic review. Ann Intern Med 2004; 140:211–9.

54. Carlsson S, Hammar N, Valdemar G, Jaakko K. Alcohol consumption and the incidence of type 2 diabetes: A 20 year follow up of the Finnish twin cohort study. Diabetes Care 2003; 26:2785–90.

55. Hu FB, Manson JE, Stampfer MJ, Colditz G, Liu S, Solomon CG, Willett WC. Diet, lifestyle, and the risk of type 2 diabetes mellitus in women. N Engl J Med 2001; 345:790–7.

56. Beulens JW, Stolk RP, van der Schouw YT, Grobbee DE, Hendriks HF, Bots ML. Alcohol consumption and risk of type 2 diabetes among older women. Diabetes Care 2005; 28:2933–8.

57. Diabetes Food Pyramid: Alcohol. American Diabetes Association Web site. Available at: http://www.diabetes.org/nutrition-and-recipes/nutrition/alcohol.jsp. Accessed March 12, 2009.

58. Fast Facts on Osteoporosis. National Osteoporosis Foundation Web site. Available at: http://www.nof.org/osteoporosis/diseasefacts.htm#top. Accessed March 12, 2009.

59. Felson DT, Kiel DP, Anderson JJ, Kannel WB. Alcohol consumption and hip fractures: the Framingham study. Am J Epidemiol 1988; 128:1102–10.

60. Kanis JA, Johansson H, Johnell O, Oden A, De Laet C, Eisman JA, Pols H, Tenenhouse A. Alcohol intake as a risk factor for fracture. Osteoporos Int 2005; 16:737–42.

61. Williams FM, Cherkas LF, Spector TD, MacGregor AJ. The effect of moderate alcohol consumption on bone mineral density: a study of female twins. Ann Rheum Dis 2005; 64:309–10.

62. Diaz NM, O'Neill TW, Silman AJ, and the European Vertebral Osteoporosis Study Group. Influence of alcohol consumption on the risk of vertebral deformity. Osteoporosis International 1997; 7:65–71.

63. Prevention. National Osteoporosis Foundation Web site. Available at: http://www.nof.org/preven-tion/risk.htm#alcoholabuse. Accessed March 12, 2009.

64. Horner MJ, Ries LAG, Krapcho M, Neyman N, Aminou R, Howlader N, Altekruse SF, Feuer EJ, Huang L, Mariotto A, Miller BA, Lewis DR, Eisner MP, Stinchcomb DG, Edwards BK (eds). SEER cancer statistics review, 1975-2006: National Cancer Institute. Bethesda, MD. Available at: http:// seer.cancer.gov/csr/1975_2006/. Accessed March 12, 2009.

65. Bandera EV, Freudenheim JL, Vena JE. Alcohol consumption and lung cancer: a review of the epidemiologic evidence. Cancer Epidemiol Biomarkers Prev. 2001; 10:813–21.

66. Pollack ES, Nomura AM, Heilbrun LK, Stemmermann GN, Green SB. Prospective study of alcohol consumption and cancer. N Engl J Med 1984; 310:617–21.

67. Djoussé L, Dorgan JF, Zhang Y, Schatzkin A, Hood M, D'Agostino RB, Copenhafer DL, Kreger BE, Ellison RC. Alcohol consumption and risk of lung cancer: The Framingham Study. J Natl Cancer Inst. 2002; 94:1877–82.

68. Centers for Disease Control and Prevention, National Center for Health Statistics. Compressed Mortality File 1999-2005. CDC WONDER On-line Database, compiled from Compressed Mortality File 1999-2005 Series 20 No. 2K, 2008. Available at: http://wonder.cdc.gov/cmf-icd10.html. Accessed March 12, 2009.

69. Fuchs CS, Stampfer MJ, Colditz GA, Giovannucci EL, Manson JE, Kawachi I, Hunter DJ, Hankinson SE, Hennekens CH, Rosner B. Alcohol consumption and mortality among women. N Engl J Med 1995; 332:1245–50.

70. Smith-Warner SA, Spiegelman D, Yaun SS, Adami HO, Beeson WL, van den Brandt PA, Folsom AR, Fraser GE, Freudenheim JL, Goldbohm RA, Graham S, Miller AB, Potter JD, Rohan TE, Speizer FE, Toniolo P, Willett WC, Wolk A, Zeleniuch-Jacquotte A, Hunter DJ. Alcohol and breast cancer in women: a pooled analysis of cohort studies. JAMA 2001; 185:769–76.

71. Willett WC, Green A, Stampfer MJ, Speizer FE, Colditz GA, Rosner B, Monson RR, Stason W, Hennekens CH. Relative and absolute excess risks of coronary heart disease among women who smoke cigarettes. N Engl J Med 1987; 317:1303–9.

72. Gapstur SM, Potter JD, Sellers TA, Folsom AR. Increased risk of breast cancer with alcohol consumption in postmenopausal women. Am J Epidemiol 1992; 136:1221–31.

73. Thun MJ, Peto R, Lopez AD, Monaco JH, Henley SJ, Heath CW, Doll R. Alcohol consumption and mortality among middle-aged and elderly U.S. adults. N Engl J Med 1997; 337:1705–14.

74. Swanson CA, Coates RJ, Malone KE, Gammon MD, Schoenberg JB, Brogan DJ, McAdams M, Potischman N, Hoover RN, Brinton LA. Alcohol consumption and breast cancer risk among women under age 45 years. Epidemiology 1997; 8:231–7.

75. Li Y, Baer D, Friedman GD Md, Udaltsova N, Shim V, Klatsky AL. Wine, liquor, beer and risk of breast cancer in a large population. Eur J Cancer 2009; 45: 843–50.

76. European Cancer Conference. Alcohol amount, not type—wine, beer, liquor—triggers breast cancer. ScienceDaily. Available from: http://www.sciencedaily.com/releases/2007/09/070927083251.htm. Accessed March 12, 2009.

77. Allen NE, Beral V, Casabonne D, Kan SW, Reeves GK, Brown A, Green J. Moderate alcohol intake and cancer incidence in women. J Natl Cancer Inst 2009; 101: 296–305.

78. Longnecker MP, Newcomb PA, Mittendorf R, Greenberg ER, Clapp RW, Bogdan GF, Baron J, MacMahon B, Willett WC. Risk of breast cancer in relation to lifetime alcohol consumption. J Natl Cancer Inst 1995; 87:923–9.

79. Swanson CA, Coates RJ, Malone KE, Gammon MD, Schoenberg JB, Brogan DJ. Alcohol consumption and

breast cancer risk among women under age 45 years. Epidemiology 1997; 8:231–7.

80. Hill HA, Austin H. Nutrition and endometrial cancer. Cancer Causes Control 1996; 7:19–32.

81. Parazzini F, La Vecchia C, D'Avanzo B, Moroni S, Chatenoud L, Ricci E. Alcohol and endometrial cancer risk: findings from an Italian case-control study. Nutr Cancer 1995; 23:55–62.

82. Purohit V. Moderate alcohol consumption and estrogen levels in postmenopausal women: a review. Alcohol Clin Exp Res 1998; 22:994–7.

83. Castellsagué X, Munóz N, De Stefani E, Victora CG, Castelletto R, Rolón PA, Quintana MJ. Independent and joint effects of tobacco smoking and alcohol drinking on the risk of esophageal cancer in men and women. Int J Cancer 1999; 82:657–64.

84. Talamini G, Bassi C, Falconi M, Sartori N, Salvia R, Rigo L, Castagnini A, Di Francesco V, Frulloni L, Bovo P, Vaona B, Angelini G, Vantini I, Cavallini G, Pederzoli P. Alcohol and smoking as risk factors in chronic pancreatitis and pancreatic cancer. Dig Dis Sci 1999; 44:1303–11.

85. Ewing JA. Detecting alcoholism: The CAGE questionnaire. JAMA 1984; 252:1905.

86. Seizes ML. The Michigan Alcoholism Screening Test: A quest for a new diagnostic instrument. Am J Psychiatry 1971; 127:89.

87. Hurt RD, Morse RM, Sorenson WM. Diagnosis of alcoholism with a self-administered alcoholism screening test: Results with 1,002 consecutive patients receiving general examinations. Mayo Clin Proc 1980; 55:365.

88. Zilberman ML, Tavares H, Blume SB, el-Guebaly N. Towards best practices in the treatment of women with addictive disorders. Addict Disord Treat 2002; 1:39–46.

89. Beckman LJ. Women alcoholics: a review of social and psychological studies. J Stud Alcohol 1975; 36: 794.

90. Ambrose JA, Barua RS. The pathophysiology of cigarette smoking and cardiovascular disease: An update. J Am Coll Cardiol 2004; 43:1731–7. Available at: http://content.onlinejacc.org/cgi/reprint/43/10/1731.pdf. Accessed March 13, 2009.

91. U.S. Department of Health and Human Services. Women and Smoking: A Report of the Surgeon General. Atlanta, GA: U.S. Department of Health and Human Services, CDC, National Center for Chronic Disease Prevention and Health Promotion, Office on Smoking and Health, 2001. Available from: http://www.cdc.gov/tobacco/data_statistics/sgr/sgr_2001/index.htm. Accessed March 13, 2009.

92. Novotny TE, Giovino GA. Tobacco Use. In: Brownson RC, Remington PW, Davis JR (eds). Chronic disease epidemiology and control. American Public Health Association 1993; Washington, DC:117–48.

93. U.S. Department of Health and Human Services. Women and smoking: a report of the surgeon general. Atlanta, GA: U.S. Department of Health and Human Services, Public Health Service, CDC, National Center for Chronic Disease Prevention and Health Promotion, Office on Smoking and Health, 2001. Available from: http://www.cdc.gov/tobacco/data_statistics/sgr/sgr_2001/index.htm. Accessed March 13, 2009.

94. Centers for Disease Control and Prevention. Perspectives in disease prevention and health promotion, smoking-attributable mortality and years of potential life lost—United States, 1984. Morbidity and Mortality Weekly Report [serial online] 1997; 46:444–51. Available at: http://www.cdc.gov/mmwr/preview/mmwrhtml/00047690.htm. Accessed March 13, 2009.

95. Parkin DM, Pisani P, Ferlay J. Global Cancer Statistics, 2002. Cancer J Clin 1999; 49:33–64, 1.

96. Centers for Disease Control and Prevention. Surgeon General's report: the health consequences of smoking. 2004. Available at: http://www.cdc.gov/tobacco/data_statistics/sgr/sgr_2004/index.htm#lights. Accessed March 13, 2009.

97. Centers for Disease Control and Prevention. Fact sheet: women and tobacco. 2006. Available at: http://www.cdc.gov/tobacco/data_statistics/Factsheets/women_tobacco.htm. Accessed March 13, 2009.

98. Radzikowska E, Glaz P, Roszkowski K. Lung cancer in women: age, smoking, histology, performance status, stage, initial treatment and survival: population-based study of 20,561 cases. Ann Oncol 2002; 13:1087–93.

99. Shriver SP, Bourdeau HA, Gubish CT, Tirpak DL, Davis AL, Luketich JD, Siegfried JM. Sex-specific expression of gastrin-releasing peptide receptor: relationship to smoking history and risk of lung cancer. J Natl Cancer Inst 2000; 92:24–33. Available at: http://jnci.oxfordjournals.org/cgi/content/abstract/92/1/24. Accessed March 12, 2009.

100. World Health Organization. Fact sheet: the top ten causes of death. November 2008. Fact Sheet No 310. Available at: http://www.who.int/mediacentre/factsheets/fs310_2008.pdf. Accessed March 12, 2009.

101. Centers for Disease Control and Prevention. National vital statistics reports. April 2008. Deaths: Final Data for 2005. Vol 56, No 10. Available online: http: //www.cdc.gov/ nchs/data/ nvsr/nvsr56/nvsr56_ 10.pdf. Accessed March 12, 2009.

102. American Thoracic Society. Cigarette smoking and health. Am J Respir Crit Care Med 1996; 153: 861–5.

103. Fletcher C, Peto R, Tinker C, Speizer FE. The natural history of chronic bronchitis and emphysema: an eight-year study of early chronic obstructive lung disease in working men in London. Oxford University Press, New York, 1976.

104. Centers for Disease Control. Mortality patterns—United States, 1993. Morbid Mortal Weekly Rep 1996; 45:161–4.

105. Scanlon PD, Connett JE, Waller LA, Altose MD, Bailey WC, Buist AS. Smoking cessation and lung function in mild-to-moderate chronic obstructive pulmonary disease: the Lung Health Study. Am J Respir Crit Care Med 2000; 161:381-90. Available at: http://ajrccm.atsjournals.org/cgi/reprint/161/2/381. Accessed March 12, 2009.

106. Hennekens CH. Coronary disease: risk intervention. In: Julian DG, Wenger NK eds. Women and heart disease (1st ed.). London: Martin Dunitz, 1997:39–48.

107. Roeters van Lennep JE, Westerveld HT, Erkelens DW, van der Wall EE. Risk factors for coronary heart disease: implications of gender. Cardiovasc Res 2002; 53:538–49. Available at: http://cardiovascres.oxfordjournals.org/cgi/reprint/53/3/538. Accessed March 12, 2009.

108. Jonas MA, Oates JA, Ockene JK, Hennekens CH. Statement on smoking and cardiovascular disease for health care professionals: American Heart Association. Circulation 1992; 86:1664–9.

109. Black HR. Smoking and cardiovascular disease. In: Laragh JH, Brenner BM, eds. Hypertension: pathophysiology, diagnosis and management (2nd ed.). New York: Raven Press Ltd., 1995:2621–47.

110. Price JF, Mowbray PI, Lee AJ, Rumley A, Lowe GD, Fowkes FG. Relationship between smoking and cardiovascular risk factors in the development of peripheral arterial disease and coronary artery disease: Edinburgh Artery study. Eur Heart J 1999; 20:344–53.

111. Negri E, Franzosi MG, La Vecchia C, Santoro L, Nobili A, Tognoni G. Tar yield of cigarettes and risk of acute myocardial infarction: GISSI-EFRIM Investigators. BMJ 1993; 306:1567–70.

112. Bolinder G, Alfredsson L, Englund A, de Faire U. Smokeless tobacco use and increased cardiovascular mortality among Swedish construction workers. Am J Public Health 1994; 84:399–404.

113. Rosenberg L, Palmer JR, Shapiro S. Decline in the risk of myocardial infarction among women who stop smoking. N Engl J Med 1990; 322:213–7.

114. Wang XL, Tam C, McCredie RM, Wilcken DE. Determinants of severity of coronary artery disease in Australian men and women. Circulation 1994; 89:1974-81. Available online: http://circ.ahajournals.org/cgi/reprint/89/5/1974. Accessed February 26 2009.

115. American Heart Association. Gender and age differences found in clotting mechanism of sudden cardiac death. Available online: http://www.eurekalert.org/pub_releases/1998-04/AHA-GAAD-270498.php. Accessed 9 March 2009.

116. Arbustini E, Dal Bello B, Morbini P, Burke AP, Bocciarelli M, Specchia G, Virmani R. Plaque erosion is a major substrate for coronary thrombosis in acute myocardial infarction. Heart 1999; 82:269–72. Available online: http://www.pubmedcentral.nih.gov/picrender.fcgi?artid=1729173&blobtype=pdf. Accessed March 12, 2009.

117. Burke AP, Farb A, Malcom GT, Liang Y, Smialek J, Virmani R. Effect of risk factors on the mechanism of acute thrombosis and sudden coronary death in women. Circulation 1998; 97:2110–6. Available at: http://circ.ahajournals.org/cgi/reprint/97/21/2110. Accessed March 12, 2009.

118. American Cancer Society. Global cancer facts & figures 2007. Available at: http://www.cancer.org/downloads/STT/Global_Facts_and_Figures_2007_rev2.pdf. Accessed March 12, 2009.

119. IARC Monographs on the evaluation of carcinogenic risks to humans. Tobacco smoke and involuntary smoking. Vol. 83. Lyon: IARC; 2004.

120. Nagata C, Mizoue T, Tanaka K, Tsuji I, Wakai K, Inoue M, Tsugane S. Tobacco smoking and breast cancer risk: an evaluation based on a systematic review of epidemiological evidence among the Japanese population. Jpn J Clin Oncol 2006; 36: 387–94. Available online: http://jjco.oxfordjournals.org/cgi/reprint/36/6/387. Accessed March 12, 2009.

121. Morabia A, Ambrosone CB, Baron JA, Phillips DH, Russo IH. What do we currently know about the epidemiological and biological plausibility of the association of smoking and breast cancer? J Womens Cancer 2001; 3:5–8.

122. Hecht SS. Tobacco smoke carcinogens and breast cancer. Environ Mol Mutagen 2002; 39:119–26.

123. Ha M, Mabuchi K, Sigurdson AJ, Freedman DM, Linet MS, Doody MM, Hauptmann M. Smoking cigarettes before first childbirth and risk of breast cancer. Am J Epidemiol 2007; 166:55–61.

124. GeneCards. N-acetyltransferase 2. Last updated Jan 2009. Available online: http://www.genecards.org/cgi-bin/carddisp.pl?gene=NAT2. Accessed March 12, 2009.

125. Ambrosone CB, Kropp S, Yang J, Yao S, Shields PG, Chang-Claude J. Cigarette smoking, N-acetyltransferase 2 genotypes, and breast cancer risk: Pooled analysis and meta-analysis. Cancer Epidemiol Biomarkers Prev 2008; 17:15–26.

126. Phillips and Garte. Smoking and breast cancer: is there really a link? Cancer Epidemiol Biomarkers Prev 2008; 17:1–2. Available online: http://cebp.aacrjournals.org/cgi/reprint/17/1/1. Accessed March 12, 2009.

127. Plummer M, Herrero R, Franceschi S, Meijer CJ, Snijders P, Bosch FX, de Sanjosé S, Muñoz N; IARC Multi-centre Cervical Cancer Study Group. Smoking and cervical cancer: pooled analysis of the IARC multicentric case-control study. Cancer Causes Control 2003; 14:805–14.

128. Vineis P, Alavanja M, Buffler P, Fontham E, Franceschi S, Gao YT, Gupta PC, Hackshaw A, Matos E, Samet J, Sitas F, Smith J, Stayner L, Straif K, Thun MJ, Wichmann HE, Wu AH, Zaridze D, Peto R, Doll R. Tobacco and cancer: recent epidemiological evidence. J Natl Cancer Inst 2004; 96:99–106. Available at: http://jnci.oxfordjournals.org/cgi/reprint/96/2/99. Accessed March 12, 2009.

129. Kjellberg L, Hallmans G, Ahren AM, Johansson R, Bergman F, Wadell G, Angstrom T, Dilliner J. Smoking, diet, pregnancy and oral contraceptive use as risk factors for cervical intra-epithelial neoplasia in relation to human papillomavirus infection. Br J Cancer 2000; 82:1332–8.

130. Green A, Purdie D, Bain C, Siskind V, Webb PM. Cigarette smoking and risk of epithelial ovarian cancer (Australia). Cancer Causes Control 2001; 12:713–19.

131. Zhang Y, Coogan PF, Palmer JR, Strom BL, Rosenberg L. Cigarette smoking and increased risk of mucinous epithelial ovarian cancer. Am J Epidemiol 2004; 159:133–9. Available at: http://aje.oxford-journals.org/cgi/reprint/159/2/133. Accessed March 12, 2009.

132. Lesko SM, Rosenberg L, Kaufman DW, Helmrich SP, Miller DR, Strom B, et al. Cigarette smoking and the risk of endometrial cancer. N Engl J Med 1985; 313: 593–6.

133. Brinton LA, Barren RJ, Berman ML, Mortel R, Twiggs LB, Wilbanks GD. Cigarette smoking and the risk of endometrial cancer. Am J Epidemiol 1993; 137:281–91.

134. Viswanathan AN, Feskanich D, De Vivo I, Hunter DJ, Barbieri RL, Rosner B, Colditz GA, Hankinson SE. Smoking and the risk of endometrial cancer: results from the Nurses' Health Study. Int J Cancer 2005; 114:996–1001. Available at: http://www3.interscience.wiley.com/cgi-bin/fulltext/109865074/PDFSTART. Accessed March 12, 2009.

135. Weiderpass E, Baron JA. Cigarette smoking, alcohol consumption, and endometrial cancer risk: a population-based study in Sweden. Cancer Causes Control 2001; 12:239–47.

136. Zhou B, Yang L, Sun Q, Cong R, Gu H, Tang N, Zhu H, Wang B. Cigarette smoking and the risk of endometrial cancer: a meta-analysis. Am J Med 2008; 121:501–8. Available at: http://download.journals.elsevierhealth.com/pdfs/journals/0002-9343/PIIS000293430800-1940.pdf. Accessed March 12, 2009.

137. Muscat JE, Stellman SD, Hoffmann D, Wynder EL. Smoking and pancreatic cancer in men and women. Cancer Epidemiol Biomarkers Prev 1997; 6:15–9. Available at: http://cebp.aacrjournals.org/cgi/reprint/6/1/15.pdf. Accessed March 12, 2009.

138. Castelao JE, Yuan JM, Skipper PL, Tannenbaum SR, Gago-Dominguez M, Crowder JS, Ross RK, Yu MC. Gender- and smoking-related bladder cancer risk. J Natl Cancer Inst 2001; 93:538–45. Available at: http://jnci.oxfordjournals.org/cgi/reprint/93/7/538. Accessed March 12, 2009.

139. Engeland A, Andersen A, Haldorsen T, Tretli S. Smoking habits and risk of cancers other than lung cancer: 28 years' follow-up of 26,000 Norwegian men and women. Cancer Causes Control 1996; 7:497–506.

140. Freedman ND, Abnet CC, Leitzmann MF, Hollenbeck AR, Schatzkin A. Prospective investigation of the cigarette smoking-head and neck cancer association by sex. Cancer 2007; 110:1593–601.

141. Enzinger PC, Mayer RJ. Esophageal cancer. N Engl J Med. 2003; 349:2241–2252. Available at: http://www.usagiedu.com/articles/esoca03/esoca03.pdf. Accessed March 12, 2009.

142. Pisani P, Parkin DM, Bray F, Ferlay J. Estimates of the worldwide mortality from 25 cancers in 1990. Int J Cancer 1999; 83:18–29. [Erratum: Int J Cancer 1999; 83:870–3.]

143. Wu AH, Wan P, Bernstein L. A multiethnic population-based study of smoking, alcohol and body size and risk of adenocarcinoma of the stomach and esophagus (United States). Cancer Causes Control 2001; 12:721–32.

144. De Stefani E, Barrios E, Fierro L. Black (air-cured) and blond (flue-cured) tobacco and cancer risk. III. Oesophageal cancer. Eur J Cancer 1993; 29A:763–6.

145. Baron JA, La Vecchia C, Levi F. The antiestrogenic effect of cigarette smoking in women. Am J Obstet Gynecol 1990; 162:502–14.

146. Augood C, Duckitt K, Templeton AA. Smoking and female infertility: a systematic review and meta-analysis. Hum Reprod 1998; 13:1532–9.

147. Hu FB, Grodstein F, Hennekens CH, Colditz GA, Johnson M, Manson JE, Rosner B, Stampfer MJ. Age at natural menopause and risk of cardiovascular disease. Arch Intern Med 1999; 159:1061–6.

148. Hollenbach KA, Barrett-Connor E, Edelstein SL, Holbrook T. Cigarette smoking and bone mineral density in older men and women. American Journal of Public Health 1993; 83:1265–1270.

149. Law MR, Hackshaw AK. A meta-analysis of cigarette smoking, bone mineral density and risk of hip fracture: recognition of a major effect. BMJ 1997; 315:841–6.

150. Department of Health and Human Services; Substance Abuse and Mental Health Services Administration, Office of Applied Studies. Results from the 2007 National Survey on Drug Use and Health: National Findings [monograph on the Internet]. Available at: http://www.oas.samhsa.gov/NSDUH/2k7NSDUH/2k7-results.cfm. Accessed March 12, 2009.

151. Manchikanti L. Prescription drug abuse: what is being done to address the new drug epidemic? Testimony before the subcommittee on criminal justice, drug policy and human resources. Pain Physician 2006; 9:287–321.

152. Educating Voices. Oxycontin facts. Available from: http://www.educatingvoices.org/OXYCONTIN.asp.

153. Educating Voices Heroin facts. Available from: http://www.educatingvoices.org/HEROIN.asp.

154. Calefati J. Heroin hits the suburbs hard amid wave of drug abuse by teens and 20-somethings. Available at: http://www.usnews.com/articles/news/national/2008/12/05/heroin-hits-the-suburbs-hard-amid-wave-of-drug-abuse-by-teens-and-20-somethings.html. Accessed March 12, 2009.

155. Simoni-Wastila L, Yang HK. Psychoactive drug abuse in older adults. Am J Geriatr Pharmacother 2006; 4:380–94.

156. Anglin MD, Hser YI, McGlothlin WH. Sex differences in addict careers. 2. Becoming addicted. Am. J. Drug Alcohol Abuse 1987; 13:59–71.

157. Arfken CL, Klein C, di Menza S, Schuster CR. Gender differences in problem severity at assessment and treatment retention. J Subst Abuse Treat 2001; 20:53–7.

158. Olsen GD, Wilson JE, Robertson GE. Respiratory and ventilatory effects of methadone in healthy women. Clin Pharmacol Ther 1981; 29:373–80.

159. Nettleton RT, Ransom TA, Abraham SL, Nelson CS, Olsen GD. Methadone-Induced Respiratory Depression in the Neonatal Guinea Pig. Pediatr Pulmonol 2007; 42:1134–43.

160. Neal RC, Olsen GD. The effects of methadone on respiration and ventilation in Pygmy goats. J Pharmacol Exp Ther1980; 215:45–52.

161. Fanoe S, Jensen GB, Sjøgren P, Korsgaard MP, Grunnet M. Oxycodone is associated with dose-dependent QTc prolongation in patients and low-affinity inhibiting of hERG activity in vitro. Br J Clin Pharmacol 2009; 67: 172–9.

162. Tóth AR, Varga T. Myocardium and striated muscle damage caused by licit or illicit drugs. Journal of Legal Medicine. In press.

163. Hosseini SY, Safarinejad MR, Amini E, Hooshyar H. Opium consumption and risk of bladder cancer: A case-control analysis. Urol Oncol 2008 Dec 24. [Epub ahead of print].

164. Aliasgari M, Kaviani A, Gachkar L, Hosseini-Nassab S. Is bladder cancer more common among opium addicts? Urol J 2004; 1:253–4.

165. Nasrollahzadeh D, Kamangar F, Aghcheli K, Sotoudeh M, Islami F, Abnet CC, Shakeri R, Pourshams A, Marjani HA, Nouraie M, Khatibian M, Semnani S, Ye W, Boffetta P, Dawsey SM, Malekzadeh R. Opium, tobacco, and alcohol use in relation to esophageal squamous cell carcinoma in a high-risk area of Iran. Br J Cancer 2008; 98:1857–63.

166. Mousavi MR, Damghani MA, Haghdoust AA, Khamesipour A. Opium and risk of laryngeal cancer. Laryngoscope 2003; 113:1939–43.

167. Ribeiro-Pinto LF, Swann PF. Opium and esophageal cancer: Effect of morphine and opium on the metabolism of N-nitrosodimethylamine and N-nitrosodiethylamine in the rat. Carcinogenesis 1997; 18:365–9.

168. Sacerdote P, Limiroli E, Gaspani L. Experimental evidence for immunomodulatory effect of opioids. In: Machelska H, Stein C, eds. Immune Mechanisms of pain and analgesia, advances in experimental medicine and biology. New York: Kluwer Academic Press, 2001; 521:106–12.

169. Sacerdote P. Opioids and the immune system. Palliat Med 2006; 20(Suppl 1):S9–15.

170. Vallejo R, de Leon-Casasola O, Benyamin R. Opioid therapy and immunosuppression: A review. Am J Ther 2004; 11:354–65.

171. Risdahl JM, Khanna KV, Peterson PK, Molitor TW. Opiates and infection. J Neuroimmunol 1998; 83:4–18.

172. Wang J, Barke RA, Charboneau R, Roy S. Morphine impairs host innate immune response and increases susceptibility to Streptococcus pneumoniae lung infection. J Immunol 2005; 174:426–34.

173. Guerra D, Sole A, Cami J, Tobena A. Neuropsychological performance in opiate addicts after rapid detoxification. Drug Alcohol Depend 1987; 20: 261–70.

174. Kamboj SK, Tookman A, Jones L, Curran HV. The effects of immediate-release morphine on cognitive functioning in patients receiving chronic opioid therapy in palliative care. Pain 2005; 117:388–95.

175. Mintzer MZ, Stitzer ML. Cognitive impairment in methadone maintenance patients. Drug Alcohol Depend 2002; 67:41–51.

176. Ornstein TJ, Iddon JL, Baldacchino AM, Sahakian BJ, London M, Everitt BJ, Robbins TW. Profiles of cognitive dysfunction in chronic amphetamine and heroin abusers. Neuropsychopharmacology 2000; 23:113–126.

177. Sjogren P, Christrup LL, Petersen MA, Hojsted J. Neuropsychological assessment of chronic non-malignant pain patients treated in a multidisciplinary pain centre. Eur J Pain 2005; 9:453–62.

178. Prosser J, Cohen LJ, Steinfeld M, Eisenberg D, London ED, Galynker I. Neuropsychological functioning in opiatedependent subjects receiving and following methadone maintenance treatment. Drug Alcohol Depend 2006; 84:240–7.

179. Lee TM, Pau CW. Impulse control differences between abstinent heroin users and matched controls. Brain Inj 2002; 16:885–9.

180. Davydov DM, Polunina AG. Heroin abusers' performance on the Tower of London Test relates to the baseline EEG alpha2 mean frequency shifts. Prog Neuropsychopharmacol Biol Psychiatry 2004; 28:1143–52.

181. Wang JH, Liu XF, Chen YM, Sun HY, Fu Y, Ma MX, He J, Wang HY, Wilson FA, Carlson S, Ma YY. Heroin impairs map-picture-following and memory tasks dependent on gender and orientation of the tasks. Behav Neurosci 2007; 121:653–64.

182. Liu N, Li B, Wilson FA, Ma Y, Hu X.Gender effect on the right-left discrimination task in a sample of heroin-dependent patients. Psychopharmacology (Berl) 2005; 181:735–40.

183. Marzuk PM, Tardiff K, Leon AC, Portera L, Weiner C. Fatal injuries after cocaine use as a leading cause of death among young adults in New York City. N Engl J Med 1995; 332:1753–57. Available at: http://content.nejm.org/cgi/content/full/332/26/1753. Accessed March 12, 2009.

184. Griffin ML, Weiss RD, Lange U. A comparison of male and female cocaine abuse. Arch Gen Psychiatry 1989; 46:122–6.

185. White KA, Brady KT, Sonne S. Gender differences in patterns of cocaine use. Am J Addict 1996; 5: 259–61.

186. Haas AL, Peters RH. Development of substance abuse problems among drug-involved offenders. Evidence for the telescoping effect. J Subst Abuse 2000; 12: 241–53.

187. Kosten TA, Gawin FH, Kosten TR, Rounsaville BJ. Gender differences in cocaine use and treatment response. J Subst Abuse Treat 1993; 10:63–6.

188. Mendelson JH, Weiss R, Griffin M, Mirin SM, Teoh SK, Mello NK, Lex BW. Some special considerations for treatment of drug abuse and dependence in women. NIDA Res Monogr 1991; 106:313–27.

189. Karch SB. Cocaine cardiovascular toxicity. South Med J 2005; 98:794.

190. Evans SM, Haney M, Fischman MW, Foltin RW. Limited sex differences in response to "Binge" smoked cocaine use in humans. Neuropsychopharmacology 1999; 21:445–54.

191. Dudish SA, Hatsukami DK. Gender differences in crack users who are research volunteers. Drug Alcohol Depend 1996; 42:55–63.

192. Ou DW, Shen ML, and Luo YD. Effects of cocaine on the immune system of Balb/C mice. Clin Immunol Immunopathol 1989; 52:305–12.

193. Baldwin, GC, Roth, MD, Tashkin, DP. Acute and chronic effects of cocaine on the immune system and the possible link to AIDS. J Neuroimmunol 1998; 83: 133–8.

194. Cook JA, Burke-Miller JK, Cohen MH, Cook RL, Vlahov D, Wilson TE, Golub ET, Schwartz RM, Howard AA, Ponath C, Plankey MW, Levine AM, Grey DD. Crack cocaine, disease progression, and mortality in a multicenter cohort of HIV-1 positive women. AIDS 2008; 22: 1355–63.

195. Barsky SH, Roth MD, Kleerup EC, Simmons M, Tashkin DP. Histopathologic and molecular alterations in bronchial epithelium in habitual smokers of marijuana, cocaine, and/or tobacco. J Natl Cancer Inst 1998; 90:1198–205. Available online: http://jnci.oxfordjournals.org/cgi/reprint/90/16/1198. Accessed March 12, 2009.

196. Slaughter DP, Southwick HW, Smejkal W. 'Field cancerization' in oral stratified squamous epithelium: clinical implications of multicentric origin. Cancer 1953; 6:963–8.

197. Braakhuis BJ, Tabor MP, Kummer JA, Leemans CR, Brakenhoff RH. A genetic explanation of Slaughter's concept of field cancerization: evidence and clinical implications. Cancer Res 2003; 63:1727–30.

198. Sofuoglu M, Dudish-Poulsen S, Nelson D, Pentel PR, Hatsukami DK. Sex and menstrual cycle differences in the subjective effects from smoked cocaine in humans. Exp Clin Psychopharmaco. 1999; 7:274–83.

199. Justice AJ, de Wit H. Acute effects of d-amphetamine during the follicular and luteal phases of the menstrual cycle in women. Psychopharmacology (Berl) 1999; 145:67–75.

200. Wisniewski AB, Brown TT, Cofranceso JM, Golub ET, Ricketts EP, Wand G, Dobs AS. Cortisol levels and depression in men and women using heroin and cocaine. Psychoneuroendocrinology 2006; 31:250–5.

201. Tjaden P, Thoennes N. Extent, nature, and consequences of intimate partner violence: findings from the National Violence Against Women Survey. Washington, DC: Department of Justice; 2000. Publication No. NCJ 181867. Available at: www.ojp.usdoj.gov/nij/pubs-sum/181867.htm. Accessed March 12, 2009.

202. Bureau of Justice Statistics Web site. Intimate homicide victims by gender. Available at: http://www.ojp.usdoj.gov/bjs/homicide/intimates.htm. Accessed March 12, 2009.

203. Caetano R, Schafer J, Cunradi CB. Alcohol-related intimate partner violence among White, Black, and Hispanic couples in the United States. Alcohol Res Health 2001; 25:58–65.

204. Kantor GK, Straus MA. Substance abuse as a precipitant of wife abuse victimization. Am J Drug Alcohol Abuse 1989; 15:173–89.

205. Leonard KE, Senchak M. Prospective prediction of husband marital aggression within newlywed couples. J Abnorm Psychol 1996; 105:369–80.

206. Miller BA, Downs WR, Gondoli DM. Spousal violence among alcoholic women as compared to a random household sample of women. J Stud Alcohol 1989; 50:533–40.

207. O'Farrell TJ, Van Hutton V, Murphy CM. Domestic violence before and after alcoholism treatment :A two-year longitudinal study. J Stud Alcohol 1999; 60: 317–21.

208. Kyriacou DN, Anglin D, Taliaferro E, Stone S, Tubb T, Linden JA, Muelleman R, Barton E, Kraus JF. Risk factors for injury to women from domestic violence. N Engl J Med 1999; 341:1892–8.

209. Toman, RM. Rosen D. Domestic violence in the lives of women receiving welfare mental health, substance dependence, and economic well-being. Violence Against Women 2001; 7:141–58.

210. Slade M, Daniel LJ, Heisler CJ. Application of forensic toxicology to the problem of domestic violence. JFS 1991; 36:708–13.

211. UNAIDS (2006). Annex 2: HIV and AIDS estimates and data, 2005 and 2003. Available at: http://data.unaids.org/pub/GlobalReport/2006/2006_GR_ANN2_en.pdf. Accessed March 12, 2009.

212. AIDSinfo (2008). HIV infection in women: overview 2006. AIDSinfo Web site. Available from: http://www.aidsinfo.nih.gov/. Accessed March 12, 2009.

213. UNAIDS Epidemic Update, Dec. 2007; UNAIDS, Report on the global AIDS epidemic, 2008; Kaiser Family

Foundation; U.S. Centers for Disease Control and Prevention, 2008.
214. Curran JW, Jaffe HW, Hardy AM, Morgan WM, Selik RM, Dondero TJ. Epidemiology of HIV infection andAIDS in the United States. Science 1988; 239:610–6.
215. Chaisson RE, Moss AR, Onishi R, Osmond D, Carlson JR. Human immunodeficiency virus infection in heterosexual intravenous drug users in San Francisco. Am J Public Health 1987; 77:169–72.
216. Marmor M, Des Jarlais DC, Cohen H, Friedman SR, Beatrice ST, Dubin N, el-Sadr W, Mildvan D, Yancovitz S, Mathur U, et al. Risk factors for infection with human immunodeficiency virus among intravenous drug users in New York City. AIDS 1987; 1:39–44.
217. Fullilove MT, Golden E, Fullilove RE 3rd, Lennon R, Porterfield D, Schwarcz S, Bolan G. Crack cocaine use and high-risk behaviors among sexually active black adolescents. Adolesc Health 1993; 4:295–300.
218. Booth RE, Watters JK,Chitwood DD. HIV risk-related sex behaviors among injection drug users, crack smokers, and injection drug users who smoke crack. Am J Public Health 1993; 83:1144–8.
219. Zenilman JM, Hook EW, 3rd, Shepherd M, Smith P, Rompalo AM, Celentano DD. Alcohol and other substance use in STD clinic patients: relationships with STDs and prevalent HIV infection. Sex Transm Dis 1994; 21: 220–5.
220. Fisher JC, Cook PA, Sam NE, Kapiga SH. Patterns of alcohol use, problem drinking, and HIV infection among high-risk African women. Sex Transm Dis 2008; 35: 537–44.
221. Hutton HE, McCaul ME, Santora PB, Erbelding EJ.The relationship between recent alcohol use and sexual behaviors: gender differences among sexually transmitted disease clinic patients. Alcohol Clin Exp Res 2008; 32:2008–15.

Ethical Issues and Addiction

Binta Lambert, MD
Melissa Scheiner, RN, NNP
Deborah Campbell, MD

ABSTRACT. The epidemic of substance abuse continues to pose a significant challenge to clinicians nationwide. Although there is a tendency to simply associate drug abuse with poverty, the problem affects every social stratum gender and race; and pregnant women are no exception. Caring for pregnant, substance-using women and their infants presents complex legal and ethical issues. Debate is ongoing about whether criminal penalties should be imposed on women based solely on their use of alcohol and other drugs during pregnancy. Furthermore, controversies persist about the rights and wishes of pregnant women versus the interests of their fetuses. For health professionals, conflict arises when the pregnant woman chooses behaviors that have the potential to harm the developing fetus. The ethical dilemma arises from competing autonomy-based and beneficence-based obligations to the maternal-fetal dyad. This chapter explores the ethics-based conflicts in the delivery of health care to drug abusing pregnant women.

SCOPE OF THE PROBLEM

The epidemic of substance abuse continues to pose a significant challenge to clinicians nationwide. Drugs of abuse range from long-known illicit substances such as cocaine and heroin to the evolving problem of methamphetamine abuse, as well as legally available but no less harmful substances such as alcohol and tobacco. Although there is a tendency to simply associate drug abuse with poverty, the problem affects every social stratum, crossing the boundaries of socioeconomic status, gender, and race. According to the 2006 U.S. National Survey of Drug Use and Health (NSDUH), of the 17.9 million current illicit drug users aged 18 or older, 13.4 million were employed fulltime or part-time.[1] Substance abusers are found among every racial and ethnic group. The reported rate of substance use among persons aged 12 years or older varies widely. Substance abuse rates reported by racial or ethnic category vary: 13.7 % for Native Americans, 9.8% for Blacks, 8.9 % for mixed (two or more) race persons, 8.5 % for Whites, 7.5% for Native Hawaiians, 6.9% for Hispanics, and 3.6% for Asians.[1] In the United States, it is reported that approximately 90% of women abusing substances are of reproductive age.[2] Although substance use during pregnancy decreases as gestation progresses, postnatal substance use, particularly cigarette smoking, increases significantly during the initial 6 months postpartum.[3–5]

Discussion of the ethical issues encountered in caring for the addicted pregnant or parenting woman requires an understanding of the impact of prenatal drug exposure on the woman, her fetus, and later the developing child, on family functioning, and on the broader community (society). Results from the 2006 NSDUH revealed that 10% of non-pregnant women in the 15 to 44 year age group admitted to illicit drug use during the preceding month. Among pregnant women, the reported rate was 4%. An estimated 11.8% of pregnant women, aged 15 to 44 years, reported current alcohol use, whereas 2.9% and 0.7% reported binge drinking and heavy alcohol consumption, respectively. Cigarette smoking (nicotine) continues to be the most frequently used substance, with 29.5% of non-pregnant and 16.5% of pregnant women in the 15 to 44 year age group acknowledging cigarette use in the previous month.[1]

WHY ARE WE CONCERNED?

Substances most commonly abused during pregnancy include cocaine, opioids, marijuana, amphetamines, alcohol, and nicotine. These drugs can have detrimental effects on the developing fetus, which are well described and best discussed within the context of the individual drug. In addition to the possibility of adverse pregnancy outcome for the fetus as well as the woman, there are significant costs, both medical and financial, associated with caring for perinatally substance-exposed infants born. Infants exposed to drugs and alcohol in utero often face a greater risk of low birth weight, preterm birth, stillbirth and neonatal death, and birth-related complications due to the consequences of placental insufficiency. These infants are more likely to require neonatal intensive care. Exposure to cocaine and its derivatives, nicotine, and opiates is associated with a higher incidence of sudden infant death syndrome.[2,6] Prevalence rates and a summary of the perinatal and longer term effects of the substances more commonly abused during pregnancy are contained in Table 1. More detailed discussion about the specific physiologic effects of these substances is provided elsewhere in this supplement.

ETHICAL CHALLENGES ENCOUNTERED IN CARING FOR PREGNANT WOMEN WHO ARE ABUSING DRUGS

In response to the continuing challenges affecting communities and families caused by substance abuse, society has increasingly assumed the role of protector of its most vulnerable members: children. In recent years, this protection has expanded to include pregnant women and their fetuses, bringing into focus the interplay between pregnant women, health care professionals, and society. Maternal-fetal conflict arises when a pregnant woman's interests as she defines them (in this case drug use or abuse) conflicts with the interests of her fetus: to be born healthy with the best possible chance of meaningful survival. Traditionally, the practice of medicine and delivery of health care are grounded in the ethical principles of respect for the individual's autonomy, beneficence, and justice (fairness). Care of the pregnant woman has the potential to create several ethical challenges, as well as create conflict between the rights of the mother and the rights of the fetus. This conflict is based on the fact that although two patients exist—the pregnant woman and the developing fetus—the fetus' existence is dependent on the well-being and actions of mother.[27] In the setting of pregnant women who are abusing substances, these challenges become particularly complex.

Selected, well-publicized tragedies attributed to the effects of maternal substance abuse on newborn infants and young children have led local jurisdictions to incarcerate and prosecute pregnant women who are chemically dependent and new mothers. Suspicion about perinatal substance use during pregnancy requires the health care professional to question the pregnant woman regarding illicit substance use, request her permission to test her urine, and to screen her infant (parental consent is not required) for evidence of exposure to drugs of abuse (urine, meconium, hair, and umbilical cord blood). Confirmation of in utero exposure to illegal drugs or alcohol in the infant requires notification of child protection services. This initiates a process during which the family circumstances are evaluated. A determination is made about the

TABLE 1. Maternal, Fetal, and Neonatal Effects of Perinatal Substance Exposure

Perinatal Exposure	Alcohol[1,6,10,21–23]	Amphetamine[1,17–19]	Cocaine[6,7,9–16]	Marijuana[1,2,6]	Nicotine[4,7,9,10]	Opiates[1,6,24,25]
Incidence during pregnancy (%)	11.8%	5%	7-15%	9.5-27%	16.5%	2.3%[24]
Maternal health effects and pregnancy complications	Increased risk of alcohol-related complications: alcohol-induced liver and brain damage, breast cancer; high co-dependence with smoking	Increased alertness, euphoria, sense of self-confidence	Increases risk of spontaneous abortion, preterm labor, premature rupture of the membranes, abruptio placenta, uterine rupture, cardiac dysrhythmia, hepatic rupture, cerebral ischemia and death	May suppress maternal ovulation; freely crosses the placenta; chronic usage may increase risk labor dysfunction; may potentiate effects maternal anesthesia and analgesia	Chronic respiratory illness, asthma, cancer; CAD, PVD; neuropsychological addiction	Risk overdose; increased risk acquired infections (HIV, hepatitis B and C); increased risk of preterm labor, premature rupture of the membranes, uterine irritability, eclampsia
Fetal effects	Fetal alcohol syndrome and fetal alcohol spectrum disorder occur in 0.5 to 2.0/1000 live births in the United States; risk is 4 to 5% with heavy alcohol consumption	Impairs fetal growth	Vasoconstriction placental and fetal blood vessels – impaired fetal growth (322 grams lighter, 1.5-2.5 cm shorter head circumference 1-1.5 cm smaller), 1 week shorter gestation, congenital anomalies (vascular disruptions)	Decreased utero-placental perfusion and impaired fetal growth with chronic use	Placental vessel vasoconstriction, fetal hypoxia, Interferes with cholinergic transmission in developing brain; higher rates of spontaneous abortions, stillbirth, abruptio placenta, preterm delivery	Fetal dependence ; stillbirth, low birth weight
Neonatal abstinence	Following maternal acute intoxication	Not described	Not described	Not described	Not described	Yes
Neonatal effects	Dysmorphic midfacial features, disproportionately smaller head circumference or microcephaly	Diaphoresis, agitation, lassitude, miosis, vomiting	Poorer arousal responses, quality of movements and self-regulation	No dysmorphism or congenital malformations described; equivocal data on neurobehavioral effects	284 gram average reduction in birth weight; poorer state regulation and neurobehavioral organization	Withdrawal symptoms include irritability, increased tone and activity, tremors, seizures, feeding difficulty and poor weight gain, autonomic instability
Childhood and adolescent outcomes	Cognitive deficits, behavioral problems; deficits in learning, memory, executive function	No confirmed causal relationship to later outcomes; outcome studies complicated by co-dependence on other substances	Increased risk SIDS; no confirmed causal relationship to later outcomes	No confirmed causal relationship to later outcomes	Respiratory illness and asthma; SIDS; cognitive deficits (verbal abilities and memory)	SIDS; Limited outcome data – studies complicated by co-dependence on other substances; reports of mild memory and perceptual defficulties[25]

mother's and family's suitability to retain custody of the newborn infant and any other children in the home. The range of criminal charges has, in the past, included criminal abuse and drug possession, delivery of a controlled substance through the umbilical cord to a minor, and involuntary manslaughter in the case of a woman who experienced a placental abruption and the early neonatal death of her infant following cocaine use.

It has been argued that the criminalization of perinatal substance abuse as a strategy to deter drug use during pregnancy is counterproductive because it instead tends to discourage pregnant and parenting women who are chemically dependent from seeking health care and treatment for their drug dependency. Even if prenatal care is sought, services are often fragmented because the woman may seek to avoid detection of her drug use by obtaining episodic care at multiple sites and by delivering her infant in a hospital not affiliated with any of her prenatal care providers. Lack of sufficient drug treatment programs and other necessary resources to assist and support women who are chemically dependent and their children, as well as inequities in the approach to women with histories of drug use based on race and socioeconomic status, have contributed to significant bias in community and state approaches to care for these women and their families. In a 1998 report by the Robert Wood Johnson Foundation's Substance Abuse Policy Research Program, it was noted that imprisoning pregnant drug abusers is not only ineffective, but also unethical and unconstitutional. However, such prosecutions continue 10 years later.[28]

The medical and legal communities have previously established an individual's autonomous right to refuse medical treatment for himself or herself and to behave as he or she chooses, irrespective of the impact on the person's own health. When pregnancy occurs, the lives of the pregnant woman and the fetus are entwined. Thus, maternal lifestyle decisions, including the choice to use substances prior to conception and during pregnancy, have long-ranging effects on the fetus and child. The premise that a fetus has interests (rights) apart from the pregnant woman and the concept of the fetus as a patient focus attention on the question of whether a fetus has independent moral status.[26] There are two perspectives that form the basis for the paradigm often used in discussions about fetal rights. One viewpoint proposes that the fetus should be accorded independent moral status while the opposing view claims that the fetus does not have independent standing, but rather has a dependent moral status.[29] Independent moral status asserts that a fetus has intrinsic characteristics, unique to the fetus, that confer full moral value on the child-to-be. The fetus therefore should be considered a separate patient, with its own interests to be protected and rights to be promoted. Controversy exists as to what these intrinsic characteristics may be and precisely when independent moral status is attained. The alternative perspective, that of the fetus having a dependent moral status, does not afford the fetus independent rights, noting instead the fetus' full dependence on the pregnant woman for its continued existence.

This viewpoint of "all or nothing" is contentious and fails to reflect the sequential developmental processes that lead to fetal viability (the ability to survive outside the womb). Concerns arise not only in the context of perinatal substance exposure, but under circumstances in which the maternal and fetal health may be jeopardized without intervention, as in cases of maternal cancer or HIV infection or when the fetus is diagnosed with a potentially life-limiting condition for which experimental treatments are available (aortic stenosis, hypoplastic left heart syndrome, o congenital diaphragmatic hernia). A pregnant woman with a newly diagnosed cancer may be asked to consider ending her pregnancy to initiate treatment for her own disease or she may choose to delay starting her own medical care in the hope of allowing the fetus to reach viability and have a greater chance for survival. The woman infected with HIV may refuse medical therapy during her pregnancy and delivery even though the risk for perinatal HIV transmission is greatly reduced by appropriate prenatal and intrapartum treatment. As the field of fetal therapy develops, women are being offered the opportunity to consider or accept intrauterine interventions with the hope that it will improve the chance for survival of the fetus or lessen the severity of the morbidity associated with the underlying fetal condition.

Another context in which to consider whether a fetus should be viewed as having moral standing is the concept of personhood. Here too, controversy exists as to the inherent qualities required for full moral standing to be given to the fetus. Some advocate that one cannot achieve full moral status (personhood) without possessing the ability to think (cognition).[30] Opposing perspectives state that personhood is achieved once biological human properties exist. For these proponents, personhood occurs at the time of conception. A third view based on a developmental perspective is that personhood is attained only after the live birth of an infant sufficiently mature to survive outside the womb. Thus, the fetus has no moral status until (s)he is capable of independent survival outside the womb. Some ethicists and clinicians who advocate for graded moral status for the fetus have further refined this perspective. Within this framework personhood can be ascribed once the fetus reaches viability even if the fetus remains in utero.

From a societal perspective, irrespective of the health care professional's views about the degree of independent moral status due a fetus, once a pregnant woman decides to continue with a pregnancy, many advocates argue that the fetus becomes a patient, with interests and rights that should be protected. However, this obligation should not ignore the fact that the mother is herself a patient, with full moral status, and independent interests outside of her obligations to her fetus. Maternal rights to privacy, bodily integrity, and decision making for herself and her fetus must be balanced against the imperative to protect the fetus. Just as parents are presumed to be in the optimal position to decide what is in their child's best interest, so too is the pregnant woman deemed to be in the optimal position to decide what is in the best interest of her fetus.

This spectrum of perspectives increasingly collides with the science of neonatal medicine. Emerging technologies and treatments now permit the survival of extremely immature infants as young as 22 to 23 weeks gestation as well as infants with previously life-limiting congenital malformations. Once an infant is born, there is a consensus that the newborn attains independent moral status that obliges both parents and health professionals to act in the infant's best interest.

However, drug abuse and addiction may diminish the pregnant woman's capacity to pursue her fetus' best interest. Although the pregnant substance abuser may want what is best for her fetus, her drug dependence or lack of resources may make her feel powerless to accomplish this end. Society's revulsion against drug abuse, its associations with criminal behavior, and its deleterious impact on individuals and communities has propelled policy makers to seek solutions including criminalization of the pregnant drug abuser. This stands in stark contrast to the non-pregnant woman using drugs for whom seeking and drug use behaviors do not carry the same penalty. Health care professionals may feel justified in instituting measures to promote the interests of the fetus while simultaneously infringing on maternal rights.

ETHICAL (MORAL) PRINCIPLES

Three moral principles provide a framework for this ethical analysis: respect for autonomy, beneficence, and justice. In the clinical care setting, an additional factor to be considered is the health care professional's moral obligation to the pregnant woman and to the fetus.

Autonomy

At a minimum, autonomy is "self-rule that is free from both controlling influence by others, and from limitations such as inadequate understanding, that prevent meaningful choice" (p. 58).[31] A physician's autonomy-based obligation to the pregnant woman includes the need to protect and promote the woman's health-related interests while simultaneously honoring (protecting and promoting) the woman's interests as she defines them. This requires that the health professional provide adequate information about the patient's condition, treatment options, and reasonable medical alternatives; elicit the woman's values and preferences; and implement the woman's wishes, unless there is a compelling reason not to do so. The pregnant woman has the right and responsibility to make informed decisions for herself and her fetus. Respect for autonomy gives the drug user the liberty to be in control of decisions affecting her own health care. One of the essential conditions of autonomy is liberty that in this context means independence from controlling influences. Drug abuse, which has the effect of altering one's thought processes, clearly violates this condition. In addition, the health professional must respect the woman's decisions regardless of impact on the woman's own health and well-being.[26] It is important to emphasize that a health professional's obligations to respect a patient's autonomy rights does not extend to individuals who are incapacitated and who are not able to make informed, independent decisions for themselves. It can therefore be argued that the impaired drug-abusing individual deserves to be considered within the category of individuals without capacity to make fully informed decisions. Nevertheless, respect for autonomy requires that, at the very least, the wishes and decisions of incapacitated individuals be acknowledged and, in an ideal situation, be protected.

Beneficence

The principle of beneficence is captured in the tenet "morality requires not only that we treat persons autonomously and refrain from harming them but that we contribute to their welfare" (p. 165).[26] In the context of pregnancy, the health care professional must consider the welfare of two patients: that of the mother and the fetus. Therefore, the health care professional has a beneficence-based obligation to both the mother and the fetus. In her or his interaction with the pregnant mother, the healthcare provider should always seek to promote clinical strategies or to encourage behaviors that favor the greater balance of good over harm for both patients. The beneficence-based obligation to the fetus can also be extended to the mother, who should also be expected to behave in a manner that protects the welfare or interests of her developing fetus.[32,33] An additional ethical principle, nonmaleficence, takes this concept one step further. Not only must the health professionals promote the well-being of their patients, they must also *do no harm*, or at the very least minimize harm to the individuals entrusted to their care. Similarly, this principle applies to the pregnant woman who chooses to continue a pregnancy. She has a moral obligation to not intentionally harm her fetus, particularly when the developing fetus has reached viability.

Justice

Justice is concerned with equal and fair access to opportunities or services that individuals are deemed to have rights. In the setting of perinatal substance abuse, this principle extends beyond the pregnant woman-health professional relationship. It requires consideration of and advocacy for the best interests of the fetus or newborn infant, as well as equity or fairness in the response to maternal drug abuse and the goal to avoid further endangerment of the child. Concerns for the child include the harmful effects of intrauterine exposure to substances (illicit and prescription drugs, alcohol, and tobacco), the short-term and long-term health and developmental consequences of these exposures, and the ramifications on the parent-child interaction and parenting abilities of the mother and other caregivers.

AUTONOMY VERSUS BENEFICENCE: CAN THE SCALE BE BALANCED?

The most obvious ethical challenge encountered by the health care professional who is caring for a pregnant woman who is abusing substances is the dichotomy created by the health professional's (physician's) autonomy-based obligations to the mother and the beneficence-based obligation to the fetus. In clinical practice, fulfilling these dual roles can become challenging and pose an additional source of conflict, as when the woman's choice of a course of action is not in her health-related best interest or has the potential to negatively impact the developing fetus she is carrying. Physicians are obligated to respect the woman's decisions regarding her own health, even if it entails behaviors that have adverse consequences (alcohol or drug abuse); however, they are also duty-bound to promote the best outcome for the fetus. Some argue that moral obligations are greater to those who are most in need,[32] suggesting that the beneficence-based obligation to the fetus overrides the autonomy-based obligation to the mother. This rationale has been the basis for several recent legal actions and policies aimed at protecting the fetus as an entity separate from the mother. Mandatory drug screening of neonates, mandated drug rehabilitation of the pregnant woman or new mother, criminal prosecution and incarceration of the pregnant or parenting woman, and removal of the child from the mother's custody have all been justified as a societal response to its obligation to protect the interests of the fetus and the child. Such punitive policies and actions are strengthened by the argument that because of the very nature of addiction, an addict is unable to be fully autonomous and by the sometimes unjustified, overly simplified, but widely believed association of drug abuse with child abuse. It is of note that in a small study of 76 children that examined the relationship between prenatal cocaine exposure and child welfare outcomes, prenatal cocaine exposure was not found to be a marker for abusive parenting after adjustment for prior maternal involvement with the child welfare system.[34]

Others hold the view that a pregnant woman's autonomy should always override the rights of her fetus, provided the woman is fully informed and is competent to make a decision.[35] This forms the argument of those proponents who believe that a fetus has no moral status. As such, the fetus has no rights or interests that require protection and therefore the physician has no obligation to advocate for fetal protections. A 1990 legal precedent established by a District of Columbia Appellate Court upheld the importance of the primacy of maternal autonomy over fetal interests or rights, as the judges wrote that, "in virtually all cases, the question of what is to be done is to be decided by the patient- the pregnant woman- on behalf of herself and the fetus" (A.C 573 A2d 1235, D.C (Ct App. 1990)). Although this ruling was not handed down specifically in response to a case of perinatal substance abuse, it does suggest implications for a range of maternal behaviors that have the potential to cause fetal harm, of which perinatal drug abuse is one example.

Health care professionals have the added ethical challenge of deciding how best to exercise their beneficence-based obligation to the mother once there is an awareness or suspicion of the pregnant woman's drug use or dependency. Physicians' attitudes vary with regard to the acceptability of mandatory drug screening, incarceration, and the use of the threat of prosecution to deter pregnant women from drug use.[36] Most physicians favor mandatory screening for alcohol abuse, while there is less consensus on the appropriateness of mandatory screening for illicit drugs. This is related to physicians' concern that fear of prosecution would cause women who are using substances to avoid prenatal care. Compelling arguments exist for mandatory drug testing (testing without maternal consent), the foremost of these being that it allows the physician to identify and appropriately treat the infant. However, this infringes on the pregnant woman's right to privacy, in addition to undermining her right to informed consent implicit in the principle of respect for autonomy.[37] Furthermore, the finding of a positive drug screen often results in child protection services being informed, with potential consequences for both the new mother and her children. It has been argued that engaging child protection services results in both serious infringement of the mother's rights and the potential for her incarceration. This was exemplified in the case of *Ferguson v. the City of Charleston*, in which the Medical University of South Carolina instituted a policy of conducting urine drug screens on selected pregnant women without their consent to look for evidence of cocaine use. Women with positive drug screens were reported to the police and subsequently arrested on charges of child abuse or drug delivery to a minor child. The Supreme Court ruled that, "drug testing of pregnant women for the purpose of criminal investigation may not be conducted without a warrant or explicit consent, even when justified by the benign purposes of protecting fetuses and promoting drug treatment" (p. 1697).[38] Although this ruling deals with the process of collecting evidence to prosecute pregnant drug users, it did not tackle the more fundamental question about the validity of prosecuting pregnant drug users.

Interestingly, in a survey conducted by Abel et al., the authors sought to identify physician attitudes about use of legal coercion of pregnant alcohol and drug abusers.[36] Approximately half of the responding physicians supported redefining child abuse laws to include maternal alcohol or drug abuse during pregnancy as a valid reason for removal of a child from the mother's custody. Even among the physicians who did not support this as an appropriate practice, there was support for legally mandated reporting of perinatal women who are abusing substances to child protective authorities or law enforcement personnel, even if this resulted in infringement of the maternal rights.

The issue of the necessity for or permissibility of criminal prosecution of pregnant women who endanger the lives of their children-to-be through drug use remains unresolved. Legal enforcement of the maternal beneficence-based obligation to her fetus through criminalization of perinatal drug abuse remains controversial. This is in large part due to our recognition that drug addiction is an illness. In this context, criminalization of the addicted pregnant woman can be considered a violation of the Eighth Amendment's prohibition against cruel and unusual punishment.[38] Currently, with the exception of South Carolina, states do not consider using drugs during pregnancy a crime. However, this has not hindered prosecutors in several states from charging pregnant women with child endangerment or abuse, illegal drug delivery to a minor, or, in some extreme cases, murder or manslaughter. In each of these instances, the fetus was equated with and given the rights of a child, as prosecutors sought to have existing murder laws applied to the mother's actions.[38] Judges, exclusive of the courts in South Carolina, have declined to expand existing state laws to punish pregnant women on the basis of a claim of fetal rights. However, several court rulings have promulgated measures aimed at punishing pregnant drug abusing women. Women have been jailed during pregnancy to safeguard the well-being of the fetus by preventing to illicit drugs.[39] Althuogh such intervention is a short-term solution to the problem, the mere knowledge that such punitive action exists can serve to further alienate the pregnant addict from seeking health services. In the long-term, that fear may cause more harm to the fetus and the mother than any potential benefit derived through incarceration.[40]

Pursuit of Justice

A dichotomy exists when society's role and responsibilities in the domain of perinatal substance abuse are considered. Federal, state, and local governments, as well as communities at large, are often criticized for their failure to address issues that plague the poor and disenfranchised: inadequate education, substandard housing, and limited access to jobs, health care, and other necessary resources. Advocates for substance abusers cite these factors as pivotal to promoting an environment that potentiates rather than reduces drug use. Proponents argue that the pregnant addict has a right to adequate health care for herself and her fetus in a non-judgmental, non-punitive setting under the premise that she is not solely responsible for her circumstances. Criminalizing perinatal substance abuse denies the mother, her fetus, and even other living children in her care this basic right. Should regulation be seen as the only solution to the problem, the execution of these laws ought to be applied fairly. Currently, although drug abuse occurs across all socioeconomic and ethnic groups, it would appear that anti-drug laws preferentially target poor and minority groups.[39,40] Important inequities also exist in the application of existing drug laws. Alcohol consumption is far more prevalent despite a well-established constellation of life-long neurodevelopmental consequences (fetal alcohol spectrum disorders). Equally well-known are the adverse consequences of nicotine on the developing fetus. However, both alcohol and nicotine are not classified as illicit drugs and therefore dependency on these substances does not carry the same stigma or fear of criminal prosecution. Promulgation of a punitive approach to perinatal substance abuse requires at the very least an equitable, fair, and validated method for identifying infants exposed to perinatal substance abuse. There remain many barriers to achieving this standard. Although mandatory universal drug screening of pregnant women or neonates has been advocated, and in some instances implemented,[38] it only identifies a subset of infants exposed to drugs prenatally and has the added disadvantage of discouraging pregnant women using substances from seeking health care for herself and her fetus or from disclosing her substance use history for fear of the repercussions against her. Furthermore, the majority of women who use drugs during pregnancy are recreational drug users and would not be classified as drug-addicted. These women often remain "under the radar screen" failing to disclose any history of perinatal or prior substance use for fear of punitive actions against them and the possibility of losing custody of their infant once the child is born.

Fairness requires that the role of the pregnant substance user's partner also be taken into account when fetal and later childhood outcomes are considered. The acute effects of passive exposure to crack/cocaine on the young infant have been well documented. However, data on a causal relationship between paternal use of nicotine, alcohol, and illicit substances and childhood biologic, developmental, and behavioral outcomes is less clear. In one study, Rubin and colleagues demonstrated a relationship between paternal smoking and birth weight after correcting for both maternal and paternal alcohol use during pregnancy.[41] A more recent investigation found an association between paternal preconception smoking and significantly elevated risk of childhood cancers among children born to non-smoking mothers.[42] This highlights the lack of established policies, punitive or otherwise, that address the ramifications of adverse paternal behaviors, specifically substance abuse. As a consequence, it can be charged that women, particularly mothers, are again unfairly singled out. Substance abuse by the father contributes to the pattern of maternal substance abuse and family dysfunction, thereby indirectly influencing adverse fetal and neonatal outcomes, which are now being solely attributed to the mother.

However, the concept of justice must also be applied to the children of drug abusing women. These children have a right to be raised in an environment that affords them an equitable share of basic necessities, such as food, shelter, and education, as well as a loving and stable home environment. It is highly likely that the addicted mother, who in many instances is a single parent, without adequate financial resources, family support, and parenting skills, may have satisfying her addiction as her primary goal rather than providing for the needs of her children. Factors associated with substance abuse, such as depression, criminality, poverty, prior physical and emotional abuse, and family violence,[27,34] increase this likelihood. However, isolated maternal cocaine use during pregnancy is not a useful marker for identifying infants at risk for abusing parenting.[27,34,37]

CONCLUSION

The complexity of the issues associated with perinatal substance abuse necessitates a comprehensive approach to the identification, assessment, and treatment of families affected by drugs and alcohol. It is important to consider perinatal substance abuse as a chronic health condition (much like diabetes mellitus or hypertensive disease of pregnancy), with the potential to cause adverse health effects in both the pregnant woman and her fetus. This entails development of public policies that will: support the expansion and enhancement of drug treatment programs for pregnant and parenting women; provide adequate social support and community services to enable the recovering addict to care for her children in a supportive home environment; support enhanced investment in programs geared at increasing awareness about the effects of substance abuse and how communities can respond to this continuing challenge; and provide ongoing evaluation of legal and societal policies toward women affected by perinatal substance abuse, including the need for research into the determinants of addiction and the developmental effects of perinatal substance exposure. In this regard, the American College of Obstetricians and Gynecologists recommends a three-pronged method of identification and treatment of substance abuse in women, comprised of universal screening during pregnancy for a history of drug use (tobacco, alcohol, prescription, and non-prescription drugs), a brief intervention, and referral to treatment.[43] These recommendations are supported by data demonstrating that rates of continued abstinence after drug treatment are comparable to the rates of medication compliance among patients with diabetes mellitus, hypertension, and other chronic diseases.[44] Furthermore, it has been shown that drug treatment saves $7 for every dollar spent.[45] Threat of incarceration has also proved ineffective in reducing the incidence of alcohol or drug abuse.[46] A final equally important factor to consider is that the removal of children from maternal custody and placement into an overstretched child welfare system has the potential to further the health and developmental risks for the children.[46] It is the responsibility of the health care and lay communities to advocate for the ethical, moral and just treatment of pregnant women and their children, including women with histories of perinatal substance use or dependency.

REFERENCES

1. Substance Abuse and Mental Health services Administration. Results from the 2006 national survey on drug use and health: national findings. Rockville, MD: Office of Applied Studies, NSDUH Series H-32, DHHS Publication No. SMA 07-4293, 2007.
2. Kuczkowski K. The effects of drug abuse on pregnancy. Curr Opin Obstet Gynecol 2007; 19:578–85.
3. Fingerhut LA, Kleinman JC, Kendrick JS. Smoking before, during and after pregnancy. Am J Public Health 1990; 80:541–4.
4. Morrison D, Spencer M, Gillmore M. Beliefs about substance use among pregnant and parenting adolescents. J Res Adoles 1998; 8:69–95.
5. Bonellie S.R. Effects of maternal age, smoking and deprivation on birth weight. Paediatr Perinatal Epidemiol 2001; 15: S19–26.
6. Shankaran S, Lester B.M, Das A, Bauer C.R, Bada H.S, LaGasse L, Higgins L. Impact of maternal substance use during pregnancy on childhood outcome. Semin Fetal Neonatal Med 2007; 12:143–50.
7. Jaddoe VW, Verburg BO, DeRidder MA, Hofman A, Mackenbach JP, Moll HA, Steegers EA, Witteman JC. Maternal smoking and fetal growth characteristics in different periods of pregnancy: the Generation R Study. Am J Epidemiol 2007; 165:1207–15.
8. Cnattingius S. The Epidemiology of Smoking during pregnancy, smoking prevalence, maternal characteristics and pregnancy outcome. Nicotin Tob Res 2004; 6(Suppl 2):S125–40.
9. Law KL, Stroud LR, LaGasse LL, Niaura R, Liu J, Lester BM. Smoking during pregnancy and newborn neurobehavior. Pediatrics 2003; 111:1318–23.
10. Bandstra ES, Accornero VH. Infants of substance abusing mothers. In: Fanaroff and Martin's Neonatal-Perinatal Medicine. Diseases of the fetus and infant, 8th ed, vol. 1. Philadelphia, Elsevier Mosby, 2006:733–57.
11. Bauer CR, Shankaran S, Bada HS, Lester B, Wright LL, Krause-Steinrauf H, Smeriglio VL, Finnegan LP, Maza PL, Verter J. The maternal lifestyle study (MLS): drug exposure during pregnancy and shot-term maternal outcomes. Am J Obstet Gynecol 2002; 186:487–95.
12. Bada HS, Das A, Bauer CR, Shankaran S, Lester B, Wright LL, Verter J, Smeriglio VL, Finnegan LP, Maza PL. Gestational cocaine exposure and intrauterine growth (Maternal Lifestyle Study). Obstet Gynecol 2002; 100: 916–24.
13. Bauer CR, Langer JC, Shankaran S, Bada HS, Lester B, Wright LL, Krause-Steinrauf H, Smeriglio VL, Finnegan LP, Maza PL, Verter J. Acute neonatal Effects of Cocaine during pregnancy. Arch Pediatr Adolesc Med 2005; 159:824–34.
14. Lester BM, Tronick EZ, LaGasse L, Seifer R, Bauer CR, Shankaran S, Bada HS, Wright LL, Smeriglio VL, Lu J, Finnegan LP, Maza PL. The Maternal Lifestyle Study: effects of substance exposure during pregnancy on neurodevelopmental outcome in 1-month-old infants. Pediatrics 2002; 110:1182–92.
15. Accornero VH, Amado AJ, Morrow CE, Xue L, Anthony JC, Bandstra ES. Impact of prenatal cocaine exposure on attention and response inhibition as assessed by continuous performance tests. J Dev Behav Pediatr 2007; 28:195–205.
16. Bada HS, Das A, Bauer CR, Shankaran S, Lester B, LaGasse L, Hammond J, Wright LL, Higgins R. Impact of prenatal cocaine exposure on child behavior problems through school age. Pediatrics 2007; 119:e348–59.
17. Smith L, Yonekura ML, Wallace T, Berman N, Kuo J, Berkowitz C. Effects of prenatal methamphetamine exposure on fetal growth and drug withdrawal symptoms in infants born at term. J Dev Behav Pediatr 2003; 24:17–23.
18. Arria AM, Derauf C, LaGasse LL, Grant P, Shah R, Smith L, Haning W, Huestis M, Strauss A, Della Grotta S, Liu J, Lester B. Methamphetamine and other substance use during pregnancy: preliminary estimates from the Infant Development, Environment and Lifestyle (IDEAL) Study. Maternal Child Health J 2006; 10:293–302.
19. Oro AS, Dixon SD. Perinatal cocaine and methamphetamine exposure: Maternal and neonatal correlates. J Pediatr. 1987; 111:571–8.
20. Mattson SN, Schoenfeld AM, Riley EP. Teratogenic effects of alcohol on brain and behavior. Alcohol Res Health 2001; 25:185–91.
21. Kodituwakku PW, Kalberg W, May PA. The effects of prenatal alcohol exposure on executive functioning. Alcohol Res Health 2001; 25:192–8.
22. Fraser RB, for the Royal College of Obstetricians and Gynaecologists, Alcohol Consumption and the Outcomes of Pregnancy. RCOG Statement, No. 5, March 2006.

Available at http://www.rcog.org.uk/index.asp? Accessed 03/22/10.

23. Lester BM, El Sohly M, Wright LL. The Maternal Lifestyle Study: drug use by meconium toxicology and maternal self-report. Pediatrics 2001; 107: 309–17.

24. Lifschitz MH, Wilson GS. Patterns of growth and development in narcotic-exposed children. NIDA Res Monogr 1991; 114:323–39.

25. Fasouliotis SJ, Schenker JG. Maternal-fetal conflict: debates and guidelines. European J Obstet Gynecol Reprod Biology 2000; 89:101–7.

26. Beauchamp TL, Childress JF. Beneficence. In: Beauchamps TL, Childress JF. Principles of biomedical ethics, 5th ed. New York, Oxford University Press, Inc., 2001:165–203.

27. Jaudes P.K, Ekwo E, VanVoorhis J. Association of drug abuse and child abuse. Child Abuse Negl 19: 1065–75.

28. Nelson LJ, Marshall MF. An Ethical and Legal Policy Analysis of State Compelled Loss of Liberty as an Intervention to Manage the Harm of Prenatal Substance Abuse and Drug Addiction. Robert Wood Johnson Foundation Substance Abuse Policy Research program Report, July, 1998.

29. Chervenak FA, McCullough LB. What is obstetric ethics? J Perinat Med 1995; 23:331–41.

30. Warren M. On the moral and legal status of abortion. In: Beauchamp TL, Walters L, eds. Contemporary issues in bioethics, 6th ed. Belmont, CA: Thomson Wadsworth Learning, 2003:298–307.

31. Beauchamp TL, Childress JF. Respect for autonomy. In: Beauchamps TL, Childress JF. Principles of biomedical ethics, 5th ed. New York: Oxford Press, Inc., 2001:57–65.

32. Tran L. Legal rights and the maternal-fetal conflict. Bio Teach J 2004; 2:76–82. Available at www.bioteach.ubc.edu. Accessed February 8, 2008

33. Beauchamp TL, Walters L. Ethical theory and bioethics. In: Beauchamp TL, Walters L, eds. Contemporary issues in bioethics, 6th ed. Belmont, CA: Thomson Wadsworth Learning, 2003:1–37.

34. Doris JL, Meguid V, Thomas M, Blatt S, Eckenrode J. Prenatal cocaine exposure and child welfare outcomes. Child Maltreat 2006; 11:326–37.

35. Isaacs D. Moral Status of the Fetus: Fetal rights or maternal autonomy? J Paediatr Child Health 2003; 39:58–9.

36. Abel EL, Kruger M. Physician attitudes concerning legal coercion of pregnant alcohol and drug abusers. Am J Obstet Gynecol 2002; 186:768–72.

37. Leventhal JM, Forsyth BWC, Qi K. Maltreatment of children born to women who used cocaine during pregnancy: a population based study. Pediatrics 1997; 100:e7.

38. Harris LH, Paltrow L. The status of pregnant women and fetuses in US criminal law. JAMA 2003; 289:1697–9.

39. Jain R, Thomasma DC, Ragas R. Ethical Challenges in the treatment of drug-abusing mothers. Camb Q Health Ethics 1999; 8:179–88.

40. Campbell DE, Fleischman AR. Ethical challenges in medical care for the pregnant substance abuser. Clin Obstet Gynecol 1992; 35:803–12.

41. Rubin DH, Krasilinikoff PA, Leventhal JM, Weile B, Berget A. Effect of passive smoking on birth weight. Lancet 1986; 2(8504):415–7.

42. Ji BT, Shu XO, Linet MS, Zheng W, Wacholder S, Gao YT, Ying DM, Jin F. Paternal cigarette smoking and risk of childhood cancer among offspring of non-smoking mothers. J Nat Cancer Inst 1997; 89:238–44.

43. At-risk Drinking and Illicit Drug Use: Ethical Issues in Obstetric and Gynecologic Practice. ACOG Committee Opinion No. 422. American College of Obstetricians and Gynecologists. Obstet Gynecol 2008: 112: 1449–60.

44. McLellan AT, Lewis DC, O'Brien CP, Kleber HD. Drug Dependence, a chronic medical illness: implications for treatment, insurance and outcomes evaluation. JAMA 2000; 284:1689–95.

45. Hubbard RL, French MT. New Perspectives on the benefit-cost and cost–effectiveness of Drug Abuse Treatment. NIDA Research Monograph 1991; 113:94–113.

46. Behrman RE, ed. Drug-exposed infants. The Future of Children 1991; 1(1):8–9.

Addiction in Pregnancy

Joan Keegan, DO
Mehdi Parva, MD
Mark Finnegan, MD
Andrew Gerson, MD
Michael Belden, MD

ABSTRACT. Substance abuse in pregnancy has increased over the past three decades in the United States, resulting in approximately 225,000 infants yearly with prenatal exposure to illicit substances. Routine screening and the education of women of child bearing age remain the most important ways to reduce addiction in pregnancy. Legal and illegal substances and their effect on pregnancy discussed in this review include opiates, cocaine, alcohol, tobacco, marijuana, and amphetamines. Most literature regarding opiate abuse is derived from clinical experience with heroin and methadone. Poor obstetric outcomes can be up to six times higher in patients abusing opiates. Neonatal care must be specialized to treat symptoms of withdrawal. Cocaine use in pregnancy can lead to spontaneous abortion, preterm births, placental abruption, and congenital anomalies. Neonatal issues include poor feeding, lethargy, and seizures. Mothers using cocaine require specialized prenatal care and the neonate may require extra supportive care. More than 50% of women in their reproductive years use alcohol. Alcohol is a teratogen and its effects can include spontaneous abortion, growth restriction, birth defects, and mental retardation. Fetal alcohol spectrum disorder can have long-term sequelae for the infant. Tobacco use is high among pregnant women, but this can be a time of great motivation to begin cessation efforts. Long-term effects of prenatal tobacco exposure include spontaneous abortion, ectopic pregnancy, placental insufficiency, low birth weight, fetal growth restriction, preterm delivery, childhood respiratory disease, and behavioral issues. Marijuana use can lead to fetal growth restriction, as well as withdrawal symptoms in the neonate. Lastly, amphetamines can lead to congenital anomalies and other poor obstetric outcomes. Once recognized, a multidisciplinary approach can lead to improved maternal and neonatal outcomes.

INTRODUCTION

Illicit drug use during pregnancy is a major risk factor for maternal morbidity and neonatal complications, but despite this fact the prevalence of illicit substance use by women of childbearing age in United States has increased markedly over the past three decades.[1]

Although substance abuse during pregnancy may be increasing, it often remains undiagnosed or under-diagnosed. A recent self-reporting survey by The National Survey on Drug Use and

Health from 2002–2003 estimated that 4.3% of pregnant women aged 15 to 44 years reported illicit drug use within the month prior to being questioned.[1,2] Approximately 250,000 women in the United States, of whom 90% are of childbearing age, meet criteria for intravenous drug abuse.[1] This suggests, conservatively, that approximately 225,000 infants born each year could be exposed to illicit drugs in the prenatal or postpartum time period.

Identifying substance misuse in pregnancy can present a significant clinical challenge. In addition, there can be difficulty evaluating the effect of substance abuse on patients' social, behavioral, psychosocial, and biological risk factors associated with both illicit drug use and adverse pregnancy outcomes. Consideration should be given to the implementation of routine antenatal education and counseling of any population identified as having an increased incidence of substance abuse.

The goal of this article is to identify the major categories of drugs and substances that are commonly abused in pregnancy and evaluate the impact these substances may have on the preconception time period, pregnancy, and the postpartum period. Neonatal issues will be addressed elsewhere in this supplement, except in those instances where a pregnancy complication is caused by a specific substance of abuse and affects the newborn directly. Tobacco, caffeine, alcohol, prescription or illicit opiates, and sedative-hypnotics/anxiolytics will be discussed. The most commonly abused illicit drugs of abuse including cocaine, amphetamines, and marijuana will also be addressed. In addition, we will review general guidelines regarding the management of high-risk pregnancies in substance abusing mothers. These guidelines primarily address the identification and management of teratogenic exposure, poor maternal nutrition, intrauterine growth restriction, placental insufficiency, labor management, and maternal/neonatal withdrawal symptoms.

TOBACCO

Preconception

Active and passive tobacco smoking presents major risks to human health. Smoking contributes to the development of various human cancers, respiratory illnesses, and other diseases.[3,4] It is estimated that 21% of American adults smoke. Each year, more than 440,000 Americans die of tobacco-related disease.[5]

Among pregnant women, there is an increased prevalence of smoking among the youngest (<20 years of age) and oldest (>35 years of age) patients. In addition, the lower the level of education achieved, the greater the risk of being a current smoker.[6,7] Studies of tobacco users have shown a 1.2 to 3.6 relative risk for infertility in the preconception period.[8] Every effort should be made to identify smokers prior to pregnancy and provide both psychosocial intervention and pharmacologic methods to enhance the likelihood of smoking cessation. Pregnancy can be a significant motivator to stop or reduce smoking.

Pregnancy

The most recent available statistics on tobacco use in pregnancy report that approximately 12% to 15% of all women continue to smoke during their pregnancy.[9] Tobacco use during pregnancy is associated with a higher rate of pregnancy complications[7] and has a clearly demonstrated dose-response relationship, which can significantly impact both maternal and fetal outcomes. In the first trimester, these risks include an increased risk of spontaneous abortion and ectopic pregnancy. In the second and third trimesters, an increased risk of placental insufficiency, low birth weight, fetal growth restriction, and preterm delivery are all potential morbidities associated with tobacco use. Several studies evaluating the role of smoking during pregnancy report a relative risk ranging from 1.5 to 2.5 for ectopic pregnancy. Spontaneous abortion is 20% to 80% higher in women who smoke in pregnancy compared to non-smokers. Maternal smoking carries a relative risk of 1.2 to 16 for preterm delivery.[8]

Nicotine is one of the 4,000 chemicals that are produced during smoking and at least 43 of these chemicals are known carcinogens.[10] Nicotine has a half life of 1 to 2 hours and is mainly metabolized by the liver and excreted by the kidneys.[8] Nicotine readily crosses the placenta, resulting in a fetal concentration that is generally 15% higher than maternal and amniotic fluid levels, and 88% higher than maternal plasma levels.[11] Women who smoke are more likely to have a low birth weight baby, with a reported relative risk of 1.3 to 10.[8,12] On average, infants born to women who smoke during pregnancy are 200 to 300 grams lighter. Furthermore, nicotine causes impaired fetal oxygen delivery, resulting in abnormal gas exchange within the placenta and activation of the sympathetic nervous system, increasing the fetal heart rate and causing a reduction in fetal breathing movements.[13]

Carbon monoxide is a major by-product of cigarette smoking that can cause harm to the mother and fetus. Carbon monoxide crosses the placenta and can be detected in the fetal circulation at a level 15% higher than in the maternal circulation.[12] Carbon monoxide diminishes tissue oxygenation via competitive inhibition with oxyhemoglobin, causing decreased availability of oxygen to the fetus.[11] Fanslow et al. concluded that smoking during pregnancy is significantly associated with violence during pregnancy.[14]

Postpartum

Approximately half of women who quit smoking during pregnancy resume smoking within 6 months postpartum and 50% to 90% have relapsed 1 year post-delivery.[12] The likely causes of relapse are stress, lack of sleep, caring for the infant, and concern about weight gain in the postpartum period.[8,12] Smoking during the postpartum period causes a significant health risk for both mother and child. To date, there are no proven effective strategies for preventing relapse during the postpartum period. Close follow-up and positive counseling may be beneficial. Crawford et al. described several strategies for prevention of postpartum relapse. Such strategies include continued counseling, focusing on the health benefits of quitting, and providing reinforcement of the patient's desire to be a good mother.[12]

CAFFEINE

Preconception

Caffeine is a widely available central nervous system (CNS) stimulant and is found in commonly consumed beverages such as coffee, soda, and tea. In addition, caffeine is also used in combination with various drugs, such as aspirin, acetaminophen, codeine, and butalbital. Caffeine has medicinal value because it can be particularly helpful in the treatment of headaches, but it is extremely popular in general use because of its appealing CNS stimulant properties. Caffeine is addictive, and physical dependence is common. Withdrawal from caffeine in adults typically causes jitteriness, a sense of non-well-being, and headaches. Because caffeine is so widely accessible and commonly used by women of childbearing age, its impact on patients in the period of preconception has been widely studied.

Caffeine does cross the placenta, but it does not appear to act as a teratogen when consumed as a component in beverages or over-the-counter medications.[15] The clinical and anecdotal evidence that supports this is relatively vast. However, there has been an ongoing concern regarding the impact of caffeine on fertility. In terms of affecting actual ovulation or causing ovulatory dysfunction, caffeinated beverages appear to be safe and do not impair ovulation.[16] There is a long-standing suspicion, however, that caffeine consumption may be associated with miscarriage or an increased risk of miscarriage. The evidence suggests that this may be the case, and a recent population-based prospective cohort trial showed that consumption of, more than 200 mg/day (about 2 to 3 standard cups of coffee or 4 12-ounce cans of cola) of caffeine may increase the risk of miscarriage.[17] There are no randomized trials to confirm this, and it is unlikely that such a study would be performed.

Pregnancy

During pregnancy, caffeine is probably safe when used in moderation. Again, there is abundant literature and anecdotal experience that suggests there is no obvious association between caffeine use and poor fetal outcomes. However, there may be some association between maternal caffeine use of more than 500 mg/day and fetal cardiac arrhythmias compared to mothers who use less than 250 mg/day.[18]

Postpartum

Caffeine use in the postpartum period will vary from patient to patient, depending on habits and personal preference. Caffeine is excreted in small amounts in breast milk, but in cases of usual moderate consumption the levels are probably too low to be clinically significant. Moderate caffeine consumption is considered to be compatible with breastfeeding.[19]

ALCOHOL

Preconception

Alcohol use is widespread among women of reproductive age. Alcohol is a well-studied teratogen, and its effects on pregnancy can include spontaneous abortion, growth restriction, and birth defects. The incidence of alcohol use in non-pregnant women ages 15 to 44 years is 53%. It is estimated that as many as 24% of young women who drink are binge drinking.[20] Oftentimes, conception occurs during times of alcohol use or abuse and women continue casual drinking into the first trimester until they are aware of their pregnancy. The development of all fetal organ systems can be affected at this early stage during the first trimester. Therefore, the preconception period is an important time to identify women at risk.[20]

In the preconception period, each encounter with patients can be an opportunity to screen for alcohol use or abuse and intervene to reduce or completely stop alcohol consumption. There are several screening tools available. Questions to ask are detailed in mnemonics such as Take, annoyed, cut down, eye opener (T-ACE), Tolerance, Worried, Eye-opener, Amnesia, and K/Cut down (TWEAK), or Alcohol Use Disorder Identification Test (AUDIT).[21] The United States Preventative Services Task Force, the American College of Obstetrics and Gynecology, and the American Academy of Pediatrics suggest using preconception and prenatal visits to discuss the benefits of abstaining from alcohol. There are no evidence-based studies to suggest any amount of alcohol use is safe during pregnancy.

Pregnancy

During pregnancy, the fetus that is exposed to alcohol can be severely affected. Fetal alcohol spectrum disorder (FASD) encompasses a wide range of disorders defined as prenatal and postnatal growth restriction, central nervous system abnormalities, and craniofacial abnormalities. Some common fetal conditions associated with alcohol abuse include facial dysmorphogenesis, cardiac septal defects, and joint abnormalities. Infrequently, other anatomic or physiologic abnormalities are found. These include abnormalities of the eyes, hearing issues, urinary problems, immune system deficiencies, and skeletal problems. FASD is permanent and has a significant affect on the baby and family. Centers for Disease Control and Prevention (CDC) studies show FASD rates ranging from 0.2 to 1.5 per 1,000 live births in different areas of the United States.

Alcohol abuse and misuse in pregnancy is the most common non-genetic cause of mental retardation.[22] There is strong medical evidence to suggest that heavy alcohol use or binge drinking can lead to high rates of fetal alcohol spectrum disorder.[22] Studies show that even small amounts of alcohol used on a daily basis can be detrimental to the fetus.[22]

Postpartum

Little data exist regarding the postpartum period and alcohol use. This time can be stressful for any mother, and particularly so if the mother is alcohol dependent. As we become more aware of the importance of identifying women at risk for postpartum depression, it may be prudent to include those mothers who are identified as using alcohol during their pregnancy as a potential focus. The postpartum visit may be a good time to screen women for alcohol abuse. The Healthy Moms Trial supports the implementation of brief alcohol intervention during the postpartum period.[23]

OPIOIDS

Preconception

The class of drug known as the opioids contains the opiates, which are natural or semi-synthetic morphine-like substances, as well as the fully synthetic opioids. Opiates include morphine, codeine, and heroin. Meperidine, fentanyl, propoxyphene, and methadone are synthetic opioids.[20] Most of the information available regarding the effects of opioids on pregnancy is derived from studies of patients who have used heroin or methadone. There has been a recent increase in the use of prescription opioid analgesics, such hydromorphone and oxycodone, during pregnancy.

The prevalence of opiate use in pregnant women ranges from 1% to 21%.[6] The higher number reflects use in at-risk populations and does not represent overall use in a more standard obstetric population. Heroin is the most commonly abused illicit opiate and crosses the placenta readily. Heroin enters the fetal tissues within 1 hour of maternal use.[19] Women who use heroin are likely to use other harmful substances, such as tobacco, alcohol, and cocaine, all of which have their own potential adverse effects on pregnancy. Therefore, it is difficult to separate the effects of heroin from these other substances. Heroin can be mixed with other substances, including amphetamines, which can have independent detrimental effects on the pregnancy and fetus. In addition, intravenous drug use is a risk factor for many infectious diseasesm, including cellulitis, endocarditis, chorioamnionitis, and human immunodeficiency virus (HIV) infection, which can further complicate pregnancy.

Pregnancy

Pregnant women who use heroin can experience a six-fold increase in maternal obstetric complications,[24] includig intrauterine growth restriction, third trimester vaginal bleeding, malpresentation, preterm delivery, and puerperal morbidity. In addition, stillbirth, decreased infant head circumference, depressed Apgar score, meconium staining of the fetus, and chorioamnionits are all increased in heroin users.[22] Neonatal abstinence syndrome is seen in 50% to 95% of infants exposed to heroin.[22] Neonatal withdrawal is well described and is the most common finding in opiate-exposed neonates is CNS irritability. Supportive care is most important for these babies.[19]

Prenatal and antepartum care for patients using heroin must be tailored to these patients' special needs. Testing for sexually transmitted infections, such as HIV, syphilis, gonorrhea, chlamydia trachomatis, and hepatitis B and C, should be included in routine care and repeated periodically throughout the pregnancy. The provider must counsel the patient regarding the effects of heroin on herself and the fetus. In addition, the physician needs to counsel the patient on the potential benefits of methadone maintenance instead of continued heroin use. Methadone is a synthetic opioid that can be taken orally, and this treatment strategy has multiple benefits. Methadone is inexpensive and can dramatically reduce the incidence of criminal behavior. It may diminish exposure to needleborn infections, including HIV and hepatitis. Typically, patients using methadone can more easily make the transition to a life that is free of heroin abuse. Methadone maintenance clinics should be made available to help patients addicted to heroin, and the obstetrician should collaborate with the clinic to facilitate comprehensive care. Each prenatal visit should be used to evaluate the patient for signs of opiate toxicity and withdrawal. Symptoms of intoxication include drowsiness, decreased respirations, miosis, constipation, and diminished drug seeking. Withdrawal signs include drug craving, lacrimation, sweating, anorexia, diarrhea and flushing.[22]

Methadone maintenance treatment of pregnant women using heroin can be beneficial, as suggested above. In a 1995 position paper, United States federal guidelines regarding the regulation of methadone recommended preferential admittance to pregnant women with heroin addiction into methadone treatment programs.[25] Women taking methadone demonstrate reduced use of illicit drugs, better compliance with prenatal care, and improved newborn birth weight.[24] In most circumstances, withdrawal from methadone is rarely appropriate during pregnancy,[25] but occasionally there may be instances when withdrawal may be helpful. Aggressive attempts at withdrawal can lead to withdrawal symptoms in the mother and fetal withdrawal and possibly intrauterine fetal death.[19] It is crucial for the obstetrician to identify patients using heroin and help them initiate a treatment program.

Opioid analgesics such as oxycodone and hydromorphone can be judiciously used in pregnancy with close supervision but are much more commonly used in the post-partum time period for post-delivery pain control following both vaginal deliveries and cesarean sections. No congenital anomalies have been reported in babies born to patients who use hydromorphone for prolonged periods. Oxycodone use in pregnancy has also not been associated with any major birth defects.[19] However, the use of both substances increases the risk of neonatal withdrawal, particularly if they are used in and around the time of delivery.

Postpartum

Patients frequently use opioid analgesics in the postpartum period. Opioids are excreted into breast milk in small quantities. Minimal, if any, effect on the newborn is clinically significant. However, the neonate should be observed for signs of adverse effects, such as gastrointestinal side effects, sedation, and feeding pattern changes. For heavy narcotic abusers and women in methadone treatment programs, the postpartum time period is an excellent time to readdress the possibility of gradual narcotic withdrawal and continued rehabilitation.

SEDATIVE-HYPNOTICS AND ANXIOLYTICS

Preconception

The classes of drugs commonly known as the barbiturates and benzodiazepines fall into the larger category of drugs called the sedative-hypnotics and anxiolytics. Barbital, first introduced in 1903, is a derivative of bartituric acid and had noteworthy sleep-inducing and anxiolytic effects tat made it instantly popular from a clinical standpoint. Other barbiturates, such as phenobarbital, have anti-convulsant properties which also make them clinically useful. These anti-convulsant barbiturates are not commonly associated with abuse or addiction. As pharmacology progressed, the separation of the anti-convulsant properties from the sedative properties of these medications led to the development of the benzodiazepines, which are widely available as prescription treatment for anxiety and insomnia, and have a high propensity for abuse.

Currently, there are only a few barbiturates remaining on the market, and they remain in use because of their depressive CNS properties, particularly in the treatment of headache. Specifically, butalbital, the active agent in fiorocet and fiorinal, remains in common use for the treatment of migraines. Migraines are more common in women, especially those of reproductive age women. Therefore, several patients will conceive while using fiorocet or fiorinal and may require these drugs for control of their migraines in pregnancy.

Fiorocet and fiorinal are both Food and Drug Administration Fetal Risk Summary category C drugs,[26] suggesting that there are no controlled studies of their teratogenic effects on the human fetus, and that these drugs should only be used if the benefits outweigh the risks. For most patients who suffer with migraines, the benefits do indeed outweigh the theoretical risks inherent in the use of barbiturate-containing medication. The literature that evaluated the safety of barbiturate use in pregnancy is somewhat dated; the work was done primarily in the 1970s and 1980s. A review of this literature suggests that no increased risk of fetal malformation was noted above expected levels of occurrence, but that severe neonatal withdrawal is a critical consideration, particularly if the mother is a heavy butalbital user close to the time of delivery.[19]

Benzodiazepine use in the preconception time period is not uncommon because of the appeal of these medicines, particularly for the treatment of anxiety. Benzodiazepines are generally category D drugs, reflecting positive evidence of fetal risk. This risk must be weighed against the seriousness of the condition for which the mother is being treated. The risk of benzodiazepine abuse is relatively high, and fetal exposure has been extensively studied. There is conflicting evidence regarding the teratogenicity of benzodiazepines, with the suggestion of an increased likelihood of multiple anomalies, including cleft lip and palate, fetal growth restriction, and intrauterine fetal death. Still, no study or meta-analysis has been able to definitively link benzodiazepine abuse with a specific neonatal syndrome or constellation of anomalies, so the overall risk to the fetus in the face of exposure may in fact be low.

Pregnancy

Barbiturate abuse is relatively uncommon, but the powerful sedative effects that initially made these drugs attractive continue to have some appeal. There are patients who, secondary to severe migraine or headache pain or because of addiction, continue to be heavy users during pregnancy. As suggested above, there appears to be no significant teratogenic effects associated with barbiturate abuse.

Benzodiazepine use in pregnancy should raise physician awareness of the potential abuse of other substances, including alcohol and tobacco. As mentioned, the risk to the exposed fetus may be minimal, but the abrupt cessation of benzodiazepine use by the mother should be avoided because of the severe withdrawal symptoms associated with rapid cessation, including suicidal ideation.

For patients who are noted to be heavy users of sedative-hypnotics in pregnancy, a rehabilitation program could be considered. In addition, an evaluation by a psychiatrist or headache/migraine specialist may help the patient make the transition away from addictive medications. It should be emphasized to the patient that there can be significant withdrawal symptoms observed in the newborns of barbiturate or benzodiazepine addicted mothers, and these babies should be identified to the neonatology team.

Postpartum

The postpartum time period can be emotionally exhausting, even for the healthiest, non-addicted mother. For patients who have known drug dependency, the postpartum period can be particularly challenging. There are also several patients who suffer with anxiety or headache/migraines and notice an exacerbation of these conditions during the post-delivery period. For sedative-hypnotic abusers, careful attention must be paid to the amount of drug used, and whether the patient is breastfeeding. Sedative-hypnotics are generally contraindicated or considered possibly unsafe in lactation because of the sedative properties of these medications are readily excreted in breast milk.

COCAINE

Preconception

According to a 2005 government survey, approximately 4% of women use illicit drugs during their pregnancy, and cocaine is one of the most commonly abused drugs.[27] Prenatal cocaine use is commonly associated with poor pregnancy and adverse birth outcomes, and cocaine abuse particularly impacts measures of fetal growth and well-being. Low birth weight, intrauterine growth restriction, and decreased head circumference are all noted to be increased in newborns of mothers who use cocaine in pregnancy. In addition, cocaine use is frequently associated with inadequate prenatal care and the frequent concomitant use of tobacco and alcohol.[28] Moreover, cocaine use is associated with psychosocial, behavioral, and biomedical risk factors, such as poverty, poor nutrition, stress, depression, physical abuse, lack of social support, and sexually transmitted infections,[28] all of which can greatly affect pregnancy outcome.[29]

Pregnancy

Maternal cocaine use may have both direct and indirect effects on the fetus. Cocaine rapidly crosses the placenta and a higher concentration occurs in the fetus. There are many adverse outcomes associated with cocaine use during pregnancy. Cocaine use during the early months of pregnancy can cause spontaneous abortion. Up to 38% of early pregnancies may result in miscarriage in cocaine-abusing mothers.[28] This increase in incidence of spontaneous abortion is probably secondary to an increase in maternal plasma norepinephrine, which increases uterine contractility, constricts placental vessels, and decreases blood flow to the fetus. Placental abruption accounts for 2% to 15% of adverse effects of cocaine use during pregnancy. Abruption is thought to be caused by vasospasm and hypoxia of the placental bed, and it is more common with cocaine binging than with regular use. As a result of maternal cocaine use and placental abruption, the incidence of stillbirth in cocaine-abusing mothers is elevated 8% above the expected level when compared to the general population.[28,30]

Cocaine stimulates uterine contractility through β-agonist action on the β_2-receptors of the uterus. The consequence of this β-agonist property is an increased risk of premature preterm rupture of membranes, preterm labor, and preterm delivery. These adverse outcomes are observed in 17% to 29% of pregnancies of cocaine-abusing mothers. Intrauterine growth restriction (IUGR) and low birth weight can be observed in 22% to 34% of all infants exposed to cocaine in utero, secondary to the constriction of the uterine blood vessels, which leads to intermittent hypoperfusion of the uterus and placenta.[31] Moreover, cocaine significantly suppresses maternal appetite which contributes to poor maternal and fetal nutrition.[30,31]

Cocaine exposure can affect embryonic and fetal development. Congenital anomalies have been reported to occur in 7% to 40% of infants exposed to cocaine in utero. Evidence of brain malformation and cardiovascular abnormalities can occur in approximately 35% and 4% to 40% of exposed fetuses, respectively.[32]

Postpartum

The mainstay of the management of the cocaine-addicted mother and newborn immediately following delivery is supportive care.[30] Although the symptoms of cocaine neurotoxicity are not often life threatening for the mother or the newborn, these symptoms are extremely unpleasant.[30–33] For the mother during the postpartum period, mood symptoms and, less commonly, hallucinations may require treatment with antipsychotic medications, particularly during the inpatient stay.

From a social-focused and family-focused standpoint, the use of cocaine is extremely problematic. Cocaine use during pregnancy is considered a significant risk factor for infant neglect and abuse. Evidence of cocaine use in pregnancy often results in the removal of the infant from maternal custody within the first 18 months of life.[34] Prospective studies have also indicated a strong link between cocaine-using mothers and child maltreatment, with high rates of care-giving disruption (43%) and child maltreatment by 2 years (9% to 23%).[34] Finally, a stable and secure home environment helps reduce the stressors associated with cocaine addiction, so any intervention in this regard may be extremely helpful.

AMPHETAMINES

Preconception

Amphetamines are powerful CNS stimulants with a profound ability to increase wakefulness and focus. The principle mechanism of action is increased release of norepinephrine, serotonin, and dopamine from neurons within the brain. At the same time, amphetamines inhibit re-uptake of these neurotransmitters. Amphetamines are commonly used as drugs of abuse, particularly methamphetamine (also known as "crystal-meth"). Drugs in the amphetamine family can also serve traditional medicinal purposes. Amphetamine/dextroamphetamine (Adderal) is an effective treatment for attention deficit hyperactivity disorder and is used frequently by women of reproductive age. Fortunately, this is not a commonly abused medication in pregnancy.

Information about amphetamine use in pregnancy and preconception is less than reliable due to the fact that the studies are retrospective or depend on voluntary maternal reporting. However, amphetamine use, particularly among young pregnant patients, appears to be increasing.[35] The effects of amphetamine use in the preconception period and pregnancy are difficult to establish because users of amphetamines will commonly use other illicit drugs while pregnant, making it difficult to separate the effects of amphetamines from those of other illicit drugs. As with virtually all other drugs of abuse, there is an important confounding effect. More important, perhaps, is the association of amphetamine use with risky sexual behaviors, teenage pregnancy, and potential increased risk of sexually transmitted infections.[36]

Pregnancy

In animal studies, cleft palate, exencephaly, growth insufficiency, retinal defects, and delayed motor development have been reported as being associated with amphetamine use during gestation.[37] There are case reports suggesting an association of increased congenital abnormalities in human fetuses exposed to amphetamines during the first trimester. These defects include heart defects, gastroschisis, small intestinal atresia, and cleft lip and palate.[38–42] Other studies have not shown any association with increased risk of fetal malformation.[43–45] Overall, amphetamine abuse does not seem to be associated with any consistent increase in congenital abnormalities above the background 3% population risk. Furthermore, there is no evidence of a consistent syndrome associated first trimester amphetamine use. Thus, current thought is that amphetamines are not human teratogens.[19,46]

Fetal growth insufficiency has been reported to be associated with amphetamine use in pregnancy. It is unclear if this is related to a direct effect of the agent on the placenta or fetus or whether this represents a nutritional problem in patients who use amphetamines.[37,44,46–48] There are also reports of fetal/neonatal cerebral cavitary lesions in patients who use amphetamines during pregnancy. It is hypothesized that this may be due to hypoxic injury related to amphetamine-induced vasoconstriction.[19]

Patients who are known to use amphetamines should be encouraged to stop, and there seems to be no detrimental effect associated with discontinuation of use during pregnancy. The patient should be referred to a substance abuse program. In addition to routine obstetric care, management of patients who are users of amphetamines should include frequent ultrasounds to assess the growth and integrity of the central nervous system of the fetus. The neonatologist needs to be alerted regarding possible maternal abuse of amphetamines at the time of birth so neonatal symptoms can be recognized and treated, if warranted.

Postpartum

Information addressing amphetamine use in the postpartum period is scant, but amphetamine use during lactation is considered possibly hazardous. Mild neonatal withdrawal has been described, including jitteriness, drowsiness, and respiratory distress.[19,49,50] Maternal methamphetamine use may have long-term detrimental effects on exposed fetuses, and exposure may result in future learning and memory impairments.[51]

MARIJUANA

Preconception

Marijuana has been reported to be used by 3% to 16% of all pregnant patients.[19,52,53] Like all substances of abuse in pregnancy, there are no prospective studies establishing the actual rate of marijuana use and the statistics cited depend on voluntary patient reporting. The effects of marijuana use on a developing fetus in the preconception time period and pregnancy are hard to establish because users of marijuana will frequently use other illicit drugs while pregnant, making it difficult to separate marijuana's effects from the effects of other drugs. Again, self-reporting is a confounder.

Delta-9-tetrahydrocannabinol is the active ingredient in marijuana and it readily crosses the placenta. However, marijuana is not a pure substance. Commonly available marijuana varies in potency and may have up to 400 other chemicals and substances admixed. Separating out the effects of these chemicals, as well as the effects of varying potency, is a confounder in any report or statistics that address marijuana use in pregnancy. There is no known increase in the risk of congenital abnormalities above the background risk of 3% in patients who smoke marijuana in the first trimester.

Pregnancy

There is no known increase in pregnancy complications for users of marijuana.[19] There has been a suspicion that patients who use marijuana during pregnancy may have longer gestations.[19] However, other studies have suggested a shorter gestation.[54] Thus, the data concerning the effect of marijuana on gestational length is contradictory. There has been some suggestion of longer, dysfunctional labors in patients who smoke marijuana around the time of delivery, but other reports fail to confirm this.[19] There is also a suggestion that there may be an association between marijuana use and an increase in low birth weight and small for gestational age infants.[55] However, other reports do not confirm this.[55–58]

Patients who are known to use marijuana during pregnancy should be counseled about the associated risks and encouraged to stop. Intervention programs should be offered. In addition to routine obstetric care, patients who use marijuana during pregnancy should have follow-up ultrasounds at 28 and 36 weeks to confirm adequacy of fetal growth. At the time of delivery, the pediatric team should be alerted regarding maternal marijuana use during pregnancy.

Postpartum

Marijuana use in the postpartum time period has not been well studied. There is limited clinical evidence to drive recommendations regarding counseling, intervention, or rehabilitation. Therefore, care for the marijuana-addicted mother must be approached on a case-by-case basis, and social work consultations should be used liberally in an attempt to stabilize the home environment as much as possible. As mentioned above, marijuana is frequently used in conjunction with other drugs and substances of abuse.

MANAGEMENT OF HIGH-RISK PREGNANCIES IN SUBSTANCE ABUSING MOTHERS

General Considerations

The substance-abusing mother by definition is considered high-risk, with significant exposure for maternal and fetal complications. In the prior discussions of the various different substances of abuse, these risks are identified individually, with particular attention paid to the most likely maternal and obstetric complications. As a general rule, teratogenicity, poor maternal nutrition, IUGR, poor placental perfusion and function (placental insufficiency), labor management, and withdrawal syndromes are the most common obstetric issues that must be addressed when considering the impact of substance abuse on pregnancy. In the case of cocaine abuse, placental abruption and stillbirth are important additional considerations.

Teratogenic Exposure

The possibility of substances of abuse causing fetal anomalies is an overriding concern, and specific considerations are mentioned for the drugs and substances of abuse discussed. Alcohol abuse in particular is highly associated with FASD, which can be manifested as structural anomalies or developmental defects, including fetal growth restriction. Mental retardation, developmental delay, and behavioral disorders are common components of FASD and can also be seen in the children of cocaine abusing mothers. Cocaine is also associated with fetal brain and cardiac malformations, and amphetamine use is associated with cavitary brain lesions. In regard to management of these problems for the expectant mother, little can be offered once the damage has been done. No prenatal test is currently available to help identify fetuses at risk for future mental retardation and developmental delay. From an obstetric standpoint, only early ultrasound identification of structural anomalies is a possibility. Once an anomaly has been identified, various pediatric specialists can be consulted for post-delivery management if this is appropriate. Serial ultrasonographic surveillance of the fetus, with the addition of frequent non-stress testing, contraction stress testing, or biophysical profiles, may have some additional value (these tests and surveillance strategies will be addressed below).

Because none of the substances of abuse discussed earlier are associated with fetal aneuploidy or chromosomal anomalies, amniocentesis or chorionic villus sampling for genetic testing should be performed only as indicated or desired by the parents—it yields no further information in regard to predicting the possibility of future retardation or developmental delay. In instances where significant fetal anatomic anomalies are observed with routine sonographic screening, it is reasonable to offer pregnancy termination to the patient, particularly if the anomaly noted would be incompatible with life. These instances must be approached in a case-by-case basis.

Nutritional Considerations

Poor maternal nutritional status is associated with many substances of abuse. Smoking, alcoholism, opiate abuse, sedative/hypnotic abuse, cocaine abuse, marijuana abuse, and amphetamine abuse have all been associated with poor maternal weight gain and nutritional status. In many cases, these substances are mixed, and most have fairly powerful appetite suppressant properties. Management of poor maternal nutrition is relatively concrete in theory but can be frustrating for the practitioner because sometimes little can be done to change established maternal behaviors in regard to nutrition. A multi-disciplinary approach incorporating nutritional counseling by trained dieticians or nutrition counselors can certainly be valuable. Frequent weight checks and fetal surveillance for IUGR should be incorporated into routine obstetric care for substance abusing mothers.

Ideally, substance abusing mothers should be counseled extensively regarding the importance of balanced nutrition, including recommendations regarding caloric intake and appropriate weight gain. Body mass index should be calculated as well because there will certainly be a significant number of substance-abusing pregnant patients who may be obese or severely underweight; both of these conditions suggest poor overall nutritional status. Nutrition counseling should focus on a well-balanced diet and the inclusion of nutritional foods. Exercise can be emphasized at these counseling sessions as well.

Dietary allowances of most vitamins and minerals increase during pregnancy, and prenatal vitamins can play an important role in supplementation. In particular, iron supplementation (27 mg of additional daily iron) should be included in the daily diet. Iron deficiency anemia is a common problem in the substance abusing population, and an additional 60 to 120 mg of iron is recommended for these individuals. Vitamin C facilitates the absorption of iron, and additional vitamin C may need to be added. Folic acid supplementation should also be addressed, particularly in the preconception period and first trimester because of the known association between folic acid supplementation and a diminution in risk of spina bifida. Caloric intake is generally calculated at 25 to 35 kcal/day of optimal body weight. An additional 100 to 300 kcal/day is recommended in pregnancy.[59]

Intrauterine Growth Restriction and Placental Insufficiency

Because of the high correlation between substance abuse and poor maternal nutrition, as well as the impact of substances of abuse on placental function, surveillance for appropriate fetal growth and placental function is an important component of care for substance-abusing mothers. Again, like many recommendations that are made to substance abusers, compliance can be an issue. Nevertheless, obstetricians should be vigilant in their attempts to follow substance-abusing mothers as closely as possible in the antenatal period, particularly in the attempt to identify suboptimal fetal growth and placental insufficiency. In many instances, IUGR and poor placental function increase the risk of stillbirth, and it is for this reason that vigilance is urged. Alcohol abuse, smoking, and illicit drug use are all strongly associated with IUGR and stillbirth, although it can be extremely difficult to differentiate the actual effect of the drug or substance of abuse on the fetus from other maternal behaviors which are associated with drug use.[59]

Recommendations regarding surveillance for fetal growth and placental function generally involve serial uterine fundal height measurements and serial ultrasound evaluation of the fetus with attention paid to fetal head circumference and biparietal diameter, abdominal circumference, amniotic fluid indices, and Doppler velocimetry. Serial ultrasound surveillance typically begins at approximately 20 weeks of gestation and continues at 4-week intervals thereafter. Non-stress testing, contraction stress testing, and the biophysical profile can be used as well, depending on the clinical situation; these tests are typically performed in the third trimester. Uterine fundal height measures can be an effective screening tool for IUGR and should be performed at every prenatal visit after 20 weeks of gestation. When a patient has a smaller than expected fundal measurement, the suspicion of IUGR should be confirmed with directed ultrasound in a timely manner. Specifically, ultrasound measures of the biparietal diameter (distance across the fetal head), head circumference, abdominal circumference, and femur length should be measured to obtain the most accurate estimated fetal weight. The amniotic fluid index should also be measured. Pockets of amniotic fluid are measured in all four quadrants of the uterus and a cumulative measure of the vertical pockets should be greater than 5 cm. A measure less than 5 cm would suggest oligohydramnios (low amniotic fluid), and this can be cause for concern because it may indicate a long-term diminution in placental function. In fact, oligohydramnios or anhydramnios (no measurable amniotic fluid pockets) may indicate a need for delivery, depending on the clinical circumstances. In general, ultrasound evaluation should occur every 2 to 4 weeks if IUGR is suspected. An interval less than 2 weeks can introduce the possibility of measurement errors.

Fetal non-stress testing or contraction stress testing may also be of value in the ongoing surveillance of substance abusing mothers, particularly if IUGR, placental insufficiency, or oligohydramnios is suspected or diagnosed. Non-stress testing can be performed on an outpatient or inpatient basis and assesses utero-placental function by evaluating the fetal heart rate over a 20-minute period of time with an external fetal heart rate monitor. The presence of accelerations of the fetal heart rate is associated with fetal movement and appropriate placental perfusion and function, and is considered reassuring. A non-stress test is reactive if there are 2 accelerations of at least 15 beats per minute above the established baseline lasting at least 15 seconds in a fetus greater than 32 weeks or 10 beats per minute above baseline lasting at least 10 seconds in a fetus less than 32 weeks within a 20-minute period. The contraction stress testing assesses utero-placental function by measuring the fetal response to induced or spontaneous contractions. A positive contraction stress testing occurs when late decelerations (an observed slowing of the fetal heart rate) occur with more than half of the contractions in a 10-minute time period. Contraction stress testing is a more cumbersome test to perform, however, and is used less commonly than the non-stress test.

The biophysical profile assesses fetal well-being using 5 biophysical components, including 4 findings determined by ultrasound in combination with a fetal heart rate non-stress test. The biophysical profile can be a useful test by itself and can also be used as an adjunct or confirmatory test if fetal non-well-being is suspected. Normal measurements are scored as 2 points and abnormal measurements are scored as 0 points. The following parameters (all observed with ultrasound) are also assigned 2 points: fetal breathing, fetal movement, fetal tone, and the amniotic fluid index. Thirty minutes of total ultrasound observation is allowed.

When IUGR is suspected and confirmed in a substance-abusing mother, the possibility of perinatal death or stillbirth becomes an important consideration. IUGR can almost never be reversed, but careful surveillance, particularly with Doppler velocimetry of the umbilical artery waveform, is associated with a reduction in perinatal death.[59] Umbilical artery Doppler velocimetry assesses umbilical artery blood flow by measuring vascular impedance. The systolic to diastolic ratio is abnormal when it is greater than the 95th percentile for gestational age or if diastolic flow is either absent or reversed.

Timing of delivery can also be a challenge in the growth-restricted fetus. The practitioner must weigh the risks of prematurity versus the ongoing risk of intrauterine fetal death if poor fetal growth or placental insufficiency is suspected. In general, absent or reversed end-diastolic flow observed with Doppler velocimetry can be an indication for delivery. Other indications for delivery included oligohydramnios and anhydramnios. Complete absence of fetal growth observed in consecutive ultrasound evaluations 2 to 4 weeks apart may also provide a strong indication for delivery. Mode of delivery (cesarean section versus vaginal delivery) should be individualized based on the patient and her obstetric considerations. For patients with a vertex fetus and reassuring fetal surveillance testing, an induction of labor with planned vaginal delivery is acceptable. A planned cesarean section may be indicated in circumstances when fetal surveillance testing is non-reassuring, the fetus is breech, or there is a low likelihood that the fetus would be able to tolerate labor.

Labor Management

Management of the substance-abusing patient in labor can present significant challenges to the obstetrical team. As a general rule, the labor and management of the substance-abusing patient should be based on widely accepted obstetric practice and recommendations, which are beyond the scope of this article. There are two issues, however, that merit special consideration—communication with the patient and management of anesthesia.

Establishing healthy and non-threatening communication with a substance-abusing mother in labor is a paramount goal for obstetrical caregivers. Nurses, physicians, and midwives must work diligently to put the patient at ease and inform her that there is a potential for many necessary obstetric interventions, all of which will be done to maximize the likelihood of a good outcome for the mother and her baby. Unfortunately, establishing lines of communication can be frustrating, particularly when addicted patients present exhibiting erratic, bizarre, angry, or uncaring behavior.[60]

Inhaled cocaine users will frequently obtain this drug when labor begins because of a fear that labor anesthesia and analgesia will not be offered or will be inadequate on presentation to the hospital. This behavior has been exhibited in narcotic abusers as well. The addicted mother can cause increased stress for the obstetrical staff, and establishing a trusting relationship with the patient by speaking in a calm voice, utilizing appropriate physical contact, and using soft lighting can all be beneficial as the caregiver attempts to gain control of a potentially chaotic situation. It must be emphasized to the patient that all indicated interventions are for her benefit. Finally, using appropriate referrals, particularly to case managers, social workers, and home nursing services, can be beneficial in helping to organize the post-delivery care for substance-abusing mothers. These referrals also provide the opportunity to keep ongoing communication with the patient intact.[60]

Considerations regarding labor anesthesia and analgesia are particularly relevant when a substance-abusing patient presents in labor. Each particular substance of abuse brings its own challenges. Tobacco use affects the pulmonary system and increases sputum and secretion production, as well as impairment of gas exchange. Cigarette smoking may also affect hepatic enzyme function and may alter metabolism of the induction agents used for general anesthesia. Therefore, regional anesthesia is preferred and can help caregivers avoid the potential problems associated with bronchospasm and airway manipulation.[61]

Alcohol-abusing patients present significant challenges when they present in labor. A blood alcohol level of 25 mg/dL is associated with significant impairment, and intoxication is typically defined as a blood alcohol level greater than 100 mg/dL. Alcohol intoxication increases gastric acidity and diminishes the ability to protect the airway. Chronic liver disease, coagulopathies, pancreatitis, and esophageal varicies must be considered based on the clinical presentation of the patient, and appropriate blood testing is indicated at the time of presentation, particularly for the evaluation of a potential coagulopathy. Regional anesthesia is usually the optimal choice for alcohol-abusing patients and is safe if the patient does not suffer with an underlying neuropathy or clotting disorder. Intravascular volume must be optimized before the administration of regional anesthesia, especially in the face of clinical dehydration. Optimal fluid resuscitation will diminish the potential adverse effects of sympathetic blockade. Alcohol withdrawal syndrome, which is common, should be managed with benzodiazepines, alpha-2 agonists, or the resumption of alcohol consumption.[61]

Opioid abuse in the laboring patient presents several problems, including respiratory depression and arrest. Regional anesthesia/analgesia is widely considered to be safe in opioid abusers. Patients who present with recent opioid use may have diminished anesthetic requirements. Conversely, chronic use may increase tolerance and chronic abusers may require higher anesthetic and analgesic doses than would be anticipated. Mothers using methadone maintenance regimens should be treated as usual; the key point is that their methadone should not be withheld unless there is a strong clinical indication to do so. There is no reason to believe that methadone maintenance patients will have lower pain requirements than other patients.[62]

Cocaine abuse in pregnancy can present life-threatening complications to both the mother and fetus, including acute myocardial infarction and placental abruption. Therefore, the cocaine-abusing mother must be given particular consideration. Hypertension, tachycardia, arrhythmias, seizures, fever, and emotional instability are all associated with cocaine abuse. Regional and general anesthesia can both be complicated in cocaine users. Cocaine-induced thrombocytopenia can present a contraindication to regional anesthesia or analgesia. Epidural or spinal placement can be further jeopardized by the agitated patient and intrathecal opioids administered in labor typically have a shorter duration in cocaine-abusing patients.[62]

General anesthesia administered to the cocaine-abusing mother presents additional challenges. Halothane should be avoided because it sensitizes the myocardium to the effects of catecholamines. Cardiac arrhythmias and increased systemic vascular resistance have been associated with the use of isoflurane. Currently, there is no information available regarding the use of sevoflurane or desflurane. Propofol, which is commonly used in the United States, is safe and effective for the induction of anesthesia in cocaine-abusing mothers.[62]

The management of hypertension in cocaine abusers can also be challenging. Beta-blockers can cause unopposed alpha stimulation and associated vasoconstriction of the coronary arteries. Labetolol, a combined alpha and beta blocker, is widely considered to be safe and does not impede uterine blood flow. Hydralazine may cause a significant maternal reflex tachycardia.[62]

Amphetamines affect the serotonin and dopamine systems, as described previously. The profound CNS findings commonly seen in amphetamine users, including increased alertness, decreased fatigue, and euphoria, can make placement of regional anesthesia difficult. Maternal hypertension, tachycardia, and arrhythmias all mimic the side-effects associated with cocaine abuse and should be treated accordingly. Inhalation agents should be used with caution, as is similar with cocaine-abusing patients.[62]

Patients presenting in labor with recent marijuana use often experience myocardial depression and tachycardia, which should be taken into consideration when anesthesia and analgesia are administered. Marijuana may also potentiate the sedative-hypnotic effects of other anesthetic agents and may cause increased tolerance of medications, including benzodiazepines and opioids, which may need to be given for medical indications. Heavy marijuana use may impair lung function, and drugs that may be likely to cause tachycardia should be avoided.[63]

Management of Withdrawal Symptoms

Issues arising as a result of maternal and fetal withdrawal must be managed on an individualized basis, taking into consideration the substance of abuse in question, along with maternal or fetal needs. For example, it may not be prudent to withdraw methadone from an addicted or abusing mother because this may increase the likelihood of stillbirth.[59] In contrast, the withdrawal of cocaine will likely diminish the possibility of catastrophic placental abruption or stillbirth. It is best to adopt a team approach regarding maternal and neonatal withdrawal, incorporating a system-based practice model involving neonatologists, psychiatrists, psychologists, and social workers. Preferably, these providers will have some expertise in the management of substance-abusing mothers and their newborns.

CONCLUSION

The opportunities for the abuse of psychoactive substances in pregnancy are vast, and there is evidence that the use and misuse of these substances may be increasing. Tobacco use has a strong association with spontaneous miscarriage, fetal growth restriction, and preterm delivery. Heavy caffeine use may be associated with first-trimester loss. The abuse of alcohol has a significant potential impact on pregnancy, the most important being fetal alcohol spectrum disorder. Heavy use of opioids and sedative-hypnotics may not be strongly associated with teratogenicity, but fetal sedation and withdrawal at the time of delivery is an extremely unfortunate consequence and the long-term effects of prolonged fetal exposure to these drugs may be potentially concerning. Methadone maintenance clinics are suggested for opiate abusing pregnant patients. Cocaine abuse is strongly associated with fetal growth restriction and potentially catastrophic placental abruption and stillbirth. Amphetamine use may be increasing, particularly in younger mothers, and is associated with poor maternal nutrition and fetal growth restriction. Like most of the other drugs and substances of abuse, marijuana use may also be associated with fetal growth restriction as well.

It remains extremely important to take a careful history when you are caring for patients with potential substance abuse issues and develop a team approach involving individuals with expertise in rehabilitation and the care of mothers and newborns with substance abuse issues. Social workers and neonatologists should be consulted as well, especially at the time of delivery and in the postpartum period. In many instances pregnancy can act as a sentinel event that can help substance-abusing mothers begin to come to terms with their highly self-destructive behaviors, which can also have an unanticipated impact on their unborn or newborn children.

REFERENCES

1. Kuczkowski KM. The effects of drug abuse on pregnancy. Curr Opin Obstet Gynecol 2007; 19:578–85.
2. Office of Applied Studies, Substance Abuse and Mental Health Services Administration. Results from the 2002 National Survey on Drug Use and Health: National findings (DHHS Publication No. SMA 03-3836, NSDUH Series H-22). Rockville, MD: Substance Abuse and Mental Health Services Administration, Office of Applied Studies, 2003. [Available at http://www.oas.samhsa.gov/p0000016.htm#2k2].
3. IARC (International Agency for Research on Cancer) Working Group on the Evaluation of Carcinogenic Risks to Humans. Tobacco smoke and involuntary smoking. IARC Monogr Eval Carcinog Risks Hum 2004; 83:1–1438.
4. Spitzer WO, Lawrence V, Dales R, Hill G, Archer MC, Clark P, Abenhaim L, Hardy J, Sampalis J, Pinfold SP, et al. Links between passive smoking and disease: a best-evidence synthesis. A report of the Working Group on Passive Smoking. Clin Invest Med 1990; 13:17–42.
5. National Institutes of Health State-of-the-Science conference statement: tobacco use: prevention, cessation, and control. Ann Intern Med 2006; 145:839–844.
6. Kandel DB, Griesler PC, Schaffran C. Educational attainment and smoking among women: risk factors and consequences for offspring. Drug Alcohol Depend 2009; 104(Suppl 1):S24–33.
7. Lumley J, Oliver SS, Chamberlain C, Oakley L. Interventions for promoting smoking cessation during pregnancy. Cochrane Database Syst Rev 2004:CD001055.
8. Einarson A, Riordan S. Smoking in pregnancy and lactation: a review of risks and cessation strategies. Eur J Clin Pharmacol 2009; 65:325–30.
9. Goodwin RD, Keyes K, Simuro N. Mental disorders and nicotine dependence among pregnant women in the United States. Obstet Gynecol 2007; 109:875–83.
10. Thielen A, Klus H, Muller L. Tobacco smoke: unraveling a controversial subject. Exp Toxicol Pathol 2008; 60:141–56.
11. Andres RL, Day MC. Perinatal complications associated with maternal tobacco use. Semin Neonatol 2000; 5:231–41.
12. Crawford JT, Tolosa JE, Goldenberg RL. Smoking cessation in pregnancy: why, how, and what next. Clin Obstet Gynecol 2008; 51:419–35.
13. Burton GJ, Palmer ME, Dalton KJ. Morphometric differences between the placental vasculature of non-smokers, smokers and ex-smokers. Br J Obstet Gynaecol 1989; 96:907–15.
14. Fanslow J, Silva M, Robinson E, Whitehead A. Violence during pregnancy: associations with pregnancy intendedness, pregnancy-related care, and alcohol and tobacco use among a representative sample of New Zealand women. Aust N Z J Obstet Gynaecol 2008; 48:398–404.
15. Rosenberg L, Mitchell AA, Shapiro S, Slone D. Selected birth defects in relation to caffeine-containing beverages. JAMA 1982; 247:1429–32.
16. Chavarro JE, Rich-Edwards JW, Rosner BA, Willett WC. Caffeinated and alcoholic beverage intake in relation to ovulatory disorder infertility. Epidemiology 2009; 20(3):374–81.
17. Weng X, Odouli R, Li DK. Maternal caffeine consumption during pregnancy and the risk of miscarriage: a prospective cohort study. Am J Obstet Gynecol 2008; 198:279 e1–8.
18. Hadeed A, Siegel S. Newborn cardiac arrhythmias associated with maternal caffeine use during pregnancy. Clin Pediatr (Phila) 1993; 32:45–7.
19. Briggs G, Freeman R, Yaffe J. Drugs in pregnancy and lactation. Philadelphia: Lippincott Williams & Wilkins, 2008.
20. Floyd RL, Jack BW, Cefalo R, Atrash H, Mahoney J, Herron A, Husten C, Sokol RJ. The clinical content of preconception care: alcohol, tobacco, and illicit drug exposures. Am J Obstet Gynecol 2008; 199:S333–9.

21. Chang G. Alcohol-screening instruments for pregnant women. Alcohol Res Health 2001; 25:204–9.

22. Creasy RK, Resnik R, Iams JD. Creasy and Resnik's maternal-fetal medicine : principles and practice. Philadelphia, PA: Saunders/Elsevier, 2009.

23. Fleming MF, Lund MR, Wilton G, Landry M, Scheets D. The Healthy Moms Study: the efficacy of brief alcohol intervention in postpartum women. Alcohol Clin Exp Res 2008; 32:1600–6.

24. Minozzi S, Amato L, Vecchi S, Davoli M. Maintenance agonist treatments for opiate dependent pregnant women. Cochrane Database Syst Rev 2008:CD006318.

25. Rettig R. Federal Regulation of Methadone: Table of Contents and Executive Summary. Washington, DC: National Academy Press, 1995.

26. Food and Drug Administration. Labelling and prescription drug advertising:content and format for labelling for human prescription drug. Fed Reg 1980; 44:37434–67.

27. NSDUH. Substance Abuse and Mental Health Administration. Results form the 2005 National Survey on Drug Use and Health: National Findings. In: Office of Applied Studies, NSH- Ed. Rockville, MD: DHHS, 2006.

28. Schempf AH, Strobino DM. Illicit drug use and adverse birth outcomes: is it drugs or context? J Urban Health 2008; 85:858–73.

29. Muhuri PK, Gfroerer JC. Substance use among women: associations with pregnancy, parenting, and race/ethnicity. Matern Child Health J 2009; 13:376–85.

30. Bhuvaneswar CG, Chang G, Epstein LA, Stern TA. Cocaine and opioid use during pregnancy: prevalence and management. Prim Care Companion J Clin Psychiatry 2008; 10:59–65.

31. Bateman DA, Chiriboga CA. Dose-response effect of cocaine on newborn head circumference. Pediatrics 2000; 106:E33.

32. Vidaeff AC, Mastrobattista JM. In utero cocaine exposure: a thorny mix of science and mythology. Am J Perinatol 2003; 20:165–72.

33. Bauer CR, Langer JC, Shankaran S, Bada HS, Lester B, Wright LL, Krause-Steinrauf H, Smeriglio VL, Finnegan LP, Maza PL, Verter J. Acute neonatal effects of cocaine exposure during pregnancy. Arch Pediatr Adolesc Med 2005; 159:824–34.

34. Minnes S, Singer LT, Humphrey-Wall R, Satayathum S. Psychosocial and behavioral factors related to the post-partum placements of infants born to cocaine-using women. Child Abuse Negl 2008; 32:353–66.

35. Cox S, Posner SF, Kourtis AP, Jamieson, DJ. Hospitalizations with amphetamine abuse among pregnant women. Obstet Gynecol 2008; 111:341–7.

36. Zapata LB, Hillis SD, Marchbanks PA, Curtis KM, Lowry R. Methamphetamine use is independently associated with recent risky sexual behaviors and adolescent pregnancy. J Sch Health 2008; 78:641–8.

37. Wouldes T, LaGasse L, Sheridan J, Lester B. Maternal methamphetamine use during pregnancy and child outcome: what do we know? N Z Med J 2004; 117: U1180.

38. Bateman DN, McElhatton PR, Dickinson D, Wren C, Matthews JN, O'Keeffe M, Thomas SH. A case control study to examine the pharmacological factors underlying ventricular septal defects in the North of England. Eur J Clin Pharmacol 2004; 60:635–41.

39. Werler MM, Sheehan JE, Mitchell AA. Association of vasoconstrictive exposures with risks of gastroschisis and small intestinal atresia. Epidemiology 2003; 14:349–54.

40. Thomas DB. Cleft palate, mortality and morbidity in infants of substance abusing mothers. J Paediatr Child Health 1995; 31:457–60.

41. Bays J. Fetal vascular disruption with prenatal exposure to cocaine or methamphetamine. Pediatrics 1991; 87:416–8.

42. Nora JJ, Vargo TA, Nora AH, Love KE, McNamara DG. Dexamphetamine: a possible environmental trigger in cardiovascular malformations. Lancet 1970; 1:1290–1.

43. Heinonen OP, Sloan D, Shapiro S. Birth defects and drugs in pregnancy. Littleton, MA: Publishing Sciences Group Inc., 1977.

44. Little BB, Snell LM, Gilstrap LC 3rd. Methamphetamine abuse during pregnancy: outcome and fetal effects. Obstet Gynecol 1988; 72:541–4.

45. Milkovich L, van der Berg BJ. Effects of antenatal exposure to anorectic drugs. Am J Obstet Gynecol 1977; 129:637–42.

46. Smith LM, LaGasse LL, Derauf C, Grant P, Shah R, Arria A, Huestis M, Haning,W, Strauss A, Della Grotta S, Liu J, Lester BM. The infant development, environment, and lifestyle study: effects of prenatal methamphetamine exposure, polydrug exposure, and poverty on intrauterine growth. Pediatrics 2006; 118:1149–56.

47. Naeye RL. Maternal use of dextroamphetamine and growth of the fetus. Pharmacology 1983; 26:117–20.

48. Ramin SM, Little BB, Trimmer KJ, Standard DI, Blakely CA, Snell LM. Methamphetamine use during pregnancy. Am J Obstet Gynecol 1992; 166:353.

49. Oro AS, Dixon SD. Perinatal cocaine and methamphetamine exposure: maternal and neonatal correlates. J Pediatr 1987; 111:571–8.

50. Smith L, Yonekura ML, Wallace T, Berman N, Kuo J, Berkowitz C. Effects of prenatal methamphetamine exposure on fetal growth and drug withdrawal symptoms in infants born at term. J Dev Behav Pediatr 2003; 24:17–23.

51. Skelton MR, Williams MT, Vorhees CV. Developmental effects of 3,4-methylenedioxymethamphetamine: a review. Behav Pharmacol 2008; 19:91–111.

52. Abel EL, Sokol RJ. Marijuana and cocaine use during pregnancy. Philadelphia: Lea & Febiger, 1988.

53. Chasnoff IJ, Landress HJ, Barrett ME. The prevalence of illicit drug or alcohol use during pregnancy and discrepancies in mandatory reporting in Phila County, Florida. N Engl J Med 1990; 322: 1202.

54. National Institute on Drug Abuse (NIDA) Research Report Series: Marijuana Abuse. July 2005. NIH Publication Number 05-3859.

55. Hatch EE, Bracken MB. Effect of marijuana use in pregnancy on fetal growth. Am J Epidemiol 1986; 124:986–93.

56. Greenland S, Richwald GA, Honda GD. The effects of marijuana use during pregnancy. II. A study in a low-risk home-delivery population. Drug Alcohol Depend 1983; 11:359–66.

57. Linn S, Schoenbaum SC, Monson RR, Rosner R, Stubblefield PC, Ryan KJ. The association of marijuana use with outcome of pregnancy. Am J Public Health 1983; 73:1161–4.

58. Shiono PH, Klebanoff MA, Nugent RP, Cotch MF, Wilkins DG, Rollins DE, Carey JC, Behrman RE. The impact of cocaine and marijuana use on low birth weight and preterm birth: a multicenter study. Am J Obstet Gynecol 1995; 172:19–27.

59. American College of Obstetricians and Gynecologists. Guidelines for Perinatal Care, Sixth Edition. Atlanta, GA: ACOG, 2007.

60. Byrne MW, Lerner HM. Communicating with addicted women in labor. MCN Am J Matern Child Nurs 1992; 17:22–6.

61. Kuczkowski KM. Labor analgesia for the tobacco and ethanol abusing pregnant patient: a routine management? Arch Gynecol Obstet 2005; 271:6–10.

62. Ludlow J, Christmas T, Paech MJ, Orr B. Drug abuse and dependency during pregnancy: anaesthetic issues. Anaesth Intensive Care 2007; 35:881–93.

63. Kuczkowski KM. Anesthetic implications of drug abuse in pregnancy. J Clin Anesth 2003; 15(5):382–94.

Human Immunodeficiency Virus Risk Behavior Among Female Substance Abusers

Susan E. Ramsey, PhD
Kathryn M. Bell, PhD
Patricia A. Engler, PhD

ABSTRACT. HIV is an increasingly critical and costly health problem for American women. Substance use plays a major role in human immunodeficiency virus (HIV) infection in women. There are several plausible explanations for the association between substance use and HIV risk behavior. Pregnant substance abusers are a population deserving special attention given the prevalence of risk behavior in this population and the added risk of perinatal transmission of HIV. Current guidelines for the screening and treatment of HIV among pregnant women and their infants are delineated. Substance abuse treatment has a limited impact on HIV risk behavior in female substance abusers. Similarly, traditional knowledge-based and skill-based HIV risk reduction interventions have modest efficacy in this population. Hence, there is a need to develop new interventions that directly target sex-related and drug-related HIV risk behavior among female substance abusers. Recent work suggests that the incorporation of motivational interviewing components into traditional HIV risk reduction interventions may be a promising new direction for the field.

INTRODUCTION

Human immunodeficiency virus (HIV) is an increasingly critical and costly health problem for American women. Women comprise the most rapidly expanding group infected by HIV in the United States.[1] Women now represent 27% of all AIDS cases in the United States, increased 17% between 2001 and 2005, with the most dramatic increases among minority women.[2,3] Although African American and Hispanic women combined comprise less than 25% of all U.S. women, they account for 82% of AIDS cases among women.[2,4] Across age groups, women between 15 and 39 years old have demonstrated the greatest proportionate increase in AIDS cases.[3] In the United States, HIV is the sixth leading cause of death for women between 25 and 34 years of age and the fifth leading cause of death for women between 35 and 44 years of age.[3] Women now encompass more than one-quarter of all newly diagnosed HIV/AIDS cases, more than three-quarters of which are acquired heterosexually.[2,3]

Supported in part by Grant #R01DA020930 from the National Institute on Drug Abuse to Susan E. Ramsey. The content is solely the responsibility of the authors and does not necessarily represent the official views of the National Institute on Drug Abuse or the National Institutes of Health.

HIV SEX-RISK AND DRUG-RISK BEHAVIOR AMONG FEMALE SUBSTANCE ABUSERS

Substance use plays a major role in HIV infection in women. As many as 29% of women contract HIV through their own injection drug use, and another 15% contract HIV through sexual contact with an injection drug user.[5] Furthermore, female injection drug users have one of the lowest rates of survival among those diagnosed with AIDS.[2]

Use of alcohol and non-injection drugs, including crack cocaine, may increase a woman's risk of sexually transmitted HIV infection through increased engagement in high-risk sexual behaviors, such as unprotected sex and sex exchange for drugs or money.[6,7] Extensive research has found that individuals who use alcohol and drugs are at higher risk for engaging in several sex risk behaviors, including reduced condom use, increased number of sexual partners, use of drugs and alcohol before and during sexual activity, engagement in sexual activity with high risk partners (e.g., sex with injection drug users), and involvement in sex exchange for drugs or money.[7–16] Rates of unprotected sex events are especially high among drug users, regardless of the type of drug used.[8,13,15,17,18] Additional findings suggest that as much as 70% of sex events among drug users involve the presence of drugs and alcohol immediately prior to and during sexual activity,[15] which is particularly troubling given that substance use has been shown to reduce intent to use condoms.[19,20]

REASONS FOR THE ASSOCIATION BETWEEN SUBSTANCE USE AND HIV RISK BEHAVIOR

The presence of drug-related HIV risk behavior among substance users is not surprising. However, the reason for the increased rate of sex-related HIV risk behavior among substance users is not as readily apparent. Several hypotheses have been proposed to account for the relationship between substance use and sex risk behavior. Some have suggested that the use of alcohol and drugs increases the probability for sex risk behavior through impairment of judgment, disinhibition, and reduced pain sensitivity during intercourse.[21–24] Indeed, findings indicate that use of alcohol prior to and during sexual activity may lead individuals to minimize their sexual risk while unrealistically inflating their perceived ability to detect sexual risk (see Norris et al.[25] for a review of findings). Additional research suggests that drug cravings and associated drug-seeking behavior may supersede women's concerns regarding unsafe sex, resulting in an increased potential for engagement in risky sexual behavior.[26] Nadeau et al.[13] also found that women's use of substances before and during sexual activity prevented them from thinking about the potentially negative consequences associated with unsafe sex. Alarmingly, one recent study found that some female substance users even falsely believed that use of drugs and alcohol protects against pregnancy.[18]

Others have argued that the relationship between substance use and sex risk behavior is complicated by additional social, interpersonal, contextual, and individual risk factors associated with risky sexual behavior.[25,27–31] For instance, research indicates that individuals who use drugs while engaging in unprotected sex also score higher on measures of impulsivity, risk taking, and sensation seeking.[32] In other instances, substance use may exacerbate the influence of other risk factors on sex risk behavior. For example, previous research indicates that alcohol use may intensify the relationship between increased sexual arousal and reduced condom use.[33]

The association between relationship characteristics/dynamics and sex risk behavior has been examined among substance users. Among substance users, condom use has been found to occur less frequently within main, long-term, cohabitating, financially interdependent, and trusted relationships.[13,15,17,34,35] Consistent with findings based on HIV risk among general populations, research on female substance users indicates that women may engage in unprotected sexual activity in order to preserve and enhance intimate relationships.

Women's requests to use condoms may be suppressed to preserve and enhance intimate relationships or because of fear of partner rejection and distrust.[13,17,36,37] Partners' willingness to use condoms, increased communication about condom use, and greater perceived control over condom use have also both been shown to increase condom use among female substance users.[15,18,34] Conversely, female substance users who have problems communicating with their partners about condom use and feel incapable of negotiating condom use are less likely to use condoms.[13,18]

Substance use appears to play a unique role in influencing the association between relationship characteristics/dynamics and sex risk behavior. Although condom use among substance users typically occurs more commonly with casual or new partners, research indicates that unprotected sex with a casual partner is more likely to occur when an individual is high or intoxicated, sexually aroused, and when condoms are unavailable.[15,32] Use of alcohol immediately prior to and during sex events can impair safe sex negotiation and refusal skills, resulting in an increased risk of unsafe sexual practices.[25] In addition, substance use can increase risk for sexual assault, which often involves unprotected sexual contact.[27] Partner's drug use behavior can further affect decisions related to female drug use and condom use,[38–41] and findings suggest that condom use is less likely to occur in relationships characterized as drug interdependent.[35] Despite the fact that increased perceptions of partner risk can increase condom use under certain circumstances,[15,42] additional research conducted by Booth et al.[8] found that drug user with an injection drug user partner were more likely than those without an injection drug user partner to engage in unprotected sexual activity.

PREGNANT SUBSTANCE ABUSERS DESERVE SPECIAL ATTENTION

Among substance abusers, sex-related HIV risk behavior has been found to remain prevalent or even increase during pregnancy. Pregnant injection drug users, relative to non-pregnant injection drug users, have been found to be just as likely to exchange sex for money or drugs but may be less likely to use condoms with regular and casual sexual partners.[43] Pregnant substance abusers may reduce their use of condoms during pregnancy given the temporary elimination of the need for birth control. Alternatively, this finding may merely reflect a pre-existing lower rate of condom use among women who became pregnant. In other words, these women were more likely to become pregnant due to lower rates of condom use. Whether condom use is reduced or merely remains low during pregnancy, low rates of condom use place these women and their unborn children at risk for contracting HIV.

In addition to sex-related risk behavior, pregnant substance abusers often engage in drug-related risk behavior. For example, pregnant injection drug users have been found to be as likely as their non-pregnant peers to engage in the sharing of injection drug use equipment.[43] These risk behaviors have also been found among pregnant women in drug treatment. Baker et al.[44] found that pregnant women in methadone maintenance treatment engaged in as much injection drug-related risk behavior as women not enrolled in treatment and more injection drug-related risk behavior than non-pregnant women in methadone maintenance treatment.

In addition to placing the women at risk for HIV, this sex-related and drug-related risk behavior poses a risk to their unborn children. Perinatal transmission of HIV accounts for nearly all new HIV infections in children.[45] Children born to women infected with HIV face the additional risk of the loss of a primary caregiver.

SCREENING AND TREATMENT OF PREGNANT WOMEN AND THEIR NEWBORNS

To minimize the risk of perinatal transmission of HIV, the Centers for Disease Control and Prevention (CDC) recommends screening for HIV early in all pregnancies.[46] The CDC recommends the inclusion of HIV testing in the panel of routine prenatal tests unless the patient declines testing. Furthermore, the CDC recommends that a second HIV test during pregnancy be considered for all pregnant women[46] as a result of work that demonstrated that, even in populations with low rates of HIV, a second HIV test during pregnancy is cost-effective[47] and work that suggests that an increasing percentage of perinatally infected infants have mothers who acquire the infection during pregnancy.[48] In addition to the consideration of a second HIV test during pregnancy for all pregnant women, the CDC recommends a second HIV test for all women who receive health care in areas with elevated incidence rates of HIV or AIDS, for women who receive health care from facilities with a prenatal screening rate of at least one HIV-infected case per 1,000 screens conducted, for women who engage in behavior that places them at elevated risk of contracting HIV, and for women who have signs or symptoms of an acute HIV infection.[46] Finally, the CDC recommends rapid HIV testing for any woman with undocumented HIV status at the time of labor unless she refuses testing.[46]

For women who are HIV-positive and have been receiving highly active antiretroviral therapy (HAART) and for women who are HIV-positive who have not been receiving antiretroviral therapy but demonstrate clinical indications for antiretroviral therapy, the current recommendation is to continue or begin a HAART regimen, avoiding drugs with teratogenic potential or with a known potential risk to pregnant women.[49] The recommendation is that the HAART regimen be continued during the intrapartum period, with a continuous infusion of zidovudine during labor and during the postpartum period. A 6-week course of zidovudine is recommended for the infant. Cesarean delivery at 38 weeks is recommended in cases in which plasma HIV RNA remains more than 1,000 copies/mL. The recommendations are very similar for pregnant women who are HIV-positive and have not been receiving antiretroviral therapy and do not display clinical indications for antiretroviral therapy.[49] For these individuals, the recommendation is to consider delaying HAART initiation until the first trimester has concluded and to evaluate need for antiretroviral therapy postpartum. All other treatment recommendations are the same as stated above. The recommendations for women who are HIV-positive who have received no antiretroviral therapy prior to labor involve prescribing some combination of zidovudine, nevaripine, and/or lamivudine to the woman during labor and possibly postpartum and administering zidovudine, nevirapine and zidovudine, or zidovudine in combination with additional drugs to the infant; however, appropriate dosing of other drugs has not been well established in neonates.[49] If no antiretroviral therapy is delivered during labor to an infant born to an HIV-infected woman, the recommendation is to administer zidovudine for 6 weeks to the infant or to use zidovudine in combination with additional drugs.[49]

IMPACT OF DRUG ABUSE TREATMENT ON HIV RISK BEHAVIOR

Unfortunately, drug abuse treatment appears to have a circumscribed impact on HIV risk behavior. In a review of 33 studies, totaling more than 17,000 subjects, Sorenson and Copeland[50] found strong support for a reduction of needle use and HIV infection among individuals in methadone maintenance treatment. However, there was less definitive evidence regarding the impact of methadone maintenance treatment on needle sharing and unsafe sexual behavior. In addition, they concluded that there is a paucity of data regarding the impact of treatment modalities other than methadone maintenance on HIV risk behavior and that it is important for future studies to include more women to determine whether gender effects are present. These findings point to the need for interventions that directly target sex-related and drug-related HIV risk behavior.

KNOWLEDGE- AND SKILL-BASED HIV RISK REDUCTION INTERVENTIONS WITH WOMEN

Given that little work has been done examining HIV interventions with female substance users, options for intervening in this population derive from non-substance using populations. Following a comprehensive review of HIV risk reduction intervention studies conducted with women, Exner et al.[51] concluded that interventions that teach self-management and interpersonal skills can be effective in decreasing HIV risk behavior, increasing risk-related knowledge and producing the desired changes in attitudes toward risk behavior. The most efficacious programs were tailored specifically for women, emphasized relationship and negotiation skills, and included multiple and sustained contacts with program participants. Although these interventions have demonstrated some efficacy, the magnitude of the effects achieved with these interventions suggests that improvements are possible.

MOTIVATIONALLY-ENHANCED HIV RISK REDUCTION INTERVENTIONS WITH WOMEN

A key way in which traditional knowledge-based and skill-based HIV risk reduction interventions have been enhanced is through the incorporation of motivational interviewing components.[52] Motivational interviewing[53,54] is an intervention approach with wide dissemination and demonstrated efficacy (see Burke et al.[55] and Dunn et al.[56]). Motivational interviewing[53,54] is a collaborative and non-confrontational approach used to discuss and facilitate behavior change. In motivational interviewing, a key tenet is that motivation is the product of the interaction between the client and the therapist rather than some personal state or trait that resides within the client. Therefore, the therapist's task is to create an environment that promotes behavior change. Ambivalence about change is considered normative within the motivational interviewing framework. The client's readiness to make changes is not assumed. Instead, an important exercise in motivational interviewing is the exploration of level of readiness to change. Therefore, the intervention is appropriate for varying levels of readiness to change.

To facilitate behavior change, motivational interviewing employs four general principles. The first is expressing empathy, which creates a therapeutic environment of acceptance, which is seen as facilitating change. The second is developing discrepancy. To achieve this, the therapist attempts to explore any discrepancies between the client's current life situation and his or her goals. The belief is that greater discrepancy will lead to more ambivalence about his or her current behavior, moving the client toward adaptive behavior change in an effort to relieve the ambivalence. The assumption is that it is most effective if the client presents the arguments for change. The third principle of motivational interviewing is rolling with resistance, in which therapists are discouraged from opposing or arguing against resistance. Client resistance is interpreted as an interpersonal phenomenon and as a signal that the therapist should change his or her behavior. Furthermore, the client is seen as a valuable source of ideas and solutions. In motivational interviewing, the therapist may invite the client to consider new perspectives; however, there is no attempt to impose alternative perspectives on the client. The fourth principle is supporting the client's self-efficacy to make changes. Self-efficacy is viewed as an important determinant of readiness to change. To increase self-efficacy, the therapist is encouraged to discuss the client's personal responsibility for making a change, to convey his or her own belief in the client's ability to change, and to highlight the client's previous adaptive changes.

The incorporation of intervention components that directly target motivation to change HIV risk behavior is consistent with leading theoretical models of HIV risk behavior change, such as the Information-Motivation-Behavior model of HIV risk behavior.[57,58] The Information-Motivation-Behavior model posits that HIV risk behavior is determined by an individual's *information* about HIV transmission and prevention, *motivation* to reduce risk for HIV infection, and mastery of *behavioral* skills necessary to reduce risk. In the area of HIV risk reduction, the Information-Motivation-Behavior model is a well-established model, and interventions based on this model have garnered strong empirical support.[58–61]

Carey et al.[59] examined the efficacy of a motivationally enhanced, 4-session HIV risk behavior intervention, relative to a waitlist control condition, among low-income urban women. They found that the women who received the intervention had greater knowledge and risk awareness, stronger intentions to employ safer sexual practices, greater communication of their intentions to their partners, less substance use that was temporally associated with sexual activity, and fewer incidents of unprotected vaginal intercourse relative to the women assigned to the control condition. These effects were found at 3-week follow-up, and most of the effects were still present at a 3-month follow-up. Furthermore, as noted by Carey et al.,[52] the motivationally enhanced intervention yielded larger effect sizes (d = 0.56) than traditional skills-based interventions (ds = 0.32 to 0.43).[62–64]

In a second study employing the same intervention, Carey et al.[60] tested the intervention against a health promotion group that equated for contact time in another sample of economically disadvantaged urban women. The women who received the HIV risk behavior intervention had greater HIV-related knowledge and reduced intentions to engage in risky behavior relative to the women in the control group. Furthermore, among the HIV risk behavior intervention women, those who reported imperfect intentions regarding risk behavior had a fourfold increase in condom use and reported more discussion about condom use and HIV testing with their partners. In addition, they were more likely to have refused to participate in unprotected sex. Carey et al.[60] interpreted these later findings as reflecting a more realistic assessment of the potential barriers to safer sex.

Belcher et al.[65] examined the efficacy of a similar intervention with low-income urban women. However, this intervention was conducted in a single 2-hour session. The control condition was an AIDS education intervention that equated for contact time. At 3-month follow-up, the women who received the HIV risk behavior intervention reported significantly higher rates of condom use during vaginal intercourse relative to women in the control condition. However, they found no treatment effects for AIDS-related knowledge and self-efficacy.

O'Neill et al.[66] conducted a randomized trial of a six-session HIV risk behavior intervention among pregnant women enrolled in methadone maintenance treatment. Their intervention consisted of motivational interviewing, psychoeducation about HIV risk, coping-skills training, and relapse prevention. The intervention in this study did not include exercises to build skills (e.g., proper condom use and cleaning of needles) to reduce sex-related and drug-related HIV risk behavior, which are typical components of HIV risk reduction interventions. At the 9-month follow-up, the intervention group displayed significantly less drug-related risk behavior compared to the standard care comparison group. The intervention did not appear to reduce sex-related risk behavior.

CONCLUSIONS

Taken together, the work in this area suggests that HIV risk reduction interventions that effectively address both sex-related and drug-related HIV risk behavior among female substance abusers are sorely needed. Interventions that incorporate motivational interviewing components may improve on the efficacy of previous interventions, at least among economically disadvantaged women.[52,60,65] Furthermore, the limited work that has been directed specifically toward female substance users highlights that motivational interviewing may not be sufficient as a stand-alone intervention to reduce HIV risk in this population and may hold more promise when coupled with the types of skill-building exercises traditionally included in HIV risk reduction interventions.[66]

REFERENCES

1. Hader SL, Smith DK, Moore JS, Holmberg SD. HIV infection in women in the United States: status at the millennium. JAMA 2001; 285:1186–93.

2. Centers for Disease Control and Prevention. HIV/AIDS surveillance report. Atlanta: US: Department of Health and Human Services, Centers for Disease Control and Prevention, 2005. Report No.: Vol 17.

3. Centers for Disease Control and Prevention. HIV/AIDS among women. Atlanta: US: Department of Health and Human Services, Centers for Disease Control and Prevention, 2007.

4. National Center for Health Statistics. Bridged-race vintage 2005 postcensal population estimates for July 1 2000-July 2005, by year, county, single-year age, bridged-race, Hispanic origin, and sex. Available at: http://www.cdc.gov/nchs/about/major/dvs/popbridge/datadochtm#vintage 2005.

5. Centers for Disease Control. HIV/AIDS surveillance in women. Available at: http://www.cdc.gov/hiv/graphics/women htm.

6. Edlin BR, Irwin KL, Faruque S, McCoy CB, Word C, Serrano Y, Inciardi JA, Bowser BP, Schilling RF, Holmberg SD for The Multicenter Crack Cocaine and HIV Infection Study Team. Intersecting epidemics-crack cocaine use and HIV infection among inner-city young adults. N Engl J Med 1994; 331:1422–7.

7. Leigh BC, Stall R. Substance use and risky sexual behavior for exposure to HIV: issues in methodology, interpretation, and prevention. Am J Psych 1993; 48:1035–45.

8. Booth RE, Kwiatkkowski CF, Chitwood DD. Sex related HIV risk behaviors: differential risks among injection drug users, crack smokers, and injection drug users who smoke crack. Drug Alc Depend 2000; 58:219–26.

9. Graves K. Risky sexual behavior and alcohol use among young adults: results from a national survey. Am J Health Promot 1995; 10:27–36.

10. Khalsa ME, Kowalewski MR, Lunn R, Anglin MD, Miller KA. AIDS-related knowledge, beliefs and risk behaviors in a sample of crack addicts. J Drug Issues 1994; 24:537–53.

11. Logan TK, Leukefeld C. Sexual and drug use behaviors among female crack users: a multi-site sample. Drug Alc Depend 2000; 58:237–45.

12. McKirnan DJ, Ostrow DG, Hope B. Sex, drugs and escape: a psychological model of HIV-risk sexual behaviors. AIDS Care 1996; 8:655–69.

13. Nadeau L, Truchon M, Biron C. High-risk sexual behaviors in a context of substance abuse: A focus group approach. J Sub Abuse Treat 2000; 19:319–28.

14. Sly D, Quadagno D, Harrison D, Eberstein I, Riehman K. The association between substance use, condom use, and sexual risk among low income women. Fam Plann Perspect 1997; 29:132–137.

15. Tortu S, McMahon J, Hamid R, Neaigus A. Drug-using women's sexual risk: an event analysis. AIDS Behav 2000; 4:329–40.

16. Wingood G, DiClemente R. The influence of psychosocial factors, alcohol, and drug use on African-American Women's high–risk sexual behavior. Am J Prev Med 1998; 15:54–9.

17. Armstrong KA, Kenen R, Samost L. Barriers to family planning services among patients in drug treatment programs. Fam Plann Perspect 1991; 23:264–71.

18. Jessup MA, Brindis CD. Issues in reproductive health and empowerment in perinatal women with substance use disorders. J Addict Nurs 2005; 16:97–105.

19. MacDonald TK, Zanna MP, Fong GT. Why common sense goes out the window: Effects of alcohol on intentions to use condoms. Pers Soc Psychol Bull 1996; 22: 763–75.

20. 20. Maisto SA, Carey MP, Carey KB, Gordon CM, Schum JL. Effects of alcohol and expectancy on HIV-related risk perception and behavioral skills in heterosexual women. Exp Clin Psychopharmacol 2004; 12:288–97.

21. Choi K, Wermuth LA. Unsafe sex and behavior change. In: Sorensen JL, Wermuth LA, Gibson DR, Choi K, Guydish JR, Batki SL, ed. Preventing AIDS in drug users and their sexual partners. New York: Guilford Press, 1991:43–74.

22. Fillmore M, Vogel-Sprott M. An alcohol model of impaired inhibitory control and its treatment in humans. Exp Clin Psychopharmacol 1999; 7:49–55.

23. Stall R, McKusick L, Wiley J, Coates T, Ostrow D. Alcohol and drug use during sexual activity and compliance with safe sex guidelines for AIDS: the AIDS Behavioral Research Project. Health Educ Q 1986; 13:359–371.

24. Stall R. The prevention of HIV infection associated with drug and alcohol use during sexual activity. Adv Alcohol Subst Abuse 1988; 7:73–88.

25. Norris J, Masters NT, Zawacki T. Cognitive mediation of women's sexual decision making: the influence of alcohol, contextual factors, and background variables. Ann Rev Sex Res 2004; 15:258–296.

26. Kearny MH, Murphy S, Rosenbaum M. Learning by losing: sex and fertility on crack cocaine. Qual Health Res 1994; 4:142–162.

27. Brown SS, Eisenberg L. The best intentions: Unintended pregnancy and the well-being of children and families. Washington, DC: National Academy Press, 1995.

28. Cooper ML. Alcohol use and risky sexual behavior among college students and youth: Evaluating the evidence. J Stud Alcohol 2002; 14:101–17.

29. Gil-Rivas V, Kooyman L. Sexual risk-taking: correlates and prevention. In: McAnulty RD, Burnette MM, eds. Sex and sexuality, Vol 1: Sexuality today: Trends and controversies. Westport, CT: Praeger Publishers/Greenwood Publishing Group, 2006:321–42.

30. Halpern Felsher BL, Millstein SG, Ellen JM. Relationship of alcohol use and risky sexual behavior: a review and analysis of findings. J Adolesc Health 1996; 19:331–336.

31. Leigh BC. Alcohol and condom use: a meta-analysis of event–level studies. Sex Transm Dis 2002; 29:476–482.

32. Schafer J, Blanchard L, Fals–Stewart W. Drug use and risky sexual behavior. Psychol Addict Behav 1994; 8(3):3–7.

33. MacDonald TK, MacDonald G, Zanna MP, Fong G. Alcohol, sexual arousal, and intentions to use condoms in young men: applying alcohol myopia theory to risky sexual behavior. Health Psychol 2000; 19:290-8.

34. Harvey SM, Bird ST, De Rosa CJ, Montgomery SB, Rohrbach LA. Sexual decision making and safer sex behavior among young female injection drug users and female partners of IDUs. J Sex Res 2003; 40:50–60.

35. Sherman SG, Latkin CA. Intimate relationship characteristics associated with condom use among drug users and their sex partners: a multilevel analysis. Drug Alcohol Depend 2001; 64:97–104.

36. Logan TK, Cole J, Leukefeld C. Women, sex, and HIV: social and contextual factors, meta-analysis of

published interventions, and implications for practice and research. Psychol Bull 2002; 128:851–85.

37. Muller R, Boyle JS. "You don't ask for trouble": women who do sex and drugs. Fam Community Health 1996; 19:35–48.

38. Amaro H. Love, sex, and power: considering women's realities in HIV prevention. Am Psychol 1995; 50:437–47.

39. Demers A, Bisson J, Palluy J. Wives' convergence with their husbands' alcohol use: Social conditions as mediators. J Stud Alcohol 1999; 60:368–377.

40. Leonard K, Das Eiden R. Husband's and wife's drinking: Unilateral or bilateral influences among newlyweds in a general population sample. J Stud Alcohol 1999; 13:130–8.

41. Roberts L, Leonard K. An empirical typology of drinking partnerships and their relationship to marital functioning and drinking consequences. J Marriage Fam 1998; 60:515–26.

42. Sheeran P, Abraham C, Orbell S. Psychosocial correlates of heterosexual condom use: a meta-analysis. Psychol Bull 1999; 125:90–132.

43. Deren S, Beardsley M, Davis R, Tortu S. HIV risk factors among pregnant and non-pregnant high-risk women in New York City. J Drug Ed 1993; 23:57–66.

44. Baker A, Heather N, Wodak A, Lewin T. Heroin use and HIV risk-taking behaviour among women injecting drug users. Drug Alcohol Rev 2001; 20:205–11.

45. Centers for Disease Control and Prevention. HIV/AIDS surveillance report. Atlanta: U.S. Department of Health and Human Services, Centers for Disease Control and Prevention, 1996, Vol 8, No 2.

46. Branson BM, Handsfield, HH, Lampe MA, Janssen RS, Taylor AW, Lyss SB, Clark JE. Revised recommendations for HIV testing of adults, adolescents, and pregnant women in health-care settings. MMWR 2006; 55(RR14):1–17.

47. Sansom SL, Jamieson DJ, Farnham PG, Bulterys M, Fowler MG. Human immunodeficiency virus testing during pregnancy: costs and effectiveness in preventing perinatal transmission. Obstet Gynecol 2003; 102:782–90.

48. Warren B, Glaros RHS. Residual perinatal HIV transmissions in 25 births occurring in New York state. Presented at the 2005 National HIV Prevention Conference, Atlanta, GA; 2005.

49. Public Health Service Task Force. Recommendations for use of antiretroviral drugs in pregnant HIV-infected women for maternal health and interventions to reduce perinatal HIV transmission in the United States. Available at: http://AIDSinfo.nih.gov.

50. Sorenson JL, Copeland AL. Drug abuse treatment as an HIV prevention strategy: a review. Drug Alcohol Deped 2000; 59:17–31.

51. Exner TM, Seal DW, Ehrhardt AA. A review of HIV interventions for at-risk women. AIDS Behav 1997; 1:93–124.

52. Carey MP, Lewis BP. Motivational strategies can enhance HIV risk reduction programs. AIDS Behav 1999; 3:269–76.

53. Miller WR, Rollnick S. Motivational interviewing: preparing people to change addictive behaviors. New York: Guilford Press, 1991.

54. Miller WR, Rollnick S. Motivational interviewing: preparing people for change, 2nd edition ed. New York: Guilford Press, 2002.

55. Burke BL, Arkowitz H, Menchola M. The efficacy of motivational interviewing: a meta-analysis of controlled clinical trials. J Consult Clin Psychol 2003; 71:843–61.

56. Dunn C, Deroo L, Rivara FP. The use of brief interventions adapted from motivational interviewing across behavioral domains: a systematic review. Addiction 2001; 96:1725–42.

57. Fisher JD, Fisher WA. Changing AIDS-risk behavior. Psychological Bulletin 1992; 111:455–74.

58. Fisher JD, Fisher WA. Theoretical approaches to individual-level change in HIV-risk behavior. In: Peterson J, DiClemente RJ, eds. HIV prevention handbook. New York: Kluwer Academic/Plenum Press, 2000:3–55.

59. Carey MP, Maisto SA, Kalichman SC, Forsyth AD, Wright EM, Johnson BT. Enhancing motivation to reduce the risk of HIV infection for economically disadvantaged urban women. J Consult Clin Psychol 1997; 65:531–41.

60. Carey MP, Braaten LS, Maisto SA, Gleason JR, Forsyth AD, Durant LE, Jaworski BC. Using information, motivational enhancement, and skills training to reduce the risk of HIV infection for low-income urban women: a second randomized clinical trial. Health Psychol 2000; 19:3–11.

61. Fisher JD, Fisher WA, Misovich SJ, Kimble DL, Malloy TE. Changing AIDS risk behavior: effects of an intervention emphasizing AIDS risk reduction information, motivation, and behavioral skills in a college student population. Health Psychol 1996; 15:114–23.

62. 62. DiClemente RJ, Wingood GM. A randomized controlled trial of an HIV sexual risk-reduction intervention for young African-American women. JAMA 1995; 274:1271–6.

63. Hobfoll SE, Jackson AP, Lavin J, Britton PJ, Shepherd JB. Reducing inner-city women's AIDS risk activities: A study of single, pregnant women. Health Psychol 1994; 13:397–403.

64. Kelly JA, Murphy DA, Washington CD, Wilson TS, Koob JJ, Davis DR, Ledezma G, Davantes B. The effects of HIV/AIDS intervention groups for high-risk women in urban clinics. Amer J Public Health 1994; 84:1918–22.

65. Belcher L, Kalichman S, Topping M et al. A randomized trial of a brief HIV risk reduction counseling intervention for women. J Consul Clin Psychol 1998; 65:531–41.

66. O'Neill K, Baker A, Cooke M, Collins E, Heather N, Wodak A. Evaluation of a cognitive-behavioural intervention for pregnant injecting drug users at risk of HIV infection. Addiction 1996; 91:1115–25.

Pharmacotherapy in the Treatment of Addiction: Methadone

Mary Jeanne Kreek, MD
Lisa Borg, MD
Elizabeth Ducat, NP
Brenda Ray, NP

ABSTRACT. Methadone maintenance treatment (MMT) is the most widely available pharmacotherapy for opioid addiction and has been shown to be an effective and safe treatment over a period of 40 years. Although women comprise approximately 40% of clients currently being treated in MMT programs, comparatively little research geared specifically toward this group has been published. This article begins with an overview of neurobiological studies on opioid addiction, including a discussion of gender differences, followed by a review of the pharmacology of methadone. The authors then examine the particular needs and differences of women being treated in MMTs, including co-dependence with other substances, women's health issues, and psychosocial needs unique to this population. Research shows that women have different substance abuse treatment needs in comparison to their male counterparts. One New York City MMT program that has attempted to address these differences is highlighted.

INTRODUCTION

During the initial development of the first effective pharmacotherapy for an addictive disease, methadone maintenance treatment (MMT) for heroin addiction, a treatment that remains the most effective and most widely used in the United States and worldwide, the initial decision was to study only very severely impaired persons and only male opiate addicts because of the potential complexities of women in their reproductive years. Therefore, in the first research completed at the Rockefeller Hospital in the then Rockefeller Institute for Medical Research in 1964 (the original work published with the transcription of the discussion at the Association of American Physicians meeting,[1] and also in the Archives of Internal Medicine[2]), no women were studied. Similarly in the 1-year follow-up of our patients admitted to the Rockefeller Hospital in 1964, along with several new patients admitted and followed for two weeks to three months at Manhattan General Hospital, no women were included.[3] We set the criteria for the admission

Supported by the National Institutes of Health (NIH)-National Institute on Drug Abuse Research Center grant P60-DA05130, the NIH- National Institute of Mental Health grant MH79880, and the New York State Office of Alcoholism and Substance Abuse Services (OASAS) grant, C003189 (Kreek).

of subjects for study, which were reviewed by the hospital ethics board at that time: all male subjects; all with a history of short-acting opiate abuse with multiple daily self-administrations for 4 years or longer; and all with failures at least three times in abstinence-based treatment or in prison with prompt relapse. It was not until 1967, after 3 years of research had taught us the effectiveness and safety of MMT, that the first women were admitted into treatment research.

Over subsequent years, the numbers of women in MMT sharply rose to the current levels of about 40% women and 60% men in most clinics, reflecting the percentages of opiate addicts in the general population and in all ethnic and cultural groups. Overall, neither we nor other groups have found important biological, pharmacokinetic, or pharmacodynamic differences between women and men in MMT studies. Furthermore, in carefully conducted basic clinical research or applied clinical research studies, few differences have been reported in terms of the clinical outcome, physiological effects, or pharmacological effects between women versus men in either MMT or in buprenorphine-naloxone treatment.

However, women have special needs, most of which are due to very discrete issues that make women different from men. The most obvious and important, and which we began to address in the early 1970s, was the fact that early on we documented that pulsatile luteinizing hormone is profoundly blunted by cycles of heroin and other short-acting opiate abuse, and that normalization of this neuroendocrine function occurs within 1 year of steady-dose MMT.[4] Also, it was quickly ascertained that women who had had hypomenorrhea or secondary amenorrhea during cycles of heroin and other short-acting opiate addiction had a low fecundity rate at that time, despite the fact that many had derived their income primarily from prostitution, and had frequent sexual exposures without protection. However, with stabilization in MMT, normal menstrual cycles returned and, with the increasing normalization of their lifestyles and social status, many women wished to become pregnant. Therefore, extensive studies were conducted to determine both the impact of MMT on women during pregnancy and on neonates, with minimal neonatal abstinence found in some, but far from all, babies born to mothers maintained on even very high doses of methadone in treatment.[5–10] The later outcome of the children appears to be normal, but these studies are complex because of the various social and environmental factors involved.

In our laboratory, we conducted several sets of studies on the metabolism of methadone during pregnancy, in which we showed an acceleration of biotransformation of methadone during the third trimester due to progesterone effects with prompt restoration to normal metabolism of methadone in the postpartum period.[6] Furthermore, we conducted two studies of the appearance of methadone in breast milk and found, as predicted, due to the very tight plasma protein binding of methadone, that very small amounts of methadone appear in breast milk, too small to have any negative impact and too small to treat any signs and symptoms of opiate withdrawal in this population. These studies are briefly reviewed in this article (and also reviewed in the article on pregnancy and methadone maintenance treatment) .[5–10]

In all of our extensive basic clinical research addressing the molecular neurobiological aspects of opiate addiction, and further in our human molecular genetic studies of opiate addiction, we have found few differences between men and women, which will be briefly outlined below. However, the additional obvious needs of women are related to their roles in society, including child bearing, child rearing, and home maintenance, along with the special needs of women brought about by the different views of the roles and value of women in different theaters of our Western society. Several of these special issues will be discussed below, along with brief presentations of the relative proportion of men and women experiencing the various special concerns commonly encountered during MMT.

MOLECULAR NEUROBIOLOGICAL STUDIES: GENDER DIFFERENCES

Over the years, our laboratory has conducted several basic clinical research studies in the context of opiate use in which we have probed the function of the brain, as well as integrated neuroendocrine physiology, by conducting a variety of rigorous tests, some of which are standard tests and others of which are provocative tests of various types that we have developed. Many of these tests have been designed to study the stress-responsive hypothalamic-pituitary-adrenal axis (reviewed in Kreek et al.[11–13]).

However, we found an interesting difference between men and women in only one of these studies. This difference occurred in a series of studies in which we used the shortened form of the dynorphin A(1-13) of the natural kappa opioid ligand dynorphin A(1-17), approved for use under an FDA investigator-initiated IND, to probe the tuberoinfundibular dopaminergic system.[14,15] In these studies, two doses of dynorphin A(1-13) were administered to healthy volunteers and, on a third day, a placebo was administered. In these studies, we used serum prolactin levels as a biological marker for dopaminergic tone in the tuberoinfundibular dopaminergic system because prolactin release is almost exclusively under tonic inhibition by dopamine in humans and non-human primates. Therefore, when dopaminergic tone is reduced, serum prolactin levels promptly increase. It has been shown that this effect is mediated primarily through the dopamine D2 receptors in the hypothalamus.

We found a dose-dependent response to the two doses of dynorphin in healthy human volunteers. However, when we looked at the results in healthy women as opposed to healthy men, even though we had a relatively small number of healthy women, we found significant differences. The women had a greater response to dynorphin administration, as shown through a greater rise, and thus a greater peak, of prolactin levels and area under the plasma concentration time curve. We therefore analyzed those studies in female subjects separately.[14] In our next set of studies, we looked at dopaminergic tone in long-term successfully maintained MMT subjects, all of whom had a history of short-acting opiate, primarily heroin, dependency.[15] Again, in these studies, because we had found a significant difference in the two genders in healthy subjects, we began our studies with men in MMT and then added another group of healthy control volunteer men. Again, we found a dose-dependent rise in serum prolactin levels, reflecting a dose-dependent lowering in dopaminergic tone. However, the peak levels in the area under the plasma concentration curve of prolactin were significantly lowered in methadone-maintained former heroin-addicted men than in normal volunteer men.[15] Currently, we are conducting gender-specific studies in methadone-maintained women as well as cocaine-dependent women. In each case, studies in each gender will be conducted.

HUMAN MOLECULAR GENETICS

Since 1994, our laboratory has been studying the human molecular genetics related to each of three different addictive diseases, opiate addiction, and cocaine addiction, without and with codependence with alcohol. To date, we have found association of many specific gene variants with a history of severe heroin dependence, with most studies conducted with long-term methadone-maintained former heroin addicts. In each of these studies, we have analyzed potential differences between men and women and have found none.[16] One of our major focuses has been genetics related to both heroin addiction and alcoholism, considering stress responsivity as a covariable. This work has been extensively reviewed recently.[17,18] We discovered, in collaboration with Lei Yu, a relatively common variant to the human mu opioid receptor in the coding region, specifically in the N-terminus where opioids and opiates bind.[19] This variant is functionally different from the prototype in molecular and cell biological studies. Later, our group and many others have shown that presence of this variant alters stress responsivity in healthy humans.[17–19] Further, we have shown that this variant is associated with heroin addiction and also alcoholism in two separate studies conducted in a relatively non-admixed population.[20,21]

In one study, we addressed a question of whether baseline levels of the stress-responsive hormones were different in healthy subjects with this variant. We found that male and female healthy control subjects with one or two copies of this A118G variant, which alters mu opioid receptor protein, had higher basal levels of cortisol when studied in a stress-minimized environment, although these levels did not exceed the upper limits of normal.[22] In these studies, we found a small but non-significant difference in women's cortisol levels compared to healthy men.[22] Specifically, there was a trend, but not a significantly higher level, of basal cortisol in women with one or two copies of this A118G variant producing a functionally different mu opioid receptor.

The only one of our specific hypothesis-driven studies of the human molecular genetics that has yielded gender differences is in the catechol-O-methyl transferase gene (*COMT*).[23] In this study, we found that a common and functional variant of the *COMT* gene is significantly associated with heroin addiction, but only in Hispanic subjects.[23] Further, this association was also found in female subjects of Hispanic origin when analyzed separately. Because this is an admixed population, further studies are essential to determine whether this finding can be replicated.

Thus, most of the differences in women discussed below are related to their basic reproductive biological differences, as well as differences in their roles in culture and society. However, it is important to continue to address this question, especially related to special needs that might be encountered by women as they enter methadone maintenance or buprenorphine maintenance treatment for short-acting opiate addiction, whether it be heroin addiction or prescription opiate addiction.

PHARMACOLOGY OF METHADONE

Methadone was approved by the U.S. Food and Drug Administration (FDA) in 1972 as a treatment for opioid addiction. Opioids are all compounds which are related in function to opium, which is derived from poppies (as reviewed in Borg et al.[24]). Opiates are those compounds with opioid-like activity and which are directly derived from natural poppy plant thebaine structure compounds, such as morphine and codeine. Methadone is a structurally dissimilar or synthetic opioid, which has two enantiomers found in equal amounts in a racemic mixture; the active *l*(R) enantiomer has a half-life of 36-48 hours and the inactive *d*(S) enantiomer has a half-life of approximately 16 hours.[25–27] Methadone is also used effectively in the treatment of chronic pain. Methadone meets the two important criteria for a maintenance treatment: high systemic bioavailability (>90%)[28] when given orally and long half-life with long-term treatment.[29] Methadone is rapidly absorbed by the oral route with a delayed onset of action, detectable in plasma at 30 minutes with peak levels at 2 to 4 hours with sustained levels maintained over 24 hours.[25,30–33] Methadone also has N-methyl-D-aspartate (NMDA) receptor antagonist properties, which affect the development of tolerance.[34]

During MMT, methadone levels are relatively constant due to slow release of methadone into the blood from hepatic stores.[35,36] Methadone is greater than 90% plasma protein bound in the bloodstream and is also redistributed into lipid stores, which are among the reasons that MMT is effective as a once per day, oral treatment for heroin addiction.[30] This is in contrast to heroin and morphine, which have a rapid onset of action and are short-acting.[37] Methadone has both low abuse liability and reward effect due to its slow onset and offset.

Due to the long half-life of methadone, an initial maintenance dose should usually start with 20 to 40 mg/daily; then the dose is gradually increased, since a dose increase greater than the rate of development of tolerance can result in accumulation which can lead to sedation and respiratory depression. Doses must be raised slowly, usually by 10 mg every 4 to 7 days. Patients in effective MMT receiving appropriate doses (80 to 150 mg per day) and adequate blood levels (250 to 400 ng/mL) still may have symptoms of withdrawal toward the end of the dosing interval.[38] These symptoms may be due to drug interactions (e.g., phenytoin, rifampin, or alcohol consumption of more than 4 drinks/day), but in this case lower plasma levels are found at the end of a 24h dosing interval.[39–42] Alternatively, early abstinence symptoms may be due to undefined pharmacodynamic factors (those determining response to the drug) or other factors such as medical or psychological comorbidity,[38] such as depression, which has been found to be more prevalent in women in MMT.[43] When relatively high doses of methadone do not result in apparent therapeutic levels, it may be due to individual genetic factors, although these have not been well elucidated, or undefined drug interactions usually due to clandestine use of alcohol.[32,44,45]

Methadone is metabolized in the liver by the cytochrome P450-related enzyme systems (mostly the CYP3A4 and, to a lesser degree, the CYP2D6, CYP2B6, and CYP1A2 systems) to two biologically inactive metabolites, a pyrroline and a pyrrolidine, which are then further metabolized.[27,46] Methadone and its metabolites are excreted nearly equally in urine and in feces.[47–51] The amount of methadone excreted in the urine is modestly affected by urine acidity. In patients with renal impairment, methadone can be metabolized almost completely by the gastrointestinal system.[47–50] This reduces potential toxicity by avoiding accumulation. In peritoneal dialysis, less than 1% of methadone is cleared, probably because it is extensively protein bound, and due to the small degree that methadone is actually found in the blood at any given time.[49] Patients with severe chronic liver disease have decreased methadone metabolism, thus slower metabolic clearance of methadone, yet lower than expected plasma methadone levels for a given dose due to lower hepatic reservoirs of methadone because of reduced liver size.[52] Methadone metabolism is relatively normal in the presence of mild to moderate liver dysfunction.[36,50]

Drug-drug interactions with methadone have been well-documented.[41] The major categories of drugs that may interact with methadone include both inducers and inhibitors of the hepatic cytochrome p450-related enzyme system, mostly CYP3A4, as well as inhibitors of CYP2D6 (reviewed in Ferrari et al.[27]). However, few of these medications (e.g., rifampin or phenytoin)[39–40] have been shown to have an actual significant drug interaction effect at the therapeutic dose of each second medication, and most medications which have been hypothesized to have an interaction, when studied, have no interaction effect (e.g., disulfiram).[53]

Pharmacokinetic interactions occur with methadone and specific antiretroviral medications prescribed in the treatment of human immunodeficiency virus (HIV-1). These interactions are usually via the CYP3A4 system and can have effects on the level of either methadone or the antiretroviral medication, which can then have actual clinical effects (reviewed in Bruce et al.[54]). Alfa-2b interferon given as treatment for hepatitis C, which is common in intravenous drug users (IVDUs), does not appear to have any clinically significant interaction in terms of subjective or objective effects, as noted in three studies;[55–57] however, interferon produces flu-like symptoms in all patients, which may mimic opioid withdrawal.

Methadone levels are affected by the regular high intake of more than 4 alcoholic drinks/day. When blood measures of ethanol are acutely elevated (more than 150 mg/dL) increased levels of methadone can be anticipated. However, whenever alcohol is no longer present in the body at these high levels and there are no longer high doses of alcohol, methadone levels may be lower due to induction of the P450 enzymes (reviewed in McHugh and Kreek[58] and Cushman and Kreek[59]).

Methadone metabolism is significantly accelerated in the third trimester of pregnancy, and methadone doses often need to be increased at that time to prevent withdrawal symptoms and drug-seeking behavior.[60] During pregnancy, methadone may need to be given twice daily (in divided doses) due to differences in elimination, absorption, and clearance.[61] Methadone crosses the placenta and is metabolized mainly by the placental enzyme aromatase/CYP19, which has large inter-individual variability in its activity. Nanovskaya[62] and Hieronymous et al.[63] suggest that this variability may be a factor related to both the presence and severity of neonatal abstinence syndrome. Studies have shown a clear relationship to time of dosing of methadone and breast milk levels of methadone, although the levels in breast milk are very low at all times because of the extensive plasma protein binding of methadone.[4–10] Breast feeding is safe for women in MMT and their babies and is supported by the American Academy of Pediatrics.[64] It is recommended that women who are HIV-1 positive should not breastfeed due to concerns about mother-to-child transmission.[65]

No cardiac or significant electrocardiographic abnormalities related to methadone treatments were noted in the early or more recent prospective or cross-sectional studies of medical safety for almost 40 years. In the past 6 to 8 years, and predicted from in vitro calcium channel focused studies of opiate effects, issues have been raised regarding possible cardiac effects of methadone. Higher doses of methadone (more than 200 to approximately 400 mg/day) in MMT and chronic pain patients have been reported to be potentially associated with prolongation (more than 500 msec) of the QTc interval on electrocardiogram and possibly with Torsades de pointes, a potentially life-threatening arrhythmia.[66] Many of these patients had other risk factors[67] including taking other medications such as antiretrovirals[68] or antidepressants,[69,70] which are known to prolong QTc, or abusing other drugs. The effect may or may not be related to dose or methadone serum concentration,[69] and may become clinically significant (generally if more than 500 ms).[70] It may be prudent for all patients requiring a chronic methadone dose of more than 150 mg to have a baseline electrocardiogram and then to be monitored periodically afterward; also high risk patients with prior QTc prolongation should be monitored.[71]

Before initiating methadone treatment, it is important to make sure that the patient is in fact opioid dependent, which can be established by history, clinical examination, and urine toxicology. Opioids have several potential side effects; however, when appropriate doses of methadone are used below the level of tolerance developed to each effect, the effects are minimal. If the dose is increased too rapidly, sedation (the major side effect observed in an opioid-tolerant patient) may occur. In an opiate-naïve patient, the initial side effects of methadone may include drowsiness, nausea, and constipation, while emesis, itching, and dizziness are less common.[72] However, in a properly managed long-term MMT patient, the two most significant side effects are constipation, to which tolerance usually occurs over the course of 3 years, and sweating, which persists in about 50% of patients.[73] Constipation and the other side effects tend to lessen due to the development of tolerance, defined as a loss of an effect over time after repeated use. Tolerance develops at different rates for the side effects of methadone, occurring over days, weeks, or years.[73] Dosing must be titrated to the tolerance of the individual patient to avoid somnolence, an early sign of central nervous system (CNS) depression. As with all opioids, methadone must be used prudently in patients with compromised respiratory function.

ACCIDENTAL METHADONE OVERDOSE AND ITS MEDICAL MANAGEMENT

Methadone should always be provided in childproof containers. However, in an opioid-naïve child or when methadone is taken illicitly by an adult who is opioid-naïve or with low tolerance, methadone overdose may occur, characterized by stupor or coma or respiratory depression, which can lead to death. Decreased response to carbon dioxide in centers of specific areas of the pons and medulla of the brain may lead to carbon dioxide retention.[74] Depression of the mental status is accompanied by suppressed gag reflex, predisposing the patient to aspiration of gastric contents into the lungs. Constriction of the pupil occurs, which is the result of parasympathetic nerve excitation.[75]

A methadone overdose can be effectively treated with an opioid antagonist; however, the pharmacokinetic profile of each drug is critical. Naloxone has a half-life of 30 minutes; thus more than one dose will be needed. When overdose occurs due to use of methadone in an opioid-naïve or mildly tolerant person, repeated intravenous doses or a constant infusion of naloxone may be needed for more than 24 hours[75] to prevent relapse into coma.[58]

RETENTION IN METHADONE TREATMENT: WOMEN'S ISSUES

A substantial body of research exists, documenting that methadone, when given as maintenance, is the most effective treatment for heroin/opiate addiction. When given in adequate daily doses, methadone will: decrease heroin use;[76–79] decrease criminal behavior;[80–82] decrease spread of HIV/sexually transmitted diseases (STDs) and other blood-borne diseases, such as hepatitis C;[83–86] decrease mortality;[82,87,88] possibly decrease secondary drug use;[89–91] increase retention in treatment;[92,93] increase stable family relationships; and increase employment and participation in job training.[94]

These benefits can only occur if patients are retained in treatment. Dr. Vincent Dole of The Rockefeller Institute reported that 80% to 90% of patients discharged or lost to treatment returned to illicit substance abuse and all its inherent risks. The early literature demonstrated that when patients are given adequate doses of methadone, then between 80 to 120 mg, they are more likely to be retained in treatment and to reduce their illicit opiate use, particularly in the first 6 months of treatment.[92,95–98] Adequate dosing, tailored to the patient's individual need, is the dose that when administered will block superimposed short-acting narcotic euphoria, prevent withdrawal symptoms, and reduce or eliminate drug craving for 24 hours or more.[99]

In the mid to late 1960s, during the first 6 years of MMT clinical trials, the Rockefeller team and their collaborators titrated more than 2,205 patients to daily doses of methadone equaling 80 to 120 mg.[100] At that dose level, overall retention in treatment was 82%, arrest rates dropped from 20% a year prior to treatment to less than 3% a year after treatment, and employment rates reached 70%, as reported by Gearing et al.[101] Nearly 20 years later, in 1983, Hargreaves[102] reviewed 22 methadone studies and concluded that a 100 mg dosage was associated with a more positive outcome than a 50 mg dosage in the first 5 to 10 months of MMT. Other studies have shown an inverse relationship between the frequency of heroin use and the dose of methadone. In the 1990s, Strain et al.[103] followed 247 intravenous opioid-dependent patients for 20 weeks. Patients were assigned to 0, 20, or 50 mg methadone groups. After 20 weeks, the 50 mg group had greater retention in MMT (52% in the 50 mg group, versus 42% in the 20 mg group, and 21% in the 0 mg group); rates of urine-positive toxicologies were 56% in the 50 mg group, 68% in the 20 mg group, and 74% in the 0 mg group. In 2002, Maxwell and Shinderman[104] reported the clinical courses of 245 MMT patients over 152 weeks. Patients prescribed methadone doses greater than 100 mg per day had better retention rates (61.1% vs. 46.3%) and lower rates of opiate-positive urine toxicologies (16% vs. 36.6%) than patients treated with less than 100 mg per day. Peles et al.[92] prospectively studied 492 patients in a MMT program in Israel and found that factors predicting retention in treatment were methadone doses of 100 mg or greater, negative urine toxicology for opiates, and being a parent.

Other confirmatory studies were conducted in Denver, Colorado, and Ireland. In the former study, Booth et al. concluded that higher methadone doses, as well as free treatment, increased retention rates in programs.[105] In the latter study, Kamal et al. found that patients enrolled in MMT with higher methadone doses were more likely to be opiate abstinent.[106]

Despite this compelling research, by the 1980s more than 40% of MMTP patients were receiving daily methadone doses of less than 40 mg. Even as late as 2005, Brady et al.[107] found that more than two-thirds of methadone patients nationwide were receiving less than 60 mg/day.

DRUG AND ALCOHOL CODEPENDENCY IN FEMALE METHADONE-MAINTAINED PATIENTS

Cocaine

Beginning in the 1980s and 1990s, a high prevalence of cocaine abuse among patients entering methadone treatment was reported in the literature.[108,109] Kosten's study reported a 74% rate of recent cocaine use among a cohort of New York City MMT admissions from 1978 to 1980 and the Drug Abuse Treatment Outcome Studies (DATOS), which tracked MMT admissions during 1990-1995 reported a 42% prevalence. The latter statistic appears steady over the past decade, as 2007 statistics obtained for New York City MMT programs show that 44% of patients self-reported cocaine as the secondary drug of abuse on admission. Interestingly, women in NYC reported a higher frequency (49.4%) than men (41.6%) (New York

State Office of Alcoholism and Substance Abuse Services Client Data System).[110] A higher rate of cocaine-positive urine samples was also observed among women (20%) as compared to men (11.3%) in Israel during the first month of admission to methadone maintenance,[111] notable in a country where cocaine abuse was not prevalent until a period of time after the clinic opened in 1993. The role of the mu-opioidergic system in cocaine craving and relapse was first elucidated by studies in rodent models demonstrating upregulation of mu-opioid receptors in rats following chronic intermittent "binge" cocaine administration and persisting throughout early withdrawal.[112,113] These findings were corroborated by positron-emission tomography (PET) studies in humans showing an increase in mu-opioid binding immediately following chronic cocaine use, and persisting for up to 4 weeks during abstinence.[114,115] Treatment outcome studies have shown that a majority of patients demonstrate significant reductions in cocaine use during long-term MMT,[81,109,116] and at least two studies have found an association between higher methadone levels and cessation of cocaine use.[91,116,117]

Despite this success, a percentage of long-term methadone-maintained patients, reported from 15% to 25%, continued chronic cocaine abuse.[108,116,118] Treatment strategies employed to reduce cocaine use in these patients vary by program with a majority of MMT programs surveyed by Kolar et al. instituting more frequent counseling and urine toxicology submission in response to positive cocaine tests.[118] However, as overall heroin abuse is mitigated and cocaine abuse reduced by MMT, it seems inappropriate to discharge patients due solely to continued cocaine use.

Alcohol

Alcohol abuse at treatment entry and during long-term methadone maintenance is more difficult to assess because data is frequently derived from patient self-report as opposed to breathalyzer or urine testing.[119] Drug Abuse Treatment Outcome Studies (DATOS) showed that 20% to 50% of all methadone maintenance patients in the United States display alcohol-related problems.[109] Overall, women in methadone maintenance have been shown to abuse alcohol to a lesser extent than men. A recent Swedish study found that 39% of women compared to 54% of men admitted to MMT had been treated for an alcohol-related diagnosis or had positive laboratory tests indicating recent moderate to high alcohol use.[119] New York City statistics for 2007 corroborate this; 5.5% of women compared to 7.7% of men self-reported alcohol as the secondary substance of abuse on admission.[110]

Early prospective studies performed on 129 long-term methadone-maintained men and women demonstrated that even with 25% of the cohort reporting consumption of four or more alcoholic drinks per day, there were no significant changes in liver enzymes or serum protein values after 3 years taking methadone.[30] Therefore, methadone maintenance does not potentiate alcohol-induced hepatotoxicity. The Swedish study found a significant association between drinking alcohol and relapse to illicit drugs, particularly benzodiazepines and cannabis among women, but no such association was found in men.[119] Thus, clinicians should make an effort to screen for alcohol abuse in MMT women on admission and plan treatment accordingly.

In contrast to the observation that methadone can reduce illicit drug use, MMT does not appear to effect rates of alcohol use from admission to 1 year follow-up.[120] Therefore, providers may want to consider treatment of MMT patients for whom heavy alcohol use is a problem. Most studies show limited efficacy of disulfiram, an acetaldehyde dehydrogenase inhibitor that, when combined with alcohol induces adverse effects, attributed to poor compliance with self-administration.[121] However, because MMT provides a favorable setting for the supervised dispensing of disulfiram, it may be a helpful adjunct for reducing alcohol intake in certain motivated MMT patients. Disulfiram is metabolized by the liver and prescribing it to patients with abnormal liver tests is not recommended. It is advised that liver enzymes be obtained prior to initiating treatment and every 2 weeks thereafter for the first 2 to 3 months.[121]

Acamprosate, an antiglutaminergic approved by the FDA in 2005, is primarily excreted by the kidneys and therefore may be a better option for patients with compromised liver function.[122] Although shown to effect complete abstinence from alcohol in only about a third of patients, female gender was not found to be associated with treatment outcome in a study where potential predictive variables were examined.[123]

Benzodiazepines

A study that examined gender-based disparities in benzodiazepine use among those in MMT did not find significant differences between men and women at admission. However, women were less likely than men (18.8% vs. 29.9%) to initiate benzodiazepine use during the first year in MMT.[111] Benzodiazepines share some of the cytochrome P450 metabolic pathway with methadone, and therefore have the potential to cause interactions. Although several studies suggested an enhanced subjective effect of methadone when taken concurrently with benzodiazepines, there has been no evidence that benzodiazepines increase serum methadone levels, and the effects are most likely due to increased CNS depression.[124] Reported interventions for benzodiazepine abuse during MMT include prescribing a single, long-acting benzodiazepine (clonazepam) to replace the patient's total daily illicit dose, which may or may not be administered by the clinic's medical staff[125] or increasing the daily methadone dose in response to patients' positive toxicology for benzodiazepines.[124] Higher methadone doses were associated with better outcomes in successful detoxification from benzodiazepines for those patients who declined clonazepam maintenance in one study.[125]

Cannabis

Information regarding the prevalence of marijuana abuse among MMT patients is less available in the literature because many MMT programs no longer include cannabis in the urine toxicology panel. This may be due in part to the publication of several studies in the 1990s, two of them derived from predominantly male cohorts, which showed no significant association between cannabis use and the use of other illicit drugs.[126,127] Studies reporting treatment outcomes with MMT have shown that overall use of cannabis, similar to that of other illicit drugs, declines with long-term MMT.[120] In addition, cannabis use was not found to decrease retention in MMT programs.[128]

MEDICAL ISSUES SPECIFIC TO WOMEN IN MMT PROGRAMS

Women entering MMT programs present with a wide range of medical issues throughout their life spans. A recent study in Israel has shown that women are more likely to enter MMT programs at a younger age than men, with more than double the percentage of total female admissions occurring in the 18 to 30 age group as compared to men.[129] Statistics obtained for admissions in 2007 to New York City MMT programs indicated that 62% of all female admissions were women between 18 to 34 years as compared to 56% of the total male admissions in this age range.

Because of the relatively young age of entry into treatment, MMT programs have an opportunity to address contraception and pregnancy planning with women during intake and throughout treatment. Few studies have examined sexual activity and contraceptive practices in methadone-maintained women. Those that specifically addressed this topic reported the number of sexually active women in MMT ranged from 61% at a rural MMTP to 84.5% at an urban clinic; however, birth control rates were similar in both MMT programs, with at least a third of sexually active women reporting no use of contraception.[130,131] In one study, Harding et al. interviewed a subset of seven women who did not use contraception and cited a perceived low risk of pregnancy due to a variety of reasons: infrequent sex, a history of infertility, difficulties with male erection due to partner drug use, and falsely assuming breastfeeding afforded protection against pregnancy. Altered menstrual cycles during drug use and in early methadone maintenance were also mentioned by several women as a significant reason why they were not using contraception.[131]

Effects of illicit opiates on the menstrual cycle are well-documented, with early studies reporting that 30% to 54% of women using heroin had secondary amenorrhea.[59,132] In comparison, the prevalence of amenorrhea in a population of healthy, adult women has been estimated to be 2% to 4%.[133,134] Few researchers have examined the effects of methadone maintenance on menstrual regulation. Early data from our laboratory demonstrated that in a cohort of methadone-maintained women, 54% had reported amenorrhea on admission, whereas 83% of the subjects were reporting normal menses after an average methadone stabilization time of 2.7 years.[59] More recently, Schmittner et al. found that 59% of women reporting pre-study secondary amenorrhea had resumed menses during a 6-month period of methadone maintenance.[135] No studies have found a correlation between methadone dose and menstrual dysfunction.[132,135]

Intravenous drug use forms the route of acquisition of up to half the cases of HIV infection among women in the United States, while having had sex with a male intravenous drug user accounts for almost 25% of new HIV cases.[136] This risk of HIV acquisition underscores the need to assess sexual history in determining appropriate contraception with female methadone patients. The World Health Organization (WHO) reported that barrier methods differ in rates of pregnancy prevention for women in general, with condoms highest at 86% to 97%, diaphragms with contraceptive gel (84% to 94%) and cervical caps (68% to 91%), with the lower number representing typical use and the higher number corresponding to perfect (correct and consistent) use.[137] Although condoms are the only method to effectively prevent HIV transmission, diaphragms and cervical caps have been found to confer low level protection against chlamydia and gonorrhea. Pregnancy prevention rates with oral hormones range from 92% to 99%, injectable hormone preparations are 97% to 99.5%, and intrauterine devices 99.5%, but none of these methods offer protection against STDs. Although there are no reports of medication interactions between the hormonal methods and methadone, the use of some medications prescribed for methadone-maintained women, such as anti-retrovirals and certain anticonvulsants, may reduce the effectiveness of hormonal preparations. In addition, certain co-morbid conditions, such as active viral hepatitis, may be a contraindication to prescribing hormonal preparations. Clinicians may access the WHO Medical Eligibility Criteria for Contraceptive Use[138] online at www.who.int/reproductive-health/publications/mec for guidance.

The substance abuse treatment population as a whole is aging and an increasing percentage of women remain in treatment into middle age. As of 2000, 60% of all women in New York City MMT programs were between the ages of 35 and 54.[110] To date, only one researcher has specifically examined menopausal symptoms in methadone-maintained women. Tuchman reported a similar prevalence of vasomotor symptoms (i.e., hot flashes and night sweats) among methadone-maintained women versus other study populations, while a much larger percentage in the methadone-maintained group complained of insomnia. In a report by Tuchman et al., ethnic differences were also noted as Hispanic methadone-maintained women had a higher degree of symptom reporting than African American or White women.[139] Thus, it is important for clinicians to differentiate menopausal symptoms from opiate withdrawal or inadequate methadone dose in mid-life women.

TREATMENT ADDRESSING SPECIFIC NEEDS OF WOMEN

A consensus exists in the addiction treatment literature that women have different substance abuse treatment needs than their male counterparts and that lack of gender-specific services is a barrier to care. A strong positive correlation exists between troubled relationships, family violence, sexual abuse and poor self esteem as integral factors in substance abuse among women.[140,141] Also, a large percentage (25% to 57%) of women in drug treatment programs reported a history of intimate partner violence,[142–145] compared to rates of 1.5% to 16% in community based samples.[146,147]

Women who use substances are more likely to report a history of emotional, sexual, or physical abuse than men who use substances; this may impede or prevent the process of recovery. Unlike women with psychiatric problems, men in treatment who have a history of abuse appear to recover at rates similar to men without a history of abuse.[148] The prevalence of diagnosed posttraumatic stress disorder ranges from 20% to 60% among women in substance abuse treatment.[149,150] Research has found an association between women experiencing IPV and heroin use.[145] Female methadone patients report more depression and anxiety than men as well as more suicidal thoughts and attempts.[140,141]

In a study that examined the different perceptions of causal factors related to their substance abuse between men and women, female substance users indicated that domestic violence or incest had a greater impact on their substance use than men.[140] Retention rates appear to be similar for men and women. Older female patients are more likely to remain in treatment longer; heroin users are less likely to be retained in a program;[92,93,129] having children and less frequent use of benzodiazepines were also associated with long term retention.[92,129] As a result of research showing that women have different substance abuse treatment needs than men, a women-only MMT program was established in 2000 within the Beth Israel Medical Center. This program is named Billie's Place in memory of Billie Holiday. Billie Holiday, an African American female, has been described as the most influential singer of the 20th century and is still considered the most famous of jazz singers. "Lady Day" was also a heroin addict and alcoholic and died in 1959 at the age of 44 in a New York City hospital of complications of her addictions.

The Beth Israel Medical Center MMT program is the largest MMT program in the nation. It operates 18 clinics in two boroughs of New York City, with a patient census of 6,500. Beth Israel Medical Center, the sponsor of the MMT program, is a full service acute care teaching hospital in Manhattan. It is accredited by the Joint Commission on the Accreditation of Healthcare Organizations because is its network of methadone clinics. The methadone clinics comply with, and are overseen by, government agencies, Substance Abuse and Mental Health Services Administration (SAMHSA), the Drug Enforcement Agency, the New York State Department of Health, and the New York State Office of Substance Abuse Services. All 18 clinics are in good standing with these agencies. All of Beth Israel Medical Center's methadone clinics serve both men and women; however, Billie's Place is the only gender-specific clinic.

The overall plan for Billie's Place was to establish a positive therapeutic relationship with the female patients, and quickly stabilize each patient's methadone dose, with the aims of decreasing or eliminating heroin use and promoting program retention and improvement in overall health status. At time of inception, and during a period of 3 years of its existence, Billie's Place provided an intensive day treatment program for predominantly African American and Hispanic/Latina women who were already in MMT, as well as new admissions who were HIV-1-positive or at high risk for HIV and other infectious diseases. Female intravenous drug users who were HIV-1-positive or at high risk for HIV had more complex medical and social problems than their male counterparts. Women's health is often complicated by obstetrical, gynecological, and family issues; women often choose to attend to their children's and partner's health care needs before their own. For minority women in particular, lay therapeutic practices combined with ethnic or cultural beliefs and attitudes may complicate their acceptance of mainstream healthcare. Also, for women with limited resources, lack of health insurance, transportation difficulties, and childcare are additional barriers to accessing substance abuse treatment and other health care.

Billie's Place was originally established through a SAMHSA grant 5H79TI12162 awarded in 1999 and opened in 2000, with an initial capacity for 50 women. Formal services provided on site included MMT, co-dependency drug treatment and counseling, counseling and testing for HIV, complete gynecological examinations with initial testing for sexually-transmitted diseases (i.e., chlamydia and gonorrhea), HIV risk reduction counseling, tuberculosis screening and group counseling in the areas of sexual abuse, domestic violence, and negotiating safer sex. Workshops in parenting, employment skills, and life skills training were provided. All services were sensitive to cultural backgrounds of patients and were offered in English and Spanish. Referrals were made to primary medical care and primary HIV medical care in clinics located in the community, or to BIMC services. Patients were screened for other sexually transmitted diseases (e.g., syphilis) and hepatitis B and C and provided prenatal and postpartum care; family planning services were also available through referral. Vocational services and educational programs were provided on-site and through referrals.

The program also focused on informal social activities. These included providing a social space where health education materials, as well as light reading, were available. A computer with Internet access was available for patients' use. In addition, the women could use this space to socialize, eat light refreshments, and participate in structured weekly events. The original staffing consisted of one program director, one case manager, two substance abuse counselors, one neighborhood outreach worker, one nurse practitioner, one registered nurse, and one administrative assistant.

Billie's Place successfully provided intensive partial day treatment, individualized case management, an inclusive and non-judgmental support network, and comprehensive, direct links to health care treatment and rehabilitation services. Although the grant from SAMSHA ended, Billie's Place continues to exist as a separate women-only clinic (with markedly reduced staffing) within the Beth Israel Medical Center MMT program. (Direct inquiries for additional information regarding Billie's Place to Dr. Randi Seewald, Medical Director, BIMC MMTP, 160 Water Street, 24th floor, New York, NY 10038 rseewald@chpnet.org.)

REFERENCES

1. Dole VP, Nyswander ME, Kreek MJ. Narcotic blockade: a medical technique for stopping heroin use by addicts. Trans Assoc Am Phys 1966; 79:122–36.

2. Dole VP, Nyswander ME, Kreek MJ. Narcotic blockade. Arch Intern Med 1966; 118:304–9.

3. Dole VP, Nyswander M.E. A medical treatment for diacetylmorphine (heroin) addiction: a clinical trial with methadone methadone hydrochloride. JAMA 1965; 193:646–50.

4. Kreek MJ. Medical complications in methadone patients. Ann NY Acad Sci 1978; 311:110–34.

5. Kreek MJ. The role of qualitative and quantitative analysis of drugs and their metabolites in maternal-neonatal studies. In: National Institute on Drug Abuse Symposium on Comprehensive Health Care for Addicted Families and Their Children, Washington, DC:Services Research Report (USGPO), #017-024-00598-3, 1977:67–73.

6. Blake DA, Chappel JN, Kreek MJ, Meyer KC, Lyon Newmann L, Stimmel B, Stryker J. Drug dependence in pregnancy: clinical management of mother and child—a guide to clinical management. Finnegan LP, ed. Washington, DC: National Institute on Drug Abuse Research Monograph ADM, (USGPO), DHEW 79–678, 1979:1–109.

7. Kreek MJ. Disposition of narcotics in the perinatal period. In: Publication of AMERSA and The Career Teacher Program in Alcohol and Drug Abuse, 1981–1982; 3:7–10.

8. Kreek MJ. Opioid disposition and effects during chronic exposure in the perinatal period in man. J Addict Dis. 1982; 1:21–53.

9. Kreek MJ. Discussion on clinical perinatal and developmental effects of methadone. In: Cooper JR, Altman F, Brown BS, Czechowicz D, eds. Washington, DC: National Institute on Drug Abuse Monograph Research in the Treatment of Narcotic Addiction: State of the Art. DHHS Pub. # (ADM) 83–1281, 1983:444–53.

10. Pond SM, Kreek MJ, Tong TG, Raghunath J, Benowitz NL. Altered methadone pharmacokinetics in methadone–maintained pregnant women. J Pharmacol Exp Ther 1985; 233:1–6.

11. Kreek MJ, LaForge KS, Butelman E. Pharmacotherapy of addictions. Nat Rev Drug Discov 2002; 1:710–26.

12. Kreek MJ, Schlussman SD, Bart G, LaForge KS, Butelman ER. Evolving perspectives on neurobiological research on the addictions: celebration of the 30th anniversary of NIDA. Neuropharmacology 2004; 47(Suppl 1):324–44.

13. Kreek MJ, Schlussman SD, Reed B, Zhang Y, Nielsen DA, Levran O, Zhou Y, Butelman ER. Bidirectional translational research: Progress in understanding addictive diseases. Neuropharmacology 2009; 56:32–43.

14. Kreek MJ, Schluger J, Borg L, Gunduz M, Ho A. Dynorphin A1-13 causes elevation of serum levels of prolactin through an opioid receptor mechanism in humans: gender differences and implications for modulation of dopaminergic tone in the treatment of addictions. J Pharmacol Exp Ther 1999; 288:260–9.

15. Bart G, Borg L, Schluger JH, Green M, Ho A, Kreek MJ. Suppressed prolactin response to dynorphin A(1-13) in methadone maintained versus control subjects. J Pharmacol Exp Ther 2003; 306:581–7.

16. Kreek MJ, Bart G, Lilly C, LaForge KS, Nielsen DA. Pharmacogenetics and human molecular genetics of opiate and cocaine addictions and their treatments. Pharmacol Rev 2005; 57:1–26.

17. Kreek MJ, LaForge KS. Stress responsivity, addiction, and a functional variant of the human mu-opioid receptor gene. Molec Interv 2007; 7:74–8.

18. Kreek MJ. Role of a functional human gene polymorphism in stress responsivity and addictions. Clin Pharmacol Ther 2008; 83:615–8.

19. Bond C, LaForge KS, Tian M, Melia D, Zhang S, Borg L, Gong J, Schluger J, Strong JA, Leal SM, Tischfield JA, Kreek MJ, Yu L. Single nucleotide polymorphism in the human mu opioid receptor gene alters beta-endorphin binding and activity: possible implications for opiate addiction. Proc Natl Acad Sci USA 1998; 95: 9608–13.

20. Bart G, Heilig M, LaForge KS, Pollak L, Leal SM, Ott J, Kreek MJ. Substantial attributable risk related to a functional mu-opioid receptor gene polymorphism in association with heroin addiction in central Sweden. Mol Psychiatry 2004; 9:547–9.

21. Bart G, Kreek MJ, Ott J, LaForge KS, Proudnikov D, Pollak L, Heilig M. Increased attributable risk related to a functional mu-opioid receptor gene polymorphism in association with alcohol dependence in central Sweden. Neuropsychopharmacology 2005; 30:417–22.

22. Bart G, LaForge KS, Borg L, Lilly C, Ho A, Kreek MJ. Altered levels of basal cortisol in healthy subjects with a 118G allele in exon 1 of the mu opioid receptor gene. Neuropsychopharmacology 2006; 31:2313–7.

23. Oosterhuis BE, LaForge KS, Proudnikov D, Ho A, Nielsen DA, Gianotti R, Barral S, Gordon D, Leal SM, Ott J, Kreek MJ. Catechol-*O*-methyltransferase (*COMT*) gene variants: possible association of the Val158Met variant with opiate addiction in Hispanic women. Am J Med Genet B: Neuropsychiatr Genet 2008; 147B:793–8.

24. Borg L, Kravets I, Kreek MJ. The pharmacology of long-acting as contrasted with short-acting opioids. In: Kosten T, Gorelick D, eds. Principles of addiction medicine, 4th edition. New York: Lippincott Williams & Wilkins, 2009; 117–31.

25. Hachey DL, Kreek MJ, Mattson DH. Quantitative analysis of methadone in biological fluids using deuterium-labeled methadone and GLC-chemical-ionization mass spectrometry. J Pharm Sci 1977; 66:1579–82.

26. Kreek MJ, Hachey DL, Klein PD. Stereoselective disposition of methadone in man. Life Sci 1979; 24:925–32.

27. Ferrari A, Coccia CP, Bertolini A, Sternieri E. Methadone: metabolism, pharmacokinetics and interactions. Pharmacol Res 2004; 50:551–9.

28. Nilsson MI, Anggård E, Holmstrand J, Gunne LM. Pharmacokinetics of methadone during maintenance treatment: adaptive changes during the induction phase. Eur J Clin Pharmacol 1982; 22:343–9.

29. Wolff K, Hay AW, Raistrick D, Calvert R. Steady-state pharmacokinetics of methadone in opioid addicts. Eur J Clin Pharmacol 1993; 44:189–94.

30. Kreek MJ. Plasma and urine levels of methadone. NY State J Med 1973; 73:2773–7.

31. Dole VP, Kreek MJ. Methadone plasma level: Sustained by a reservoir of drug in tissue. Proc Natl Acad Sci USA 1973; 70:10.

32. Eap CB, Buclin T, Baumann P. Interindividual variability of the clinical pharmacokinetics of methadone: implications for the treatment of opioid dependence. Clin Pharmacokinet 2002; 41:1153–93.

33. Kling MA, Carson RE, Borg L, Zametkin A, Matochik JA, Schluger J, Herscovitch P, Rice KC, Ho A, Eckelman WC, Kreek MJ. Opioid receptor imaging with PET and [^{18}F]cyclofoxy in long-term methadone-treated former heroin addicts. J Pharmacol Exp Ther 2000; 295: 1070–6.

34. Davis AM, Inturrisi CE. d-Methadone blocks morphine tolerance and N-methyl-D-aspartate-induced hyperalgesia. J Pharmacol Exp Ther 1999; 289:1048–53.

35. Kreek MJ, Oratz M, Rothschild MA. Hepatic extraction of long- and short-acting narcotics in the isolated perfused rabbit liver. Gastroenterology 1978; 75:88–94.

36. Novick DM, Kreek MJ, Fanizza AM, Yancovitz SR, Gelb AM, Stenger RJ. Methadone disposition in patients with chronic liver disease. Clin Pharmacol Ther 1981; 30:353–62.

37. Inturrisi CE, Max MB, Foley KM, Schultz M, Shin S-U, Houde RW. The pharmacokinetics of heroin in patients with chronic pain. N Engl J Med 1984; 310:1213–7.

38. Borg L, Ho A, Peters JE, Kreek MJ. Availability of reliable serum methadone determination for management of symptomatic patients. J Addict Dis 1995; 14:83–96.

39. Tong TG, Pond SM, Kreek MJ, Jaffery NF, Benowitz NL. Phenytoin-induced methadone withdrawal. Ann Intern Med 1981; 94:349–51.

40. Kreek MJ, Garfield JW, Gutjahr CL, Giusti LM. Rifampin-induced methadone withdrawal. N Engl J Med 1976; 294:1104–6.

41. Kreek MJ, Gutjahr CL, Garfield JW, Bowen DV, Field FH. Drug interactions with methadone. Ann NY Acad Sci 1976; 281:350–71.

42. Cushman P, Kreek MJ, Gordis E. Ethanol and methadone in man: a possible drug interaction. Drug Alcohol Depend 1978; 3:35–42.

43. Peles E, Schreiber S, Naumovsky Y, Adelson M. Depression in methadone maintenance treatment patients: rate and risk factors. J Affect Disord 2007; 99:213–20.

44. Eap CB, Broly F, Mino A, Hämmig R, Déglon JJ, Uehlinger C, Meili D, Chevalley AF, Bertschy G, Zullino D, Kosel M, Preisig M, Baumann P. Cytochrome 450 2D6 genotype and methadone steady-state concentrations. J Clin Psychopharmacol 2001; 21:229–34.

45. Levran O, O'Hara K, Peles E, Li D, Barral S, Ray B, Borg L, Ott J, Adelson M, Kreek MJ. *ABCB1* (*MDR1*) genetic variants are associated with methadone doses required for effective treatment of heroin dependence. Hum Mol Genet 2008; 17:2219–27.

46. Lugo RA, Satterfield KL, Kern SE. Pharmacokinetics of methadone. J Pain Palliat Care Pharmacother 2005; 19:13–24.

47. Bowen DV, Smit ALC, Kreek MJ. Fecal excretion of methadone and its metabolites in man: application of GC-MS. In: Daly NR, ed. Advances in mass spectrometry. Philadelphia: Heyden & Son, Inc, 1978; 7B:1634–9.

48. Kreek MJ, Kalisman M, Irwin M, Jaffery NF, Scheflan M. Biliary secretion of methadone and methadone metabolites in man. Res Commun Chem Pathol Pharmacol 1980; 29:67–78.

49. Kreek MJ, Schecter AJ, Gutjahr CL, Hecht M. Methadone use in patients with chronic renal disease. Drug Alcohol Depend 1980; 5:197–205.

50. Kreek MJ, Bencsath FA, Field FH. Effects of liver disease on urinary excretion of methadone and metabolites in maintenance patients: quantitation by direct probe chemical ionization mass spectrometry. Biomed Mass Spectrom 1980; 7:385–95.

51. Chan GL, Matzke GR. Effects of renal insufficiency on the pharmacokinetics and pharmacodynamics of opioid analgesics. Drug Intell Clin Pharm 1987; 21: 773–83.

52. Novick DM, Kreek MJ, Arns PA, Lau LL, Yancovitz SR, Gelb AM. Effect of severe alcoholic liver disease on the disposition of methadone in maintenance patients. Alcohol Clin Exp Res 1985; 9:349–54.

53. Tong TG, Benowitz NL, Kreek MJ. Methadone-disulfiram interaction during methadone maintenance. J Clin Pharmacol 1980; 20:506–13.

54. Bruce RD, Altice FL, Gourevitch MN, Friedland GH. Pharmacokinetic drug interactions between opioid agonist therapy and antiretroviral medications: implications and management for clinical practice. J Acquire Immune Def Syndr 2006; 41:563–72.

55. Gupta SK, Sellers E, Somoza E, Angles L, Kolz K, Cutler DL. The effect of multiple doses of peginterferon alfa-2b on the steady-state pharmacokinetics of methadone in patients with chronic hepatitis C undergoing methadone maintenance therapy. J Clin Pharmacol 2007; 47: 604–12.

56. Berk SI, Litwin AH, Arnsten JH, Du E, Soloway I, Gourevitch MN. Effects of pegylated interferon alfa-2b on the pharmacokinetic and pharmacodynamic properties of methadone: a prospective, nonrandomized, crossover study in patients coinfected with hepatitis C and HIV receiving methadone maintenance treatment. Clin Ther 2007; 29:131–8.

57. Sulkowski M, Wright T, Rossi S, Arora S, Lamb M, Wang K, Gries JM, Yalamanchili S. Peginterferon alfa-2a does not alter the pharmacokinetics of methadone in patients with chronic hepatitis C undergoing methadone maintenance therapy. Clin Pharmacol Ther 2005; 77:214–24.

58. McHugh PF, Kreek MJ. The medical consequences of opiate abuse and addiction, and methadone pharmacotherapy. In: Brick J, ed. Handbook of the medical consequences of alcohol and drug abuse, 2nd ed. New York: Haworth Press, 2008:303–40.

59. Cushman P, Kreek MJ. Some endocrinologic observations in narcotic addicts. In: Zimmerman E, George R, eds. Narcotics and the hypothalamus. New York: Raven Press, 1974:161–73.

60. Pond SM, Kreek MJ, Tong TG, Benowitz NL. Changes in methadone pharmacokinetics during pregnancy. Clin Res 1982; 30:257A.

61. Jarvis MA, Wu-Pong S, Kniseley JS, Schnoll SH. Alterations in methadone metabolism during late pregnancy. J Addict Dis 1999; 18:51–61.

62. Nanovskaya TN, Deshmukh SV, Nekhayeva IA, Zharikova OL, Hankins GD, Ahmed MS. Methadone metabolism by human placenta. Biochem Pharmacol 2004; 68:583–91.

63. Hieronymous TL, Nanovskaya TN, Deshmukh SV, Vargas R, Hankins GD, Ahmed MS. Methadone metabolism by early gestational age placentas. Am J Perinatol 2006; 23:287–94.

64. American Academy of Pediatrics: Committee on Drugs: The transfer of drugs and other chemicals into human milk. Pediatrics 2001:108; 776–89.

65. American Academy of Pediatrics: Committee on Pediatric AIDS. HIV testing and prophylaxis to prevent mother-to-child transmission in the United States. Pediatrics 2008:122; 1127–34.

66. Krantz MJ, Lewkowiez L, Hays H, Woodroffe MA, Robertson AD, Mehler PS. Torsade de pointes associated with very-high-dose methadone. Ann Intern Med 2002; 137:501–4.

67. Martell BA, Arnsten JH, Ray B, Gourevitch MN. The impact of methadone induction on cardiac conduction in opiate users. Ann Intern Med 2003; 139:154–5.

68. Gil M, Sala M, Anguera I, Chapinal O, Cervantes M, Guma JR, Segura F. QT prolongation and Torsades de Pointes in patients with human immunodeficiency virus and treated with methadone. Am J Cardiol 2003; 92: 995–7.

69. Martell BA, Arnsten JH, Krantz M, Gourevitch MN. Impact of methadone treatment of cardiac repolarization and conduction in opioid users. Am J Cardiol 2005; 95:915–8.

70. Krantz MJ, Lowery CM, Martell BA, Gourevitch MN, Arnsten JH. Effects of methadone on QT-interval dispersion. Pharmacotherapy 2005; 25:1523–9.

71. Peles E, Bodner G, Kreek MJ, Rados V, Adelson M. Corrected-QT intervals as related to methadonedose and serum level in methadone maintenance treatment (MMT) patients: a cross-sectional study. Addiction 2007; 102:289–300.

72. Gutstein HB, Akil H. Opioid analgesics. In: Brunton L, Lazo JS, Parker KL, eds. Goodman and Gilman's the pharmacological basis of therapeutics, 11th Ed. New York: McGraw-Hill, 2005:547–90.

73. Kreek MJ. Medical safety and side effects of methadone in tolerant individuals. JAMA 1973; 223:665–8.

74. Shook JE, Watkins WD, Camporesi EM. Differential roles of opioid receptors in respiration, respiratory disease, and opiate-induced respiratory depression. Am Rev Respir Dis 1990; 142:895–909.

75. Kleinschmidt KC, Wainscott M, Ford MD. Opioids. In: Ford MD, Delaney KA, Ling LJ, Erickson T, eds. Ford: clinical toxicology, 1st ed. Philadelphia:WB Saunders, 2001:627–39.

76. Hartel DM, Schoenbaum EE, Selwyn PA, Kline J, Davenny K, Klein RS, Friedland GH. Heroin use during methadone maintenance treatment: the importance of methadone dose and cocaine use. Am J Public Health 1995; 85:83–8.

77. Maremmani I, Pani PP, Pacini M, Perugi G. Substance use and quality of life over 12 months among buprenorphine maintenance-treated and methadone maintenance-treated heroin-addicted patients. J Subst Abuse Treat 2007; 33:91–8.

78. Deren S, Kang SY, Colón HM, Robles RR. Predictors of injection drug use cessation among Puerto Rican drug injectors in New York and Puerto Rico. Am J Drug Alcohol Abuse 2007; 33:291–9.

79. Gruber VA, Delucchi KL, Kielstein A, Batki SL. A randomized trial of 6-month methadone maintenance with standard or minimal counseling versus 21-day methadone detoxification. Drug Alcohol Depend 2008; 94:199–206.

80. Dole VP, Nyswander ME, Warner A. Successful treatment of 750 criminal addicts. JAMA 1968; 206:2708–11.

81. Ball JC, Ross A. The effectiveness of methadone maintenance treatment: patients, programs, services, and outcomes. New York: Springer-Verlag, 1991.

82. Dolan KA, Shearer J, White B, Zhou J, Kaldor J, Wodak AD. Four-year follow-up of imprisoned male heroin user users and methadone treatment: mortality, re-incarceration and hepatitis C infection. Addiction 2005; 100:820–8.

83. National Institutes of Health. National Institutes of Health Consensus Development Statement (CDS): management of hepatitis C: 2002, June 10-12, 2002. Bethesda, MD: National Institutes of Health, p. 13. http://consensus.nih.gov/cons/116/cdc.statement.htm.

84. Novick DM, Stenger RJ, Gelb AM, Most J, Yancovitz SR, Kreek, MJ. Chronic liver disease in abusers of alcohol and parenteral drugs: a report of 204 consecutive biopsy-proven cases. Alcohol Clin Exp Res 1986; 10: 500–5.

85. Des Jarlais DC, Marmor M, Cohen H, Yancovitz S, Garber J, Friedman S, Kreek MJ, Miescher A, Khuri E, Friedman SM, Rothenberg R, Echenberg D, O'Malley PO, Braff E, Chin J, Burtenol P, Sikes RK. Antibodies to a retrovirus etiologically associated with Acquired Immunodeficiency Syndrome (AIDS) in populations with increased incidences of the syndrome. Morb Mortal Wkly Rep 1984; 33:377–9.

86. Novick DM, Khan I, Kreek MJ. Acquired immunodeficiency syndrome and infection with hepatitis viruses in individuals abusing drugs by injection. United Nations Bulletin on Narcotics 1986; 38:15–25.

87. Gibson A, Degenhardt L, Mattick RP, Ali R, White J, O'Brien S. Exposure to opioid maintenance treatment reduces long-term mortality. Addiction 2008; 103:462–8.

88. Zanis DA, Woody GE. One-year mortality rates following methadone treatment discharge. Drug Alcohol Depend 1998; 52:257–60.

89. Magura S, Kang SY, Nwakeze PC, Demsky S. Temporal patterns of heroin and cocaine use among methadone patients. Subst Use Misuse 1998; 33:2441–67.

90. Des Jarlais DC, Wenston J, Friedman SR, Sotheran JL, Maslansky R, Marmor M. Crack cocaine use in a cohort of methadone maintenance patients. J Subst Abuse Treat 1992; 9:319–25.

91. Peles E, Kreek MJ, Kellogg S, Adelson M. High methadone dose significantly reduces cocaine use in methadone maintenance treatment (MMT) patients. J Addict Dis 2006; 25:43–50.

92. Peles E, Schreiber S, Adelson M. Factors predicting retention in treatment: 10-year experience of a methadone maintenance treatment (MMT) clinic in Israel. Drug Alcohol Depend 2006; 82:211–7.

93. Davstad I, Stenbacka M, Leifman A, Beck O, Korkmaz S, Romelsjö A. Patterns of illicit drug use and retention in a methadone program: a longitudinal study. J Opioid Manag 2007; 3:27–34.

94. Novick DM, Richman BL, Friedman JM, Friedman JE, Fried C, Wilson JP, Townley A, Kreek, MJ. The medical status of methadone maintenance patients in treatment for 11-18 years. Drug Alcohol Depend 1993; 33: 235–45.

95. Dole VP, Nyswander ME. Methadone maintenance and its implication for theories of narcotic addiction. In: Addictive States. Association for Research in Nervous and Mental Disease. Baltimore:Williams & Wilkins Company, 1968:359–66.

96. Kreek MJ. The addict as a patient. In: Lowinson JH, Ruiz P, Millman RB, Langrod JG, eds. Substance abuse: a comprehensive textbook. Baltimore:Williams & Wilkins, 1992:997–1009.

97. Hiltunen AJ, Beck O, Hjemdahl P, Liljeberg P, Almström U, Brodin K, von Wachenfeldt J, Borg S. Rated well-being in relation to plasma concentrations of *l*- and *d*-methadone in satisfied and dissatisfied patients on methadone maintenance treatment. Psychopharmacology (Berl) 1999; 143:385–93.

98. Donny EC, Brasser SM, Bigelow GE, Stitzer ML, Walsh SL. Methadone doses of 100mg or greater are more effective than lower doses at suppressing heroin self-administration in opioid-dependent volunteers. Addiction 2005; 100:1496–509.

99. Kreek MJ. Tolerance and dependence: implications for the pharmacological treatment of addiction. In: Harris LS, ed. Problems of drug dependence, 1986; Proceedings of the 48th Annual Scientific Meeting of the Committee on Problems of Drug Dependence. National Institute of Drug Abuse Research Monograph Series, Washington, DC: Supt of Docs, US Govt Print Off, DHHS Pub No(ADM) 87-1508. 1987; 76:53–61.

100. Dole VP. Blockade with methadone. In: Clouet DH, ed. Narcotic drugs biochemical pharmacology. New York:Plenum Press 1971:478–483.

101. Gearing FR, Schweitzer MD. An epidemiologic evaluation of long-term methadone maintenance treatment for heroin addiction. Am J Epidemiol 1974; 100:101–12.

102. Hargreaves WA. Methadone dosage and duration for maintenance treatment. In: Cooper J, Altman F, Brown B, Czechowicz D, eds. Research on the treatment of narcotic addiction: state of the art. Rockville, MD:National Institute on Drug Abuse, 1983:19–79.

103. Strain EC, Stitzer ML, Liebson IA, Bigelow GE. Methadone dose and treatment outcome. Drug Alcohol Depend 1993; 33:105–17.

104. Maxwell S, Shinderman MS. Optimizing long-term response to methadone maintenance treatment: a 152-week follow-up using higher-dose methadone. J Addict Dis 2002; 21:1–12.

105. Booth RE, Corsi KF, Mikulich-Gilbertson SK. Factors associated with methadone maintenance treatment retention among street-recruited injection drug users. Drug Alcohol Depend 2004; 74:177–85.

106. Kamal F, Flavin S, Campbell F, Behan C, Fagan J, Smyth R. Factors affecting the outcome of methadone maintenance treatment in opiate dependence. Ir Med J 2007; 100:393–7.

107. Brady TM, Salvucci S, Sverdlov LS, Male SA, Kyeyune H, Sikali E, DeSale S, Yu P. Methadone dosage and retention: an examination of the 60 mg/day threshold. J Addict Dis 2005; 24:23–47.

108. Kosten TR, Gawin FH, Rounsaville BJ, Kleber HD. Cocaine abuse among opioid addicts: demographic and diagnostic factors in treatment. Am J Drug Alcohol Abuse 1986; 12:1–16.

109. Hubbard RL, Craddock SG, Anderson J. Overview of 5-year followup outcomes in the drug abuse treatment outcome studies (DATOS). J Subst Abuse Treat 2003; 25:125–34.

110. New York State Office of Alcoholism and Substance Abuse Services Client Data System (CDS) extract 09/2008.

111. Peles E, Adelson M. Gender differences and pregnant women in a methadone maintenance treatment (MMT) clinic. J Addict Dis 2006; 25:39–45.

112. Unterwald E, Horne-King J, Kreek MJ. Chronic cocaine alters brain mu opioid receptors. Brain Res 1992; 584:314–18.

113. Bailey A, Gianotti R, Ho A, Kreek MJ. Persistent upregulation of mu-opioid, but not adenosine, receptors in brains of long-term withdrawn escalating dose "binge" cocaine-treated rats. Synapse 2005; 57:160–6.

114. Zubieta JK, Gorelick DA, Stauffer R, Ravert HT, Dannals RF, Frost JJ. Increased mu opioid receptor binding detected by PET in cocaine-dependent men is associated with cocaine craving. Nat Med 1996; 2:1225–9.

115. Gorelick DA, Kim YK, Bencherif B, Boyd SJ, Nelson R, Copersino M, Endres CJ, Dannals RF, Frost JJ. Imaging brain mu-opioid receptors in abstinent cocaine users: time course and relation to cocaine craving. Biol Psych 2005; 57:1573–82.

116. Borg L, Broe DM, Ho A, Kreek MJ. Cocaine abuse sharply reduced in an effective methadone maintenance program. J Addict Dis 1999; 18:63–75.

117. Tennant F, Shannon J. Cocaine abuse in methadone maintenance patients is associated with low serum methadone concentrations. J Addict Dis 1995; 14:67–74.

118. Kolar AF, Brown BS, Weddington WW, Ball JC. A treatment crisis: cocaine use by clients in methadone maintenance programs. J Subst Abuse Treat 1990; 7:101–7.

119. Stenbacka M, Beck O, Leifman A, Romelsjö A, Helander A. Problem drinking in relation to treatment outcome among opiate addicts in methadone maintenance treatment. Drug Alcohol Rev 2007; 26:55–63.

120. Fairbank JA, Dunteman GH, Condelli WS. Do methadone patients substitute other drugs for heroin? Predicting substance use at 1-year follow-up. Am J Drug Alcohol Abuse 1993; 19:465–74.

121. Fuller RK, Gordis E. Does disulfiram have a role in alcoholism treatment today? Addict 2004; 99:21–4.

122. Kenna GA, Nielsen DM, Mello P, Schiesl A, Swift RM. Pharmacotherapy of dual substance abuse and dependence. CNS Drugs 2007; 21:213–37.

123. Verheul R, Lehert P, Geerlings PJ, Koeter MW, van den Brink W. Predictors of acamprosate efficacy: results from a pooled analysis of seven European trials including 1485 alcohol-dependent patients. Psychopharmacology (Berl) 2005; 178:167–73.

124. Maxwell S, Shinderman M. Optimizing response to methadone maintenance treatment: use of higher dose methadone. J Psychoactive Drugs 1999; 31:95–102.

125. Weizman T, Gelkopf M, Melamed Y, Adelson M, Bleich A. Treatment of benzodiazepine dependence in methadone maintenance treatment patients: a comparison of two therapeutic modalities and the role of psychiatric comorbidity. Aust N Z J Psychiatry 2003; 37: 458–63.

126. Saxon AJ, Calsyn DA, Greenberg D, Blaes P, Haver VM, Stanton V. Urine screening for marijuana among methadone-maintained patients. J Addict 1993; 1:207–11.

127. Nirenberg TD, Cellucci T, Liepman MR, Swift RM, Sirota AD. Cannabis versus other illicit drug use among methadone maintenance patients. Psych Addict Beh 1996; 10:222–7.

128. Epstein DH, Preston KL. Does cannabis use predict poor outcome for heroin-dependent patients on maintenance treatment? Past findings and more evidence against. Addiction 2003; 98:269–79.

129. Schiff M, Levit S, Moreno RC. Retention and illicit drug use among methadone patients in Israel: a gender comparison. Addictive Behaviors 2007; 32:2108–19.

130. Morrison C, Ruben S, Beeching, N. Female sexual health problems in a drug dependency unit. Int J STD AIDS 1995; 6:201–3.

131. Harding C, Ritchie, J. Contraceptive practice of women with opiate addiction in a rural centre. Aust J Rural Health 2003; 11:2–6.

132. Bai J, Greenwald E, Caternini H, Kaminetzky HA. Drug-related menstrual aberrations. Obstet Gynecol 1974; 44:713–9.

133. Chrousos GP, Torpy DJ, Gold PW. Interactions between the hypothalamic-pituitary-adrenal axis and the female reproductive system: clinical implications. Ann Intern Med 1998; 129:229–40.

134. Warren, MP. Clinical review 77: Evaluation of secondary amenorrhea. J Clin Endocrinol Metab 1996; 81:437–42.

135. Schmittner J, Schroeder JR, Epstein DH, Preston KL. Menstrual cycle length during methadone maintenance. Addiction 2005; 100:829–36.

136. Fordyce EJ, Blum S, Balanon A, Stoneburner RL. A method for estimating HIV transmission rates among female sex partners of male intravenous drug users. Am J Epidemiol 1991; 133:590–8.

137. World Health Organization. Selected practice recommendations for contraceptive use, 2nd ed. 2004. Available at www.who.int/reproductive-health/publications/spr/index.htm.

138. World Health Organization. Medical eligibility criteria for contraceptive use, 3rd ed. 2004. Available at www.who.int/reproductive-health/publication/mec.

139. Tuchman E. Exploring the prevalence of menopause symptoms in midlife women in methadone maintenance treatment. Soc Work Health Care 2007; 45:43–62.

140. Lev-Wiesel R, Shuval R. Perceived causal and treatment factors related to substance abuse: gender differences. Eur Addict Res 2006; 12:109–12.

141. Rowan-Szal GA, Chatham LR, Joe GW, Simpson DD. Services provided during methadone treatment: a gender comparison. J Subst Abuse Treat 2000; 19:7–14.

142. Brewer DD, Fleming CB, Haggerty KP, Catalano RF. Drug use predictors of partner violence in opiate-dependent women. Violence Vict 1998; 13:107–15.

143. Chermack ST, Fuller BE, Blow FC. Predictors of expressed partner and non-partner violence among patients in substance abuse treatment. Drug Alcohol Depend 2000; 58:43–54.

144. El-Bassel N, Gilbert L, Frye V, Wu E, Go H, Hill J, Richman BL. Physical and sexual intimate partner violence among women in methadone maintenance treatment. Psychol Addict Behav 2004; 18:180–3.

145. El-Bassel N, Gilbert L, Wu E, Go H, Hill J. Relationship between drug abuse and intimate partner violence: a longitudinal study among women receiving methadone. Am J Public Health 2005; 95:465–70.

146. Caetano R, Nelson S, Cunradi C. Intimate partner violence, dependence symptoms and social consequences from drinking among white, black and Hispanic couples in the United States. Am J Addict 2001(Suppl); 60–9.

147. Tjaden P, Thoennes N. Extent, nature, and consequences of intimate partner violence: findings from the National Violence Against Women Survey. Research in Brief. Washington, DC: United States Department of Justice, 2000:7.

148. Branstetter SA, Bower EH, Kamien J, Amass L. A history of sexual, emotional, or physical abuse predicts adjustment during opioid maintenance treatment. J Subst Abuse Treat 2008; 34:208–14.

149. Clark HW, Masson CL, Delucchi KL, Hall SM, Sees KL. Violent traumatic events and drug abuse severity. J Subst Abuse Treat 2001; 20:121–7.

150. Lincoln AK, Liebschutz JM, Chernoff M, Nguyen D, Amaro H. Brief screening for co-occurring disorders among women entering substance abuse treatment. Subst Abuse Treat Prev Policy 2006; 1:1–9.

Gender Issues in the Pharmacotherapy of Opioid-Addicted Women: Buprenorphine

Annemarie Unger, MD
Erika Jung, MD
Bernadette Winklbaur, PhD
Gabriele Fischer, MD

ABSTRACT. Gender, a biological determinant of mental health and illness, plays a critical role in determining patients' susceptibility, exposure to mental health risks, and related outcomes. Regarding sex differences in the epidemiology of opioid dependence, one third of the patients are women of childbearing age. Women have an earlier age of initiation of substance use and a more rapid progression to drug involvement and dependence than men. Generally few studies exist which focus on the special needs of women in opioid maintenance therapy. The aim of this paper is to provide an overview of treatment options for opioid-dependent women, with a special focus on buprenorphine, and to look at recent findings related to other factors that should be taken into consideration in optimizing the treatment of opioid-dependent women. Issues addressed include the role of gender in the choice of medication assisted treatment, sex differences in pharmacodynamics and pharmacokinetics of buprenorphine drug interactions, cardiac interactions, induction of buprenorphine in pregnant patients, the neonatal abstinence syndrome and breastfeeding. This paper aims to heighten the awareness for the need to take gender into consideration when making treatment decisions in an effort to optimize services and enhance the quality of life of women suffering from substance abuse.

INTRODUCTION: GENDER DIFFERENCES

In 2002, the World Health Organization passed its first Gender Policy, acknowledging gender as a fundamental human concern. At about the same time, the World Health Organization began using the UN's Millenium Development Goals, specifying more particularly that gender equality and the empowerment of women should be main goals worldwide.

Gender, a biological determinant of mental health and illness, intersects with and enlarges the differences associated with other important socioeconomic factors such as income, employment, and social position. Gender also differentially affects the power and control men and women have over these socioeconomic factors,

The authors thank the Austrian OENB (Project No. 9669) and the NIH (Grant Nr. 1R01 DA018417-01) for supporting our research.

their access to resources, and their status, roles, options, and treatment in society.

Gender plays a critical role in determining patients' susceptibility, exposure to mental health risks, and related outcomes.[1] Gender differences in rates of overall mental health are negligible, but they are highly significant for depression, anxiety and somatic complaints, as well as substance abuse disorders.[1] Lifetime prevalence rates of alcohol dependence are higher for men (20%) than for women (8%);[2] more generally, in 2003 men were found to be twice as likely to abuse an illicit drug than were women.[2] Gender differences are also found in patterns of help-seeking for psychological disorders. Men prefer to seek specialized mental health care and more frequently receive inpatient treatment than women, whereas women are more likely to seek help from their primary health care physician. Women are more likely to disclose emotional problems than men, whereas men are more likely to admit having an alcohol problem.[1]

Regarding gender differences in the epidemiology of opioid dependence, one-third of the patients are women of childbearing age.[3] Women have an earlier age of initiation of substance use and a more rapid progression to drug involvement and dependence than men.[4] Women expose themselves to more health risk factors, such as prostitution to secure drugs and sharing syringes, leading to a higher rate of new infections with HIV and other infectious diseases such as hepatitis.[5] Both opioid-dependent men and women show mortality rates 13 to 17 times higher than the general population, with slightly higher rates for men.[6] On the other hand, due to a higher vulnerability to the adverse consequences of these disorders, women also show a more rapid progression to treatment entry and consequently a lower number of years of active illicit substance abuse than men; however, despite this, women are still underrepresented in addiction treatment.[7]

Several gender-related issues related to the use of maintenance therapy for opioids dependence should be considered. It has been shown that women have a different opioid binding capacity than men, which will influence dosing regimens in opioid pharmacotherapy.[8] Additionally, specific dose changes have to be considered if the opioid-dependent patient becomes pregnant, especially in the last trimester, when hormonal enzyme induction often requires an elevation or splitting of the daily administered opioid dose.[9] In general, the more complicated hormonal status in women with individual levels of oestrogen/progesterone in the premenopausal (even considering the changes between pre- and post-ovulation) and postmenopausal women needs to be taken into account regarding interaction in the metabolism of medication. Detailed dosing information has been provided so far in the treatment of depression,[10] but not in the treatment of opioid dependence. It should also be noted that improved treatment approaches will lead to an aging population being on opioid pharmacotherapy for decades.[11]

Generally few studies exist which focus on the special needs of women in opioid maintenance therapy. The aim of this paper is to provide an overview of treatment options for opioid-dependent women, with a special focus on buprenorphine, and to look at recent findings related to other factors that should be taken into consideration in optimizing the treatment of opioid-dependent women.

THE ROLE OF GENDER IN THE CHOICE OF MEDICATION ASSISTED TREATMENT

Lack of data may explain why gender has rarely been considered a determinant when considering the choice of medication-assisted treatment for a specific patient. Jones et al. provided data derived from a randomized controlled study of gender differences in response to opioid agonist medications.[12] Opioid-dependent males (n = 104) and females (n = 61) were assigned to receive either levomethadyl acetate (LAAM) (75 to 115 mg), methadone (60 to 100 mg), or buprenorphine (16 to 32 mg) in flexible dosing schedules. Outcome measures included retention in treatment, percentage of positive illicit opioid urine samples, self-reported opioid use, and patient's rating of the current global severity of his or her opioid problem at the last interview before either discontinuation of the study medication or completing the study protocol. Although no significant disparities were observed in the study population among the three medication groups, some gender differences previously shown in the literature were verified.

In former studies, female opioid-dependent patients entering opioid agonist therapy were significantly more likely to be unemployed,[13–16] had a shorter duration of opioid addiction before starting treatment, and showed more psychiatric and family problems compared to males.[15,17,18] Co-occurring psychiatric problems, such as mood disorders and past and present sexual abuse, were seen more frequently in drug-dependent pregnant women compared to a control female population. Between 56% and 73% of opioid-dependent pregnant women suffer from a major psychiatric disorder according to DSM-IV.[19–22] In the substance-dependent patient, the effects of mood disorders are usually detrimental, resulting in patterns of harmful health behavior during pregnancy, post-partum depression, and consequences on mother-child interaction.[23,24] For women with a history of sexual trauma, key treatment times such as induction or delivery may lead to the occurrence of flashbacks and emotional instability; appropriately trained staff should be present to help patients cope with traumatic memories.[25] The high prevalence of co-occurring psychiatric disorders indicates that opioid-dependent women need to be examined and provided with appropriate and specific medications and other treatments.

Regarding illicit opioid consumption Jones et al.[12] showed that women receiving buprenorphine had significantly fewer opioid-positive urine samples compared to their male counterparts. Females receiving buprenorphine also had significantly fewer illicit opioid-positive urine samples than females receiving methadone. These results support the reported superior effects of buprenorphine in decreasing illicit opioid use.[13] In contrast to this, however, another study conducted by Johnson et al.[26] reported opposite results; women maintained on buprenorphine showed greater rates of illicit opioid use than men. These differences could be partially explained by different study designs, particularly different durations of assessment periods; Johnson et al.[26] investigated the patients for 14 days whereas Jones et al.[12] and Schottenfeld et al.[13] assessed the participants for 17 and 24 weeks, respectively.

One explanation for the findings of Jones et al.,[12] who found improved outcomes in women maintained on buprenorphine compared to men in regard to illicit opioid consumption, could be the superior effects of the unique pharmacology of buprenorphine (a partial mu-agonist/kappa-antagonist) combined with basic pharmacodynamic sex differences. Specifically, women of reproductive age may respond better to buprenorphine due to their higher mu-opiod and kappa-opioid receptor concentrations or unique differences in signal transduction compared to men.[12] Therefore, women in their reproductive years may predictably be more sensitive to mu-opiod and kappa-opioid medications than men.[8,27–29] Because levels of estradiol and progesterone both may influence the opioid mechanisms,[30–32] factors such as the phase of the menstrual cycle and age (i.e., menopause) may play an important role.[27,33]

GENDER DIFFERENCES IN THE PHARMACODYNAMICS AND PHARMACOKINETICS OF BUPRENORPHINE/DRUG INTERACTIONS

The pharmacokinetics and pharmacodynamics of psychotropic medications show substantial differences between male and female patients.[34–37] Many confounding factors (e.g., body weight, fat distribution, gastric absorption and emptying, and colonic transit times) seem to influence the metabolism of these drugs, but a complete understanding of these results remains elusive.[36] Most studies have shown that cytochrome P-450 (CYP) 3A4 activity is higher in women than in men,[38] while the activity of many other systems involved in drug metabolism (e.g., CYP2C19) seem to be higher in men than in women.[37] Furthermore, other studies have reported higher plasma levels of drugs metabolized by CYP1A2 in women.[37] In general, buprenorphine appears to have fewer significant drug interactions than methadone because it has low affinity for the 3A4 isoenzyme that is responsible for the metabolism of many drugs by the Cytochrome P-450 system.[39–41] When drug interactions do occur, they appear to increase the effects of buprenorphine (i.e., decreasing buprenorphine metabolism) and can be alleviated by a buprenorphine dose reduction. Similar to methadone,[42] concurrent intravenous or very high-dose use of buprenorphine and benzodiazepines is associated with overdose deaths.[43–46] The interaction mechanism does not appear to be pharmacokinetic but is more likely to be pharmacodynamic due to the fact that buprenorphine has a weak ability to inhibit the Cytochrom P-450 3A4 system.[47] Because the exact interaction of sublingually taken buprenorphine and orally consumed benzodiazepines is unclear, women put themselves at higher risk for medical complications because they are more likely to misuse benzodiazepines.[48]

BUPRENORPHINE AND CARDIAC INTERACTION

Special attention should be given to the recent discussion regarding cardiac complications of opioid medications, particularly taking gender differences into account.[49,50] QT-interval prolongation is a cardiac disorder characterized by abnormalities in cardiac repolarization resulting in prolongation of the QTc interval, T-wave changes, and torsade de pointes ventricular tachycardia (TdP).[50] TdP poses serious medical risks due to the risks of recurrence and sudden cardiac death. Women have a higher risk of developing a long QT syndrome (LQTS) because of the effect of the reproductive hormones on the electrophysiological structure of the heart.[49] While four membrane proteins produce electrical cardiac muscle activity, the KCNH2 channel binds with pharmacological substances to produce QTc interval prolongation.[50] Various prescription drugs, such as certain antipsychotics, antiarrhythmics, antibiotics, tricyclic antidepressants, and antifungals, are associated with risk of QTc interval prolongation due to the interference with the rapid component of the delayed rectifier potassium current, Ikr.[51,52] The human ether-à-go-go related gene (hERG) encodes for the major channel protein underlying IKr, and in vitro studies with hERG cell lines have successfully evaluated drugs suspected of leading to interval prolongation, especially in cardiac repolarization.[53] Methadone, buprenorphine, and many structurally diverse drugs can block the hERG,[51,54] resulting in a prolonged QTc interval.[55] Special caution is required in the prescription of drugs associated with QTc interval prolongation, especially if a combination of several is used.

LQTS can be either congenital or acquired due to medical conditions or drug exposure. Specific to drug-exposure, genetic polymorphisms may play a role in substance-induced LQTS.[56] Buprenorphine is less potent in blocking the hERG channel than methadone,[51] but nonetheless has been associated with QTc prolongation in electrocardiographic studies.[57] To date, two published direct comparisons of buprenorphine and methadone on QT interval prolongation exist. None of the 43 buprenorphine-maintained patients had prolonged QTc, whereas of 407 methadone-maintained patients, 28% of the men and 32% of the women showed QTc prolongation ($P = .002$).[57] Similarly, the second study showed that no buprenorphine-treated patients versus 23% of methadone-maintained patients had a QTc greater than 470 ms (men) or 490 ms (women) ($P < .001$). When compared with pre-drug baseline values, fewer buprenorphine (2%) than methadone (12%) participants had increases in QTc of more than 60ms ($P < .001$).[58] Prolonged QT intervals were also not found in a study of opioid-dependent subjects receiving Suboxone.[59]

INDUCTION OF BUPRENORPHINE IN PREGNANT PATIENTS

Buprenorphine treatment during pregnancy seems not to be associated with greater risk to the mother or embryo/fetus than treatment with methadone.[60–62] However, management of patients with buprenorphine can be more difficult, given the different pharmacology of the two medications. Unlike methadone, buprenorphine has the added complexity of possibly precipitating withdrawal. Methadone and buprenorphine cannot be used interchangeably and patients that are maintained on methadone are usually not good candidates for buprenorphine.[63]

For safety reasons, the use of the combination product (buprenorhpine/naloxone) cannot be recommended to pregnant patients. Pre-clinical data suggest that fetal naloxone exposure leads to maternal and subsequently fetal hormonal changes,[64,65] and that when buprenorphine/naloxone is crushed and injected the resulting maternal and fetal withdrawal symptoms are unfavorable to neonatal outcome. For patients stabilized on Suboxone, guidelines recommend transfer to Subutex following confirmation of pregnancy.[66] Only the combination product buprenorphine/naloxone (Suboxone) has been available in the United States for office-based prescription; the only exception to this has been for treatment of opioids-dependent pregnant women to whom the mono-product buprenorphine (Subutex) is administered.[67]

Due to the more complex pharmacology (mu partial agonist/kappa antagonist) of buprenorphine, induction may be more challenging than with methadone, especially if the patient is concomitantly consuming illicit drugs at the time of first assessment. A substantial risk of precipitating significant withdrawal exists if the first dose of buprenorphine is too high or if it is administered too soon after the last opioid intake (prior to manifestation of clinical symptoms of opioids withdrawal, which may be many hours if long acting opioids were used). As with methadone, it is important to ensure that the buprenorphine dose is not too low; an inadequate dose will not alleviate or prevent withdrawal symptoms before the next dose is due.[63,68]

Transition from slow-release oral morphine or methadone to buprenorphine in opioid-dependent pregnant patients has resulted in a "transient dysphoric mood status," which lasted 2 days.[69] Waiting at least 6 hours following short-acting opioid cessation to administer buprenorphine (usually some objective signs of opioid withdrawal can be found) has been found to improve the tolerability of induction onto buprenorphine.[70]

Finding the right timing for the initial buprenorphine dose is more difficult for patients taking long-acting opioids (e.g., slow-release oral morphine and methadone). Although only a few reports have been published, it is possible (but not recommended) to transition pregnant women from methadone directly to buprenorphine.[63] When women in the second or third trimester were transferred from oral methadone (up to 85 mg) doses to sublingual buprenorphine (up to 12 mg), the most frequent adverse effects reported were dysphoric mood[71,72] and "clear headed" status.[73]

Experience with pregnant women has demonstrated that rapid induction onto 12 to 14 mg of buprenorphine in 2 to 3 days can be accomplished in pregnant women.[60,61] Administering rapid-release morphine for a period of 3 days prior to buprenorphine induction seems to be beneficial for patients previously maintained on methadone. An optimal dose should be administered based on the severity of withdrawal symptoms. The fact that buprenorphine is less likely to cause sedation makes it safer for clinical use.

Complementary medications such as certain antihistamines (i.e., hydroxyzin or diphenhydramine) can be administered to ease most symptoms of withdrawal regardless of whether patients are inducted onto methadone or buprenorphine.

BUPRENORPHINE AND PREGNANCY

Because the majority of women treated for opioid addiction in maintenance programs are of childbearing age, the use of opioids during pregnancy is continuing to be a clinical challenge. Both methadone and buprenorphine are approved to treat opioid addiction in non-pregnant patients, but sufficient data regarding the use of both buprenorphine and methadone during pregnancy are currently lacking. Because of the absence of sufficient randomized clinical trial data in pregnant women to document safety and efficacy, both methadone and buprenorphine are classified as FDA pregnancy category C medications (e.g., well-controlled pregnancy studies are not available, so medication should be used during pregnancy only if the potential benefit justifies the potential fetal risk).[74] The benefits of methadone maintenance during pregnancy compared to detoxification have been well established.[75] Detoxification is usually associated with relapse and marked fluctuations of serum methadone levels, both of which are unfavorable to fetal outcome.

Methadone maintenance treatment (MMT) has been shown to reduce complications of pregnancy, childbirth, and infant development in the treatment of pregnant opiate-dependent women, and detoxification is generally not indicated.[76] The clinical effectiveness of MMT for opioid dependent non-pregnant adults is conclusive; reductions in HIV risk behaviors, mortality, levels of crime rates, and positive outcomes on drug use have been demonstrated.[77,78] Despite compelling evidence supporting the use of methadone in pregnancy, MMT during pregnancy is not without side effects. Methadone administration appears to alter fetal activity and heart rate,[79,80] and neonatal abstinence syndrome following methadone exposure is more common than with heroin exposure.[81]

With the increased use of buprenorphine maintenance in women, data supporting its efficacy have now been published. In addition to short retrospective reports, most of the evidence-based studies involve direct comparisons of buprenorphine and methadone, as well as other retrospective reports. The first open-label study with buprenorphine during pregnancy was performed by Fischer et al. in 2000;[71] 15 opioid dependent inpatient pregnant women underwent induction with 1 to 10 mg of sublingual buprenorphine followed by outpatient management. Efficacy in terms of maternal and fetal safety, as well as positive results on all birth outcome measures, were demonstrated. Neonatal abstinence was not observed in 8 infants, was mild with no treatment in 4 infants, and moderate requiring treatment in the remaining 3 infants. These promising results should be considered in light of study imitations, such as open design, lack of controls, and small patient sample.[71] In a prospective study design, research supporting the safety of buprenorphine during pregnancy was published by Schindler et al. detailing two pregnancies from conception through the postpartum period. Neither of the infants exposed to buprenophine experienced pregnancy-related complications, the birth outcomes were considered normal, and neither infant developed neonatal abstinence signs (NAS).[82]

A comparative, multicenter clinical study of high-dose buprenorphine versus methadone maintenance (259 pregnant women; 101 [39%] methadone maintenance and 158 [61%] high-dose buprenorphine) by LeJeune et al.[62] found no major difference between the groups in perinatal prognosis. The only differences found were a higher rate of prematurity in the methadone group that could also be explained by other confounding factors and a mean age at onset of neonatal withdrawal syndrome for the methadone group of 81 hours versus 66 hours ($P = .066$) for the buprenorphine group.[62]

Ebner et al. prospectively compared three groups of neonates following intrauterine exposure to either methadone, buprenorphine or slow-release morphine with no concomitant use: 32 of 53 neonates required treatment for NAS (15 of 22 in the methadone-maintained group, 14 of 17 in the morphine-maintained group, and 3 of 14 in the buprenorphine-maintained group). The mean duration from birth to requirement of NAS treatment was 33 hours for the morphine-exposed group, 34 hours for the buprenorphine-exposed group, and 58 hours for the methadone-exposed group. Buprenorphine had a significant lower incidence of NAS appearance compared to the other groups.[83]

Buprenorphine has been successfully used in this population over the past decade, and although reports in more than 500 neonates exposed prenatally (0.4 to 24 mg sublingually) have been published showing no increased risk of teratogenic effects and a low rate of prematurity,[74] randomized controlled trials of buprenorphine in pregnant women with a large enough sample size have not been conducted yet. A summary of 31 published reports of buprenorphine exposure during pregnancy is shown in Table 1.[74]

The data are limited in their significance, however, by several confounding factors: (1) although 86% of reports noted other maternal drug use, the use of concomitant medication or abuse of other substances was rarely reported in detail, making it difficult to assess the impact of buprenorphine on the neonatal abstinence syndrome; (2) the type of treatment

TABLE 1. Summary of Studies of Buprenorphine Exposure During Pregnancy (Multiple publications of the same neonates combined as one report) (Jones et al.)

Author, Year	Type of Study	Number of Buprenorphine-Exposed Neonates Reported	Number Treated for NAS	Other Drug Use[a]
Fischer et al., 2000	Prospective	15	3	Yes
Johnson et al., 2001	Prospective	3	0	No
Rohrmeister et al., 2001	Prospective	16	3	Not reported
Gourarier et al., 2001 Lejeune et al., 2001 Lejeune et al., 2002 LeJeune et al., 2005	Prospective	159	83	Yes
Schindler et al., 2003	Prospective	2	0	No
Lacroix et al., 2004	Prospective	31	8	Yes
Jones et al., 2005	Prospective	10	2	Yes
Gordon et al., 2005	Prospective	32	18	Yes
Fischer et al., 2006	Prospective	8	5	Yes
Reisinger 1995	Case Reports	4	0	No
Mazurier et al., 1996	Case Reports	6	6	Yes
Marquet et al., 1997 Marquet et al., 1998	Case Reports	6	2	Yes
Dos Santos et al., 1998	Case Reports	12	11	Yes
Regini et al., 1998	Case Reports	1	1	Yes
Herve & Quernum 1998	Case Reports	1	1	Yes
Jernite et al., 1998 Jernite et al., 1999	Case Reports	24	16	Yes
Burlet et al., 1999	Case Reports	14	8	Yes
Auriacombe et al., 1999 Loustauneau et al., 2000 Auriacombe et al., 2001	Case Reports	16	5	Yes
Marquet et al., 2002	Case Reports	21	10	Yes
Kayemba-Kay 2003	Case Reports	13	10	Yes
Siedentopf, 2004	Case Reports	33	20	Yes
Noblet 2000	Case Reports	27	?	Not reported
Ross, 2004	Case Reports	1	?	Not reported
TOTAL		455	212 of 427 (50%)	

[a]Such as self-reported or verified by urine toxicology.

setting and length of fetal drug exposure were not homogeneous, and most reports were retrospective, open-label, and had no appropriate control groups; most important, the lack of details regarding neonatal treatment and the small sample size limit the applicability of any conclusions. Moreover, different scoring systems (e.g., see Finnegan[84]or Lipsitz[85]), were used to assess NAS treatment efficacy.[87]

With the ultimate goal of establishing international, state of the art, standardized treatment recommendations for pregnant opioid-dependent women, research trials have focused on neonatal outcomes for neonates exposed to methadone/buprenorphine. The two previous small sample size, randomized controlled trials comparing methadone and buprenorphine in a double-blind double-dummy design[60,61] show a shorter intensity and duration of NAS for buprenorphine. As a result of these two randomized controlled trials, a new multisite study has been designed: The Maternal Opioid Treatment: Human Experimental Research (MOTHER) project, which is an eight-site randomized, double-blind, double-dummy, flexible dosing, and parallel group clinical trial that is currently in progress.[74] Five primary outcome measures were chosen for examination based on the results of the pilot studies: (1) NAS; (2) number of neonates requiring treatment; (3)

amount of medication needed to treat NAS; (4) head circumference; and, (5) length of hospital stay. Based on the pilot studies, the MOTHER study hypothesizes that buprenorphine will produce a superior outcome for all five variables. Because the influence of pregnancy on the pharmacokinetics and pharmacodynamics of buprenorphine and methadone is not yet fully understood, detailed research questions such as the effects of co-morbid substance abuse, concomitant medications, and nicotine on NAS and breastfeeding will be addressed in the MOTHER study.

NEONATAL ABSTINENCE SYNDROME

Intrauterine exposure to opioids or other psychopharmacological medications can produce NAS in the neonate in the first hours and days after delivery. Signs of NAS are usually seen in the central nervous system, autonomic nervous system, gastrointestinal tract, and respiratory system. Intrauterine exposure to buprenorphine during pregnancy also results in NAS in more than 50% of exposed newborns.[62] The onset, nature, and treatment of buprenorphine-associated NAS are comparable but somewhat milder than that associated with methadone.[62,86]

The severity and duration of NAS should be assessed by close clinical observation and monitoring of the newborn using an "abstinence scoring system." This system assigns points to each abstinence-associated sign and serves as a guide to treatment. Once a predetermined minimum score is reached, treatment is begun, usually with replacement opiate therapy. Weaning can begin once the neonate is assessed to be clinically stable on a set dosage for at least 48 hours.[60] Seminal work with regards to perinatal addiction has been published over decades by Finnegan et al. with an in-depth focus on the neonatal consequences of intrauterine substance exposure, resulting in the widespread adoption of the "Finnegan-scoring-system" for neonates.[87] The concomitant use of legal and illegal substances such as opiates, nicotine, cocaine, alcohol, and other specific medications, such as antidepressants, play a key role among the factors influencing NAS appearance, severity and duration.

The onset of buprenorphine-associated NAS is usually observed within the first 12 to 72 hours after delivery, reaching its peak severity within 66 to 96 hours and lasting approximately 120 to 168 hours. Considerable individual variability in abstinence exists; a reported protracted withdrawal syndrome has been seen in a few infants who exhibited withdrawal signs for 6 to 10 weeks following delivery. This extended withdrawal could be due to both the NAS medication and the regimen used to treat withdrawal rather than a direct effect of buprenorphine.[74]

The debate as to whether a correlation exists between the maternal maintenance dosage of opioids and the occurrence and severity of NAS began in the late 1960s, when methadone was first accepted as a method of treatment for opioid-dependent pregnant women. Based on existing data, Ostrea et al. made the recommendation in 1976 that at least 1 month before delivery mothers should be placed on a low-dose regiment of less than 20 mg methadone per day to help prevent serious neonatal withdrawal.[88] The controversy continued, and in 2002, Dashe et al. reported that 90% of infants whose mothers had taken more than 40 mg/day of methadone required treatment for NAS, compared to 44% of infants whose mothers had taken 20 to 39 mg/day of methadone and 12% of infants whose mothers took less than 20 mg/day.[89] However, this finding lacked a clear research design, was retrospective, and no standardized urine toxicology was performed to examine the concomitant consumption of illicit drugs. In contrast, Berghella et al. published a report on 100 methadone-maintained pregnant women and their neonates that found no correlation between methadone dosage (doses of more than 80 mg/day and less than 80 mg/day) and both the need for and duration of NAS treatment.[90] As in many previous studies, however, results should not be considered conclusive because concomitant use of legal and illegal substances was not taken into account.

In a recent retrospective study of 66 methadone-maintained patients, Lim studied the relationship between maternal dosage at delivery and neonatal abstinence.[91] Dosage groups included <70 mg in 23 women, 71 to 139 mg in 26 women, and >140 mg in 17 women. A higher dosage of methadone was associated with a higher incidence and duration of NAS; every increase of 5.5 mg of methadone in the mother was coupled statistically with 1 additional day of NAS treatment for the infant. Studies suggest that the main variable affected by higher dosage may not be appearance of NAS itself but rather its duration, and that both the occurrence and duration of NAS may be mitigated by a reduction of methadone dosages in motivated mothers.[91] However, conclusions drawn from this study are also limited because it is retrospective and no standardized urine toxicology was collected for assessing concomitant substances consumed.

The debate over maternal methadone treatment may be considered in one major context: which has the greater impact on NAS—high dosages of maternal maintenance opioids or the often-seen concomitant illicit use of other substances when women are treated with an inadequate dose of methadone to achieve clinical stability? In one study, McCarthy et al.[92] reported that pregnant patients receiving mean daily methadone doses of 132 mg had less illicit drug use at delivery and their neonates had no more severe NAS than expectant mothers receiving mean doses of 62 mg of methadone. Higher incidences of illicit drug abuse occurred in women who were receiving less than 80 mg/day than in women receiving more than 80 mg/day. It is generally felt that concomitant use of illicit drugs increases the severity of NAS, one factor cited in promoting the use of higher maintenance dosages for pregnant women.

Few reports exist on the correlation between maternal buprenophine dosages and the incidence, severity, and duration of NAS in exposed neonates. In a recent population-based comparison of 47 consecutive, prospectively followed buprenorphine-exposed pregnancies to 35 retrospectively analyzed consecutive methadone-exposed pregnancies, Kakko et al.[93] reported significant advantages with buprenorphine treatment in terms of birth weight and incidence of NAS requiring pharmacological treatment compared to methadone. The average maternal dosage was 15.4 ± 6.4 mg of buprenorphine and 71.3 ± 27.3 mg of methadone; 14.9% of the buprenorphine-exposed group and 52.8% of the methadone maintained group developed NAS requiring pharmacological treatment. Kakko et al. argued that the key to lowering NAS rates was the successful clinical management of substance use, which usually involved higher maintenance dosage.[93] Further supporting this viewpoint, a Finnish study of 67 women maintained on buprenorphine where tapering doses or even abstinence from buprenorpine was encouraged (mean dose of buprenorphine at time of birth, 4.3 mg), resulted in a NAS incidence of 76%, with 57% requiring treatment.[94] This low maintenance dosage was linked to a low retention rate and higher rates of illicit use, both of which are unfavorable to NAS occurrence. To date, only one report has found a positive correlation between maternal buprenorphine dose and the severity of the NAS;[95] this finding pertained only to the maximum Lipsitz score. Other more recent reports[60,61] and one that included a large sample size[62] have reported no such correlation.

All of these results strongly suggest that pregnant women should be treated with dosages of methadone or buprenorphine that adequately treat their addiction. Concerns regarding the impact of higher therapeutic dosages on NAS do not seem to be warranted based on available clinical data. The variability of NAS, however, mandates that close clinical surveillance of the neonate and infant should be maintained. It is hoped that the MOTHER study comparing methadone and buprenorphine in pregnant women, will shed further light on this subject.

BUPRENORPHINE AND BREAST FEEDING

An issue naturally related to opioid treatment during pregnancy is that of breastfeeding. The plasma to milk ratio for buprenorphine is approximately 1 because it is excreted in breast milk and levels are similar or higher than levels found in the blood.[96] Given this information, the total daily amount of buprenorphine consumed by the infant can be estimated. Due to the low oral bioavailability of buprenorphine, the actual infant exposure is only 1/5 to 1/10 of the total amount of buprenorphine ingested. The low oral bioavailability of buprenorphine also explains why levels in breast milk may have little effects on NAS.[97]

For methadone, recent reports have confirmed earlier findings that breastfeeding could serve as a means of diminishing duration of methadone associated NAS,[98,99] both from comfort obtained through mother/child bonding[91]and from the oral bioavailability of methadone. If methadone-maintained women wish to breastfeed and no specific contraindicationexist, such as certain infectious diseases and illicit drug use, physicians should support their decision.[100] For buprenorphine, although similar recommendations might be valid, these guidelines are based on shorter periods of observation and smaller numbers of investigated cases.[61,71]

CONCLUSION

Because data governing the use of buprenorphine are limited, significant gender-related differences in the epidemiology of opioid dependence and maintenance treatment, the pharmacodynamics and pharmacokinetics of buprenorphine, and its effects on cardiac physiology require future investigation. Promising evidence has suggested that neonatal abstinence following intrauterine exposure to buprenorphine may be less severe than that associated with methadone and that breastfeeding may be safely accomplished with buprenorphine maintenance, but more evidence is required to support these findings. Data obtained from the international MOTHER study will soon be available to shed light on whether methadone or buprenorphine should be the preferred treatment of choice for pregnant opioid-dependent women.

Buprenorphine is gaining recognition as an effective treatment for opioid dependence. The drug is well tolerated, and due to its partial agonist properties, appears to be a safe therapeutic option, especially because the severe side effects, such as respiratory depression seen with other opioids, develop only with severe overdosing with buprenorphine.[101] Individuals who have been well stabilized on buprenorphine face the risk of clinical destabilization if that medication is changed during pregnancy. The same concern applies to the fetus, which is dependent on maternal medications for intrauterine homeostasis.

The fact that relatively few gender studies exist in the field of drug dependence may be partially explained by the fact that men have had a higher rate of substance abuse than women, although the gap has been closing in recent years.[102] In addition, women are more expensive and difficult to study due to the added complexity of hormonal interactions in the reproductive years, the special requirements of postmenopausal medication response, and the unique condition of pregnancy.

The understanding of gender issues is important in the treatment of opioid dependence for several reasons. Optimizing treatment outcomes in terms of retention and completion requires consideration of barriers to treatment access and entry that are specific to women, such as lack of child care, lack of services for pregnant women, fear of losing custody when the baby is born, fear of prosecution, voyeurism, and sexual harassment.[103] In addition, treatment settings that are designed for a predominantly male population may not adequately deal with gender-specific social factors such as intimate partner violence by a co-dependent partner, unplanned pregnancy, and higher rates of sex-related risk behavior with a consequence of infectious disease.[104–106] Significant psychiatric co-morbidity, such as affective disorders, eating disorders, and posttraumatic stress disorders following sexual trauma, add to the complex challenge of attaining treatment success in women with substance abuse problems.[103,107–109]

Critical assessment of the current regimens of pharmacological treatment of opioids dependence is needed because gender and age considerations have often been neglected in treatment decision making. Public-funded studies and pharmaceutical supported drug trials are urgently needed to provide a better understanding of the gender-related differences in response to psychopharmacological medication. Women constitute a unique study group, especially under circumstances of pregnancy and child care. Optimizing treatment effectiveness for opioid-dependent women across the life cycle of teenage, child bearing age, midlife, and old age should be a goal for the international community of opioid maintenance treatment researchers, improving services and enhancing the quality of life for women suffering from substance abuse.

REFERENCES

1. World Health Organization, Department of Mental Health and Substance Dependence. Gender disparities in mental health: 2002. Available at: www.who.int/mental_health/media/en/242.pdf.

2. National Survey on Drug Use and Health. Gender differences in substance dependence and abuse. SAMHSA 2003. Available at: http://oas.samhsa.gov/2k4/genderDependence/genderDependence.htm.

3. Fischer G, Eder H. Interdisciplinary therapeutic approaches with substance abusers taking into consideration gender differences. Wien Med Wochensch 1999; 149: 331–6.

4. Zilberman M, Tavares H, el-Guebaly, N. Gender similarities and differences: the prevalence and course of alcohol- and other substance-related disorders. J Addict Dis 2003; 22:61–74.

5. Maher L, Jalaludin B, Chant KG, Jayasuriya R, Sladden T, Kaldor JM, Sargent PL. Incidence and risk factors for hepatitis C seroconvulsion in injection drug users in Australia. Addiction 2006; 10:1499–1508.

6. Bauer SM, Loipl R, Jagsch R, Gruber D, Risser D, Thau K, FischerG. Mortality in opioid-maintained patients after release from an addiction clinic. Eur Addict Res 2008; 14:82–91.

7. Hernandez-Avila C, Rounsaville B, Kranzler H. Opioid-, cannabis- and alcohol-dependent women show more rapid progression to substance abuse treatment. Drug Alcohol Depend 2004; 74:265–72.

8. Zubieta JK, Dannals RF, Frost JJ. Gender and age differences on human brain mu-opioid receptor binding measured by PET. Am J Psychiatry 1999; 156:842–48.

9. Pond SM, Kreek MJ, Tong TG, Raghunath J, Benowitz NL. Altered methadone pharmacokinetics in methadone-maintained pregnant women. J Pharmacol Exp Ther 1985; 233:1–6.

10. Kornstein SG, Schatzberg AF, Thase ME, Yonkers KA McCullough JP, Keitner GI, Gelenberg AJ, Davis SM, Harrison WM, Keller MB. Gender differences in treatment response to sertraline versus imipramine in chronic depression. Am J Psychiatry 2000; 157:1445–52.

11. Goldberg RJ, Grabowski R. Methadone maintenance: its future in skilled nursing facilities. J Am Med Dir Assoc 2003; 4:98–100.

12. Jones HE, Fitzgerald Heather, Johnson Rolley E. Males and females differ in response to opioid agonist medications. Am J Addict 2005; 14:223–33.

13. Schottenfeld RS, Pakes JR, Kosten TR. Prognostic factors in buprenorphine- versus methadone-maintained patients. J Nerv Ment Dis 1998; 186:35–43.

14. Petry NM, Bickel WK. Gender differences in hostility of opioid-dependent outpatients: role in early treatment termination. Drug Alcohol Depend 2000; 58:27–33.

15. Karuntzos GT, Caddell JM, Dennis ML. Gender differences in vocational needs and outcomes for methadone treatment clients. J Psychoactive Drugs 1994; 26:173–80.

16. Hser YI, Anglin MD, Liu Y. A survival analysis of gender and ethnic differences in responsiveness to methadone maintenance treatment. Int J Addict 1990–1991; 25:1295–315.

17. Anglin MD, Hser YI, Booth MW. Sex differences in addict careers: 4. Treatment. Am J Drug Alcohol Aubse 1987; 13:253–80.

18. Zhang Z, Friedmann PD, Gerstein DR. Does retention matter? Treatment duration and improvement in drug use. Addiction 2003; 98:673–84.

19. Burns K, Melamed J, Burns W, Chasnoff I, Hatcher R. Chemical dependence and clinical depression in pregnancy. Journal of Clinical Psychology 1985; 41:851–4.

20. Fitzsimons HE, Tuten M, Vaidya V, Jones HE. Mood disorders affect drug treatment success of drug-dependent pregnant women. J Subst Abuse Treat 2007; 32:19–25.

21. Haller DL, Kinsley JS, Dawson KS. Perinatal substance abusers. Psychological and social characteristics. J Nerv Ment Dis 1993;181:509–513.

22. Regan D, Leifer B, Matteucci, T, Finnegan L. Depression in pregnant drug dependent women. NIDA Research Monograph 1982; 41:466–72.

23. Bonari L, Pinto N, Ahn E, Einarson A, Steiner M, Koren G. Perinatal risks of untreated depression during pregnancy. Can J Psychiat 2004; 49:726–35.

24. Cohen LS, Nonacs R, Viguera AC, Reminick A. Diagnosis and treatment of depression during pregnancy. CNS Spectrums 2004; 9:209–15.

25. Records K, Rice MJ. A comparative study of postpartum depression in abused and nonabused women. Arch Psychiat Nurs 2005; 19:281–90.

26. Johnson RE, Eissenberg T, Stitzer ML, Strain EC, Liebson IA, Gibelow GE. Buprenorphine treatment of opioid dependence : clinical trial of daily versus alternate-day dosing. Drug Alcohol Depend 1995; 40:27–35.

27. Zubieta JK, Smith YR, Bueller JA, Xu Y, Kilbourn MR, Jewett DM, Meyer CR, Koeppe RA, Stohler CS. Mu-opioid receptro-mediated antinociceptive responses differ in men and women. J Neurosc 2002; 22:5100–7.

28. Gear RW, Miaskowski C, Gordon NC, Paul SM, Heller PH, Levine JD. Kappa–opioids produce significantly greater analgesia in women than in men. Nat Med 1996; 2:1248–50.

29. Kreek MJ, Schluger J, Borg L, Gunduz M, Ho A. Dynorphin A1-13 causes elevation of serum levels of prolactin through an opioid receptor mechanism in humans: gender differences and implications for modulation

of dopaminergic tone in the treatment of addictions. J Pharmacol Exp Ther 1999; 288:260–9.

30. Eckersell C, Popper P, Micevych P. Estrogen-induced alteration of mu-opioid receptor immunoreactivity in the medial preoptic nucleus and medial amygdale. J Neurosci 1998; 18:3967–76.

31. Smith Y, Zubieta J, Del Carmen M, Dannals R, Ravert H, Zacur H, Frost J. Brain μ-opioid receptor measurements by posiron eission tomography in normal cycling women: relationship to LH pulsatility and gonadal steroid hormones. J Clin Endocrinol Metab 1998; 83: 4498–505.

32. Sinchak K, Micevych P. Progesterone blockade of estrogen activation of μ-opioid receptors regulates reproductive behavior. J Neurosci 2001; 21:5723–9.

33. Craft RM. Sex differences in opioid analgesia: "from mouse to men." Clin J Pain 2003; 19:161–86.

34. Dawkins K, Potter WZ. Gender differences in pharmacokinetics and pharmacodynamics of psychotropics: focus on women. Psychophrmacol Bull 1991; 27: 417–26.

35. Kornstein SG, Wojcik BA. Gender effects in the treatment of depression. Psychiatr Clin North Am 2000; 7:23–57.

36. Frackiewicz EJ, Sramek JJ, Cutler NR. Gender differences in depression and antidepressant pharmacokinetics and adverse events. Ann Pharmacother 2000; 34:80–8.

37. Yonkers KA, Kando JC, Cole JO, Blumenthal S. Gender differences in pharmacokinetics and pharmacodynamics of psychotropic medication. Am J Psychiatry 1992; 149:587–95.

38. Harris RZ, Benet LZ, Schwartz JB. Gender effects in pharmacokinetics and pharmacodynamics. Drugs 1995; 50:222–39.

39. Iribarne C, Dreano Y, Bardou LG, Menes JF, Berthou F. Interaction of methadone with substrates of human hepatic cytochrome P450 3A4. Toxicology 1997; 117:13–23.

40. Iribarne C, Picart D, Dreano Y, Berthou F. In vitro interactions between fluoxetine or fluvoxamine and methadone or buprenorphine. Fundam Clin Pharmacol 1998; 12:194–9.

41. Iribarne C, Berthou F, Carlhant D, Dreano Y, Picart D, Lohezic F, Riche C. Inhibition of methadone and buprenorphine N-dealkylations by three HIV-1 protease inhibitors. Drg Metab Dispos 1998; 26:257–60.

42. Ernst E, Bartu A, Popescu A, Ileutt KF, Hansson R, Plumley N. Methadone-related deaths in Western Australia 1993-99. Aust NZ J Publ Heal 2002;26,364–370.

43. Kintz P. A new series of 13 buprenorphine-related deaths. Clin Biochem 2002; 35:513–6.

44. Kintz P. Buprenorphine-related deaths. In: Kintz P, Marquet P, eds. Buprenorphine therapy of opiate addiction. Totowa: Humana Press, 2002:109–18.

45. Reynaud M, Petit G, Potard D, Courty P. Six deaths linked to concomitant use of buprenorphine and benzodiazepines. Addiction 1998; 93:1385–92.

46. Singh RA, Mattoo, SK, Malhotra A, Varma VK. Cases of buprenorphine abuse in India. Acta Psychiatry Scandinavia 1992; 86:46–8.

47. Kilicarslan T, Sellers EM. Lack of interaction of buprenorphine with flunitrazepam metabolism. Am J Psychiat 2000; 157:1164–6.

48. Kornstein S, Clayton AH (Eds.). Women's mental health: A comprehensive textbook. New York: The Guilford Press, 2002.

49. Bailey MS, Curtis AB. The effects of hormones on arrhythmias in women. Curr Womens Health Rep 2002; 2:83–8.

50. Ehret GB, Esmeules JA, Broers B. Methadone-associated long QT syndrome: improving pharmacotherapy for dependence on illegal opioids and lessons learned for pharmacology. Expert Opin Drug Saf 2007; 6:289–303.

51. Katchman AN, McGroary KA, Kilborn MJ, Kornick CA, Manfredi PL, Woosley RL, Ebert SN. Influence of opioid agonists on cardiac human ether-a-go-go-related gene K(+) currents. J Pharmacol Exp Ther 2002; 303:688–94.

52. Tseng GN. I(Kr): the hERG channel. J Mol Cell Cardiol 2001; 33:835–49.

53. Ferreira S, Crumb WJ Jr, Carlton CG, Clarkson CW. Effects of cocaine and its major metabolites on the HERG-encoded potassium channel. J Pharmacol Exp Ther 2001; 299:220–6.

54. Kornick CA, Kilborn MJ, Santiago-Palma J, Schulman G, Thaler HT, Keefe DL, Katchman AN, Pezzullo JC, Ebert SN, Woosley RL, Payne R, Manfredi PL. QTc interval prolongation associated with intravenous methadone. Pain 2003; 105:499–506.

55. Sanguinetti MC, Jiang C, Curran ME, Keating MT. A mechanistic link between an inherited and an acquired cardiac arrhythmia: HERG encodes the IKr potassium channel. Cell 1995; 81:299–307.

56. Roden DM. Taking the "idio" out of "idiosyncratic": Predicting torsades de pointes. Pacing Clin Electrophysiol 1998; 21:1029–34.

57. Fanoe S, Hvidt C, Ege P, Jensen GB. Syncope and QT prolongation among patients treated with methadone for heroin dependence in the city of Copenhagen. Heart 2007; 93:1051–5.

58. Wedam EF, Bigelow GE, Johnson RE, Nuzzo PA, Haigney MC. QT-Interval Effects of Methadone, Levomethadyl, and Buprenorphine in a Randomized Trial. Arch Intern Med 2007; 167:2469–75.

59. Baker JR, Best AM, Pade PA, McCance-Katz EF. Effect of buprenorphine and antiretroviral agents on the QT interval in opioid-dependent patients. Ann Pharmacother 2006;40:392–396.

60. Jones HE, Johnson RE, Jasinski DR, O'Grady KE, Chisholm CA, Choo RE, Crocetti M, Dudas R, Harrow C, Huestis MA, Jansson LM, Lantz M, Lester BM, Milio L. Buprenorphine versus methadone in the treatment of pregnant opioid-dependent patients: effects on the neonatal abstinence syndrome. Drug Alcohol Depen 2005; 79:1–10.

61. Fischer G, Ortner R, Rohrmeister K, Jagsch R, Baewert A, Langer M, Aschauer H. Methadone versus buprenorphine in pregnant addicts: a double-blind, double-dummy comparison study. Addiction 2006; 101:275–81.

62. LeJeune C, Simmat-Durand L, Gourarier L, Aubisson S, Groupe d'Etudes Grossesse et Addictions (GEGA). Prospective multicenter observational study of 260 infants born to 259 opiate-dependent mothers on methadone or high–dose buprenorphine substitution. Drug Alcohol Depend 2006; 82: 250–7.

63. Jones HE, Martin PR, Heil SH, Stine SM, Kaltenbach K, Selby P, Coyle MG, O'Grady KE, Arria AM, Fischer G. Treatment of opioid dependent pregnant women: clinical and research issues. J Subst Abuse Treat 2008; 35: 245–9.

64. Brunton PJ, Meddle SL, Ma S, Ochedalski T, Douglas AJ, Russell JA. Endogenous opioids and attenuated hypothalamic pituitary-adrenal axis responses to immune challenge in pregnant rats. J Neurosci 2005;2 5:5117–26.

65. Douglas AJ, Meddle SL, Toschi N, Bosch OJ, Neumann ID. Reduced activity of the noradrenergic system in the paraventricular nucleus at the end of pregnancy: implications for stress hyporesponsiveness. J Neuroendocrinol 2005; 17:40–8.

66. Center for Substance Abuse Treatment. Clinical guidelines for the use of buprenorphine in the treatment of opioid addiction. TIP series 40. DHHS Pub 04–3939. Rockville, MD: SAMHSA, 2004.

67. Center for Substance Abuse Treatment. US Department of Health and Human Services, Substance Abuse and Mental Health Services Administration 2000. Available at: www.buprenorphine.samsha.gov.

68. Lintzeris N, Ritter A, Dunlop A, Muhleisen P. Training primary health care professionals to provide buprenorphine and LAAM treatment. Substance Abuse 2002; 23:245–54.

69. Eder H, Fischer G, Gombas W, Jagsch R, Stuhlinger G, Kasper S. Comparison of buprenorphine and methadone maintenance in opiate addicts. European Addiction Research 1998; 4(Suppl 1):3–7.

70. Jones HE, Johnson RE, Jasinski DR, Milio L. Randomized controlled study transitioning opioid-dependent pregnant women from short-acting morphine to buprenorphine or methadone. Drug Alcohol Depend 2005; 78:33–8.

71. Fischer G, Johnson RE, Eder H, Jagsch R, Peternell A, Weninger M, Langer M, Aschauer HN. Treatment of opioid-dependent pregnant women with buprenorphine. Addiction 2000; 95:239–44.

72. Fischer G, Etzersdorfer P, Eder H, Jagsch R, Langer M, Weninger M. Buprenorphine maintenance in pregnant opiate addicts. Eur Addict Res 1998; 4(Suppl 1);32–6.

73. Jones HE, Suess P, Jasinski DR, Johnson RE. Transferring methadone-stabilized pregnant patients to buprenorphine using an immediate release morphine transition: an open-label exploratory study. Am J Addiction 2006; 15:61–70.

74. Jones HE, Arria AM, Baewert A, Heil SH, Kaltenbach K, Martin PR, Coyle MG, Selby P, Stine SM. Evolution and innovation in the agonist treatment of opioid-dependent pregnant women: development of a multi-center randomized controlled clinical trial maintenance in the addictions. J Opioid Management, in press.

75. Kandall SR, Doberczak TM, Jantunen M, Stein J. The methadone maintained pregnancy. Clin Perinatol 1999; 26:173–83.

76. Finnegan LP, Hagan T, Kaltenbach K. Scientific foundation of clinical practice: opiate use in pregnant women. Bull N Y Acad Med 1991; 67: 223–39.

77. Corsi KF, Lehman WK, Booth RE. The effect of methadone maintenance on positive outcomes for opiate inject drug users. J Subst Abuse Treat; doi:10.1016/j.jsat.2008.11.004.

78. Connock M, Juarez-Garcia A, Jowett S, Frew E, Liu Z, Taylor RJ, Fry-Smith A, Day E, Lintzeris N, Roberts T, Burls A, Taylor RS. Methadone and buprenorphine for the management of opioid dependence: a systematic review and economic evaluation. Health Technol Assess 2007; 11(9):1–171, iii-iv.

79. Jansson LM, Dipietro J, Elko A. Fetal response to maternal methadone administration. Am J Obstet Gynecol 2005; 193(3 Pt 1):611–7.

80. Ramirez-Cacho WA, Flores S, Schrader RM, McKay J, Rayburn WF. Effect of chronic maternal methadone therapy on intrapartum fetal heart rate patterns. J Soc Gynecol Invest 2006; 13: 108–11.

81. Chasnoff IJ, Landress HJ, Barrett ME. The prevalence of illicit drug-use during pregnancy and discrepancies in mandatory reporting in Pineitas County Florida. New Engl J Med 1990; 322:1202–6.

82. Schindler SD, Eder H, Ortner R, Rohrmeister K, Langer M. Neonatal outcome following buprenorphine maintenance during conception and throughout pregnancy. Addiction 2003; 98:103–10.

83. Ebner N, Rohrmeister K, Winklbaur B, Baewart A, Jagsch R, Peternell A, Thau K, Fischer G. Management of neonatal abstinence syndrome in neonates born to opioid maintained women. Drug Alcohol Depend 2007; 87(2-3):131–8.

84. Finnegan LP, Kron RE, Connaughton JF, Emich JP. Assessment and treatment of abstinence in the infant of the drug-dependent mother. Int J Clin Pharm Biophar 1975; 12:19–32.

85. Lipsitz PJ. A proposed narcotic withdrawal score for use with newborn infants: a pragmatic evaluation of its efficacy. Clin Pediatr 1961; 14:592–4.

86. Kaltenbach K. Exposure to opiates: behavioral outcomes in preschool and school age children. National Institute on Drug Abuse Monograph 164 1996; DHHS:230–41.

87. Finnegan LP, Kaltenbach K. Neonatal abstinence syndrome. In: Hoeckelman RA, Nelson NM, eds. Primary pediatric care, 2nd ed. St. Louis: Mosby Yearbook Inc., 1991:1367–78.

88. Ostrea EM, Chavez CJ, Strauss ME. A study of factors that influence the severity of neonatal narcotic withdrawal. J Pediatr 1976; 88:642–5.

89. Dashe JS, Sheffield JS, Olscher DA, ToddSJ, Jackson GL, Wendel GD. Relationship between maternal methadone dosage and neonatal withdrawal. Obstet Gynecol 2002; 200:1244–9.

90. Berghella V, Lim PJ, Hill MK, Cerpes J, Chennat J, Kaltenbach K. Maternal methadone dose and neonatal withdrawal. Am J Obstet Gynecol 2003; 189:312–7.

91. Lim S, Prasad M, Samuels P, Gardner D, Cordero L. High-dose methadone in pregnant women and its effect on duration of neonatal abstinence syndrome. Am J Obstet Gynecol 2009; 200(1): 70.e1–70.e5.

92. McCarthy JJ, Leamon MH, Parr MS, Anania B. High dose methadone maintenance in pregnancy: maternal and neonatal outcomes. Am J Obstet Gynecol 2005; 193:606–10.

93. Kakko J, Heilig M, Sarman I. Buprenorphine and methadone treatment of opiate dependence during pregnancy: Comparison of fetal growth and neonatal outcomes in two consecutive case series. Drug Alcohol Depend 2008; 96:69–78.

94. Kahila H, Saisto T, Kivitie-Kallio S, Haukkamaa M, Halmesmaki E. A prospective study on buprenorphine use during pregnancy: effects on maternal and neonatal outcome. Acta Obstet Gynecol Scand 2007; 86:185–90.

95. Marquet P, Lavignasse P, Gaulier J-M, Lachatre G. Case study of neonates born to mothers undergoing buprenorphine maintenance treatment. In: Kintz P, Marquet P, eds. Buprenorphine therapy of opiate addiction. Totowa, NJ: Human Press, 2002:125–35.

96. Johnson RE, Jones HE, Jasinski DR, Svikis DS, Haug NA, Jansson LM, Kissin WB, Alpan G, Lantz ME, Cone EJ, Wilkins DG, Golden AS, Huggins GR, Lester BM. Buprenorphine treatment of opioid dependent women: maternal and neonatal outcomes. Drug Alcohol Depend 2001; 63:97–103.

97. Auriacombe M, Loustauneau A. Medical treatment of the pregnant heroin addict: review of the literature. In: Pregnancy and drug misuse update, 2000. Proceedings: Seminar organized by the Co-operation Group to Combat Drup Abuse and Illicit Trafficking in Drugs (Pompidou Group), Strasbourg, France, May 29–30, 2000. Drugs and Addiction Council of Europe 2000;39–74.

98. Jansson L, Choo R, Velez ML, Harrow, C, Schroeder J, Shakleya D, Huestis M. Methadone maintenance and breastfeeding in the neonatal period. Pediatrics 2008; 121:106–14.

99. Abdel-Latif ME, Pinner J, Clews S, Cooke F, Lui K, Oei J. Effects of breast milk on the severity and outcome of neonatal abstinence syndrome among infants of drug-dependent mothers. Pediatrics 2006; 117:1163–9.

100. The American Academy of Physicians. Breastfeeding and infant nutrition. In: 1994-1995 Compendium of AAFP positions on selected health issues. Kansas City, MO: Author, 1996.

101. Davids E, Gastpar M. Buprenorphine in the treatment of opioid dependence. Eur Neuropsychopharm 2004; 14:209–16.

102. NSDUH report 2004, National Survey on Drug Use and Health Report, Office of Applied Studies, Substance Abuse and Mental Health Services Administration (SAMHSA). Available at: http://www.oas.samhsa.gov.

103. Tuchman E. Women and addiction: the importance of gender issues in substance abuse research. J Addict Dis 2010; 29:127–38.

104. Paltrow LM. Punishing women for their behavior during pregnancy: an approach that undermines the health of women and children. In: Wetherington CL, Roman AB, eds. Drug addiction research and the health of women. NIH Publication, No. 98–4290.Rockville, MD: National Institute on Drug Abuse; 1998:467–502.

105. Ayyagari S, Boles S, Johnson P, Kleber H. Difficulties in recruiting pregnant substance abusing women into treatment: problems encountered during the cocaine alternative treatment study. Assoc Health Serv Res 1999; 16:80–1.

106. DeAngelis T. Better research, more help needed for pregnant addicts. APA Monitor 1993; 24(9):7–8.

107. Denier CA, Thevos AK, Latham PK, Randall CL. Psychosocial and psychopathology differences in hospitalized male and female cocaine abusers: a retrospective chart review. Addict Behav 1991; 16:489–96.

108. Fornari VM, Kent J, Kabo L, Goodman B. Anorexia nervosa: "thirty something." J Subst Abuse Treat 1994; 11:45–54.

109. Najavits LM, Weiss RD, Shaw SR. The link between substance abuse and posttraumatic stress disorder in women. Am J Addict 1997; 6:273–83.

Punishing Pregnant Drug-Using Women: Defying Law, Medicine, and Common Sense

Jeanne Flavin, PhD
Lynn M. Paltrow, JD

ABSTRACT. The arrests, detentions, prosecutions, and other legal actions taken against drug-dependent pregnant women distract attention from significant social problems, such as our lack of universal health care, the dearth of policies to support pregnant and parenting women, the absence of social supports for children, and the overall failure of the drug war. The attempts to "protect the fetus" undertaken through the criminal justice system (as well as in family and drug courts) actually undermine maternal and fetal health and discourage efforts to identify and implement effective strategies for addressing the needs of pregnant drug users and their families. In this article, the authors seek to expose some of the flawed premises on which the arrests, detentions, and prosecutions are based. The authors highlight the inherent unfairness of a system that expects low-income and drug-dependent pregnant women to provide their fetuses with the health care and safety that these women themselves are not provided and have not been guaranteed.

INTRODUCTION

No human being, not even a parent or a twin, is required to sacrifice his or her life or health for the benefit of another individual.[i] Although the state may require sacrifices for the benefit of the community at large (e.g., vaccinations), U.S. courts have steadfastly refused to use state power to weigh the value of two individual lives and require one person to sacrifice his or her life, health, or liberty for another.[1] Nonetheless, claims made on behalf of individual fetuses have been used to justify deprivations of women's liberty,[ii] bodily integrity,[iii] and even their lives.[iv] Such actions reflect increasing and highly contested claims that not only does a fetus have "rights" that must be protected, but that these rights are superior to those of pregnant women and, for that matter, all human beings.

Significantly, these claims of fetal rights are often coupled with and strengthened by drug war propaganda which makes grossly exaggerated claims about the risks posed by prenatal exposure to certain substances. Indeed, the vast majority of punitive interventions based on claims of fetal rights involve the arrest and detention of

---

The research upon which this article was based was made possible in part with funding from the Reproductive Justice Fund of the Tides Foundation and the Ms. Foundation for Women. Some material for this article is drawn from the first author's book, *Our Bodies, Our Crimes: The Policing of Women's Reproduction in America* (New York: New York University Press, 2009), and the second author's previous writings including Pregnant Drug Users, Fetal Persons, and the Threat to *Roe v. Wade*, 62 ALBANY L. REV. 999-1055 (1999).

pregnant women alleged to have used an illegal drug or alcohol. These cases assert that pregnant women are obliged to subordinate themselves to state claims of fetal rights. In addition, these cases reinforce false and misleading ideas about addiction and its treatment and the availability of appropriate health services.

The arrests and other punitive measures levied against pregnant drug-using women also serve a larger political purpose: they distract attention from significant social problems, such as our lack of universal health care, the dearth of policies to support pregnant and parenting women, the absence of social supports for children, and the overall failure of the drug war.[2] Relying on punitive approaches undermines efforts to develop effective responses to the problematic aspects of drug use and pregnancy. In this article, we draw on information from hundreds of cases that National Advocates for Pregnant Women has compiled. We seek to expose some of the flawed premises on which these arrests, detentions, and prosecutions are based. In so doing, we highlight the injustice of expecting low-income and drug-dependent pregnant women to provide their fetuses with the health care and safety to which women themselves are not deemed to be entitled.

THE PANIC OVER DRUG-DEPENDENT WOMEN AND THEIR PREGNANCIES

The fear-mongering tenor of discourse surrounding women's drug use cannot be justified by women's rates of illicit drug use, drinking, and smoking. Most women in the United States use some type of drug on a regular basis. We use prescription and over-the-counter drugs to help us sleep, stay awake, alleviate pain, lose weight, cope with depression and anxiety, and so forth. We drink coffee and tea and eat chocolate, all substances that contain caffeine. We consume alcoholic beverages, and we smoke cigarettes. However, when we think of "women and drugs" what comes to mind are users of illegal drugs even though fewer than 1 in 10 women and only approximately 4 in 100 pregnant women use illicit drugs and even fewer are dependent on them.[v,3–5]

The drug war of the 1980s and 1990s included women who used illicit drugs among its targets. A national panic ensued over "crack mothers" giving birth to "crack babies."[6] Women who used illicit drugs (including marijuana, heroin, and methamphetamine, but particularly cocaine) were portrayed as hypersexual, out-of-control women who would "do anything" for drugs. They were characterized as being completely indifferent to any harm they might cause to themselves or others, especially the children they would give birth to.[6,7] At a time when evidence existed that there was no such thing as "crack babies" and that poverty explained many of the health problems that some children were experiencing, *Time* magazine, the *New York Times*, and other leading news outlets continued to describe cocaine use during pregnancy as an epidemic destroying a generation of young people. Even respected organizations such as Columbia University's Center on Addiction and Substance Abuse discussed the exposure of newborns to alcohol and cocaine in extraordinarily exaggerated and unjustified terms, describing it as "a slaughter of innocents of biblical proportions" (p. 7).[8]

As a consequence of this moral panic surrounding women using drugs, thousands of women were and continue to be ensnared in the criminal justice system for non-violent offenses related to their use of illegal drugs; hundreds more have been singled out specifically for being pregnant and using an illegal drug or alcohol.

Consider the case of Cornelia Whitner. On April 7, 1992, Cornelia Whitner was indicted for violating South Carolina's criminal child neglect statute for her alleged unlawful neglect of a "child."[vi] Ms. Whitner, an African American woman, was born and raised in South Carolina. At the age of 14, her mother suddenly died, an event which Ms. Whitner described as the worst thing that ever happened to her. After her mother's death, Ms. Whitner dropped out of school and started smoking pot and drinking. By age 15, she was pregnant with the first of her three children. Her youngest child, Tevin, was born in good health on February 2, 1992. When a test indicated that Tevin had been exposed prenatally to cocaine, Ms. Whitner was arrested and charged with criminal child neglect, even though she was not accused of actually abusing or endangering Tevin. Instead, the prosecutors introduced a new interpretation of an existing child neglect statute, asserting that the statute also criminalized a woman's failure "to provide proper medical care for her unborn child."[vii]

Like virtually all women who have been prosecuted under similar circumstances, Ms. Whitner could not afford private counsel. Instead, she was represented by a court-appointed attorney who did not meet with her until the day of her scheduled court hearing.[viii] Her defense attorney had recently worked in the prosecutor's office, where she had previously prosecuted pregnant addicted women.[9]

Ms. Whitner was never counseled about her substance abuse problem nor was she offered drug treatment as a way of avoiding arrest. When she was indicted, there was not a single residential drug treatment program in the entire state designed to treat pregnant drug users.[ix] Believing that an admission of guilt would help her get access to inpatient treatment, Ms. Whitner pled guilty to the charge of child abuse.[x] At her sentencing hearing, she admitted that she was chemically dependent and requested assistance from the court, stating in part "I need some help, Your Honor." She stressed her need and desire for inpatient treatment. The judge responded, "I think I'll just let her go to jail." The court then sentenced Ms. Whitner to 8 years in prison. Although another court later ruled that there was no basis for the conviction, the South Carolina Supreme reversed that decision, effectively rewriting state law to make the word "child" in the state's child endangerment statute include a viable fetus.[xi]

The panic over women's use of cocaine abated somewhat in the late 1990s. Today, leading federal government agencies confirm that "the phenomena of 'crack babies'... is essentially a myth."[xii] As the National Institute for Drug Abuse has reported, "Many recall that 'crack babies,' or babies born to mothers who used crack cocaine while pregnant, were at one time written off by many as a lost generation. ... It was later found that this was a gross exaggeration" (p. 6).[10] The U.S. Sentencing Commission concluded: "[t]he negative effects of prenatal cocaine exposure are significantly less severe than previously believed" and those negative effects "do not differ from the effects of prenatal exposure to other drugs, both legal and illegal" (pp. 21–22).[11]

Nevertheless, in recent years, we have witnessed the reanimation of deeply rooted prejudice against women who use drugs, again targeting those who are pregnant and continue to term. National Advocates for Pregnant Women has and documented hundreds of known cases in at least 40 states where pregnant women who are identified as drug users have been arrested; dozens of known arrests came to light in 2005 and 2006 alone.[12] Our analysis shows that the brunt of the criminal justice system's intrusions into women's pregnancies has been borne by low-income minority women.

White, Black, and Hispanic women have comparable rates of drug use and substance dependence; the percent of White, Black, and Hispanic women in metropolitan areas who have used an illicit drug in the past month is 8.6%, 8.4%, and 5.6%, respectively.[xiii,18,19] However, a 1992 survey of arrests and prosecutions of pregnant women found overwhelming evidence that low-income Black and Hispanic women were singled out. An analysis of more recent cases is underway; the evidence so far suggests ongoing racial bias and an undeniable focus on low-income women.[12]

In addition to racial and class bias, the uncritical acceptance of medical misinformation about drugs and the stereotyping of the people who use them are being revisited today in the methamphetamine scare.[xiv,13] Concern about methamphetamine has jumped to the fore much like concern about crack cocaine did in the 1980s. For example, in April 2004 Theresa Lee Hernandez of Oklahoma was charged with first degree murder despite community opposition to her prosecution. The state claimed that the stillbirth that Ms. Hernandez had suffered was caused by her use of methamphetamine, even though research has not found an association between methamphetamine use and stillbirths.[14,15] In 2007, Ms. Hernandez plead guilty to second degree murder rather than risk a trial by jury and a life sentence. Ms. Hernandez was sentenced to 15 years in prison.[16–17] In an apparent response to extensive community education and opposition to the arrest and prosecution, Ms. Hernandez was released a year after being sentenced.

Is current media coverage of women's illicit drug use and drug dependency as sensational as it was in the late 1980s and 1990s? On one hand, leading researchers and medical professionals themselves have insisted that media coverage about drugs and pregnancy be grounded in science, not sensation, asking that experts (rather than the local pediatrician or the local sheriff) are given the opportunity to address what, if any, risks have been linked to prenatal exposure to cocaine, methamphetamine and other drugs.[20–21] On the other hand, the public is still fed a regular diet of accounts that distort and misrepresent the effects of illicit drug use (including presenting the effects of drug use on populations of mice as if they are applicable to humans), rely on non-experts, and demonize the people who use illicit drugs.[xv,22,23] Popular media accounts continue to falsely decry an "epidemic" and a "scourge" of drug use despite evidence that rates of methamphetamine use have stabilized since 1999 and have been declining since 2002.[24,25] Many reports play on exaggerated fears about the impact and addictiveness of methamphetamine and wrongly assert that we lack any effective treatments for methamphetamine addiction.[24]

The front page story of the July 11, 2005, *New York Times,* "A Drug Scourge Creates its Own Form of Orphan," typifies the problematic ways in which women who use illicit drugs are presented to the public, as well as the biases found among workers in the helping professions.[26] As with earlier media coverage of the crack epidemic, the story discussed methamphetamine's "highly sexualized" users and depicted the "children of methamphetamine" as lost causes "with so many behavioral problems." The article twice mentioned that some of the children had lice. The article's sources were harried social workers, a lawyer for a department of human services, a pediatrician involved in a state program that was run in conjunction with the Department of Justice, and other professionals with a stake in convincing the public of the gravity of the methamphetamine "scourge." Not one parent was quoted nor were any researchers actually qualified to express an opinion about the effects of prenatal exposure or trends in methamphetamine use, as distinct from trends in child welfare system intervention. The article's sources provided opinions that fell outside their areas of expertise (i.e., a pediatrician's "professional" opinion that "The parents are basically worthless."). A state attorney general urged an audience of hundreds to become foster parents, "Because we're just seeing so many kids being taken from these homes." The article never questioned whether taking so many children away from their parents and their homes was justified or even in the best interests of the children. The National Coalition for Child Protection Reform and others convincingly conclude that it is not.[27]

THE PROBLEMS WITH PUNISHMENT

The misinformed public, of course, includes not only journalists, but also police and prosecutors. Operating under false assumptions that a woman's drug dependency is inevitably and irreversibly harming her future child, police and prosecutors have persisted in arresting and pursuing charges against pregnant women. They typically claim that prosecution (or the threat of prosecution) is an effective tool in deterring pregnant women from using drugs, and that it is a useful device for forcing women to get treatment they would otherwise avoid. In reality, these measures are more likely to deter women from seeking prenatal care or from being completely forthcoming with their health care providers.[28]

Achieving total abstinence from drugs when one is addicted to them is generally a difficult and long-term process that is unlikely to occur in the relatively short term of a pregnancy. If a woman who is already addicted to drugs becomes pregnant and is not able to completely abstain from using drugs, the only way she can be assured of avoiding criminal charges for such crimes as child abuse, drug delivery to minors, and homicide is to get an abortion. Even though proponents of arrests and prosecution articulate the problem as one of a woman who uses drugs while she is pregnant, their perspective is more accurately characterized as an objection to a woman becoming and remaining pregnant.

In another South Carolina case, a woman was charged with and convicted of homicide by child abuse based on the claim that she suffered an unintentional stillbirth as a result of her cocaine use. Despite the medical evidence that Regina McKnight's pregnancy loss was the result of an infection and research studies finding no link between cocaine use and an increased incidence of stillbirths, Ms. McKnight was convicted and given a 20-year sentence that was reduced to 12-years incarceration. If she had had an early abortion, there would have been no crime. Even if she had intentionally ended her pregnancy through an illegal third-trimester abortion she would have received, at most, a 3-year sentence.

After having served almost 8 years, Ms. McKnight's conviction was finally overturned. As a result of ongoing post-conviction relief efforts, the court was finally persuaded that the conviction was based on inaccurate science. The Court ruled that Ms. McKnight had not received a fair trial and that her trial counsel was "ineffective in her preparation of McKnight's defense through expert testimony and cross-examination." Specifically, the court noted that the research the state relied on was "outdated" and that trial counsel failed to call experts who would have testified about "recent studies showing that cocaine is no more harmful to a fetus than nicotine use, poor nutrition, lack of prenatal care, or other conditions commonly associated with the urban poor."[xvi] However, to avoid a re-trial and a lengthy legal battle, Ms. McKnight plead guilty to manslaughter, permitting her release from prison and removing the threat of reincarceration.[29]

In our ongoing review of this and similar cases, we find that women are often charged with felonies, including murder or manslaughter, child abuse or neglect, and drug delivery (through the umbilical cord) and drug possession, based on evidence of pregnancy and drug use. Women have been sentenced to incarceration or given probation with numerous and sometimes impossible conditions imposed for many years.

Brenda Vaughan, a 30-year-old African American woman from Temple Hills, Maryland, pleaded guilty to felony charges for forging $721.98 in checks. The prosecutor recommended that Ms. Vaughan receive probation instead of jail time. During her sentencing hearing, Ms. Vaughan told the judge she was pregnant. The judge then ordered a drug test. When Ms. Vaughan tested positive, allegedly for cocaine, the judge ordered her to jail for 30 days, pending a decision on whether to admit her to a special intensive probation program. When it turned out that she was not eligible for the intensified probation program because she was not a District of Columbia resident, the judge sentenced her to 6 more months in jail, subject to a motion to reduce the sentence after the baby was born. At her sentencing hearing, the judge explained: "I'm going to keep her locked up until the baby is born because she's tested positive for cocaine when she came before me. . . . She's apparently an addictive personality and I'll be darned if I'm going to have a baby born that way." The judge added, "I can't trust you, Ms. Vaughan, and that's a hell of a thing to say." There was no trial or conviction on any charge relating to possession or use of an illegal drug.[xvii,30] As noted previously, in many cases women have pleaded guilty or accepted plea bargains rather than risk a protracted legal challenge that could result in an even longer period of incarceration.

When the arrests, detentions, and prosecutions of women have been challenged, they are nearly always found, eventually, to be without legal basis or to be unconstitutional. There has been near unanimity among the country's appellate courts; all but one have dismissed charges or overturned convictions of women who used drugs or experienced an addiction and sought to continue their pregnancies to term.[xviii] Courts faced with challenges to such prosecutions have routinely ruled that a plain reading of the applicable criminal statute and the absence of legislative intent to address the issue of drug using pregnant women through the criminal justice system require that the charges be dropped. Many of these courts have recognized that the application of existing criminal laws (such as those prohibiting child abuse, drug delivery, and homicide) to pregnant women in relationship to the fetuses they carry raises significant constitutional issues, including due process principles of notice, vagueness, and overbreadth, as well as privacy and sex discrimination. Numerous courts have also acknowledged the extraordinary consensus among medical groups condemning these prosecutions as counterproductive and dangerous. That is why the Supreme Court of Florida, in overturning Jennifer Johnson's conviction for drug delivery, declared: "The Court declines the State's invitation to walk down a path that the law, public policy, reason and common sense forbid it to tread."[xix]

In addition to state appellate courts, in 2001 the U.S. Supreme Court, in a landmark decision, held that health care providers who secretly search pregnant women for evidence of drug use and turn that information over to the police are violating the 4th Amendment's prohibition on illegal searches and seizures and may be held personally liable for such actions.[xx] In reaching this conclusion, the Court observed that the numerous *amici* in the case pointed to "a near consensus in the medical community that programs of the sort at issue, by discouraging women who use drugs from seeking prenatal care, harm, rather than advance, the cause of prenatal health."[xxi]

In the remainder of this article, we propose three principles that should guide our responses to pregnant drug-using women: (1) rely on the best available research and the principles of evidence-based medicine and social science rather than flawed assumptions about drug use by pregnant women and its effects; (2) distinguish, as we do with alcohol, between use and addiction and recognize that drug addiction is a chronic, relapsing health condition rather than a crime; and (3) provide support for low-income pregnant women rather than rely on policing and punishment.

Rely on Science Rather than Sensation About Maternal Drug Use

If a child is born prematurely or has a low birthweight or if a woman miscarries or delivers a stillborn baby, many hospital staff, medical examiners, social workers, and other officials blame the woman for the outcome. This is especially true if a woman has ingested any amount of an illegal drug, used too much alcohol, or in some way, such as by her race, class, or personality, offended the hospital or agency staff or officials. Also, some health care providers see drug testing as part of defensive medicine. That is, if something has gone wrong with the birth raising the specter of a lawsuit, a positive drug test provides staff with a powerful defense regardless of what actually caused the bad birth outcome.

The use of methamphetamine, cocaine, and other illicit drugs certainly presents a valid public health concern. But medical and scientific evidence suggests that the harms associated with illicit drug use have been greatly overstated. In contrast, not only are alcohol and tobacco more widely used, but the evidence of potential harm to fetuses and children from tobacco use and heavy alcohol use are far better established as a matter of scientific research.[31,32] However, our harshest responses have been reserved for those women who consume illicit drugs.

The relationship between using a substance and fetal or infant health is not straightforward. Although a correlation may exist between the use of some substances (and some medical conditions) and some pregnancy outcomes, a causal relationship does not necessarily exist. For example, two well-constructed, independent studies tried to determine whether cocaine could be linked to an increased risk of stillbirths. The authors found that it could not.[33,34] A recent article published in the peer-reviewed *American Journal of Obstetrics and Gynecology* concluded that "despite widespread reports linking methamphetamine use during pregnancy with preterm birth and growth restriction, *evidence confirming its association with an increased risk of stillbirth remains lacking*" (p. 438, emphasis added).[35] Most pregnant women who use substances such as cocaine, methamphetamine, nicotine, caffeine, or alcohol will give birth to healthy babies. Additionally, most pregnancy losses and other negative birth outcomes cannot be traced solely, or even mainly, to the use of an illicit substance, especially when it is likely that substance use is accompanied by other risk factors such as violence, heavy alcohol consumption, cigarette smoking, the use of prescription drugs, poverty, and environmental risks.

The best available medical evidence indicates that the use of illicit drugs and other substances is but one of many other factors which may affect pregnancy outcome. Recognizing this, a wide spectrum of respected medical and public health organizations, including the American Medical Association, the American Society of Addiction Medicine, the American Public Health Association, the American College of Physicians, the American College of Obstetricians and Gynecologists, the American Academy of Pediatrics, the March of Dimes, and the National Council on Alcoholism and Drug Dependence, have voiced their opposition to the arrests and prosecutions of pregnant women who use illicit drugs.

Treat Addiction as a Public Health Concern, Not a Crime

Being pregnant is not a crime, nor is being addicted to an illicit substance, as the Supreme Court held in the 1962 case, *Robinson v. California.* Because of the very nature of addiction and dependency, not every person who uses a substance "chooses" or "intends" to continue to use it or can even be said to be indifferent to its consequences. Prolonged drug use can cause dramatic changes in brain function, making it difficult for people to overcome drug dependence on their own without treatment.[xxii,36–38] The National Institute on Drug Abuse[39] (which, in 2007, began to consider a name change to "The National Institute of Diseases of Addiction") defines addiction as "a chronic, relapsing brain disease that is characterized by compulsive drug seeking and use, despite harmful consequences." The American Psychiatric Association's *Diagnostic and Statistical Manual of Mental Disorders* (DSM-IV) recognizes that an "inability to control drug use" is often a key feature of chemical dependency.[40]

Women's attempts to cease using drugs completely during pregnancy are common.[41,42] Indeed, pregnancy and motherhood have been identified as catalysts for change among women who use drugs.[xxiii,41–43] Although many women can and do stop or reduce their consumption and tolerance of potentially harmful substances while they are pregnant, permanent abstinence is no more attainable for low-income pregnant women than it is for other people, including affluent White men, such as conservative shock jock Rush Limbaugh. Wanting or intending to stop is an important element of recovery, but the physical, behavioral, and social aspects of dependence are such that it is rarely sufficient.

A woman's continued drug use should not be assumed to reflect a lack of desire to quit using drugs. Along similar lines, women who do not receive treatment for drug dependence cannot be assumed to have rejected treatment. In a country where 47 million people have no health insurance coverage, where most private insurance programs offer limited coverage for the expenses of mental health and drug treatment services, where state and federal funding for such programs is exceedingly limited, and where the most successful treatment modalities (such as methadone treatment) are deliberately limited, it is simply wrong to assume that lack of treatment is a question of personal intention or desire.[xxiv,44] Many pregnant women do not enter drug treatment because they cannot afford to, there are no spaces available, or the programs do not provide childcare or account for the fact that most women have family responsibilities. A 1993 study of 294 drug treatment programs in five major cities showed that, although most programs accepted pregnant women on some basis, the method of payment accepted and the availability of child care significantly limited access.[45] Only 55% of residential/detoxification programs accepted pregnant women on Medicaid or for free. Only one-fifth of all programs accepted pregnant women *and* provided child care, even though past research has found that lack of child care precludes addicted women's participation in treatment.[46] A survey conducted in 2007 found that only 19 states have created drug treatment programs specifically for pregnant women, and only seven states give pregnant women priority access to state-funded drug treatment programs.[47] Even in these states, the demand exceeds the number of available spaces in treatment programs. Moreover, programs touted as allowing women to bring their children typically limit the number and age of the children. This means that many women must separate from their family to get help. Also, while there is strong evidence that treatment for drug addiction is as effective, if not more effective, than treatment for other chronic relapsing conditions such as diabetes mellitus, asthma, and high blood pressure, treatment often fails patients.[48,49] As a result, it is inappropriate to assume that simply entering treatment will be sufficient to "cure" a woman of her dependency on drugs.

Women who *do* enter treatment are not necessarily insulated from inappropriate or punitive state responses. For example, women already in treatment became the subject of a South Carolina prosecutor's decision to seek out and punish pregnant drug-using women.[50] National Advocates for Pregnant Women also has documented several cases in which women who were in successful methadone treatment programs became targets of child welfare interventions to remove the child at birth because of a belief that the methadone treatment proved that they had once been drug users and therefore posed a threat to their children.

Incarcerating pregnant women to "protect the fetus" is based on similarly false assumptions that jails and prisons consistently offer high-quality prenatal care programs, nutritional diets, and reproductive health care.[51,52] Although pregnancy receives more attention than most other health concerns of incarcerated women, the quality of incarcerated women's care before, during, and after delivery typically leaves much to be desired. Incarcerated women routinely receive little to no education about prenatal care and nutrition, do not receive regular pelvic exams or sonograms, and cannot alter their diets to meet their changing caloric needs. Prison medical staff and administrators may ignore orders from outside OB/GYNs. In most states, pregnant women, even those who pose no security risk, may be shackled or otherwise restrained during transport to the hospital and during labor and delivery.

As we should have learned from the crack panic, the distrust that stigma and prejudice engender among drug-using women may pose greater dangers to maternal and fetal health than the use of an illicit drug itself. Reporting pregnant women to child protection agencies and the police or locking them up in the name of "protecting the fetus" can be expected to have a chilling impact on women's willingness to seek care and on physicians' relationships with their patients. Health care workers and hospital social workers, in particular, should play important roles in finding out from the women what services and support they need and, when appropriate, securing drug treatment for women who are addicted to drugs. Frequently, however, a hospital worker's report of a pregnant woman's drug use leads, directly or indirectly, to the mobilization of the criminal justice system and highly intrusive interventions by child welfare authorities.[31]

Pregnant women's fears of being judged by those who are assigned with helping them are not without foundation. Survey results suggest a sizable proportion of hospital medical staff and social workers already support defining illicit drug use as "child abuse" and coercive approaches to addressing a woman's drug use (e.g., incarceration or threatening women with loss of custody of their children to "encourage" them to complete drug treatment).[31,53,54] At the same time, some health care providers may refrain from asking women in their care about drug use for fear they will have to turn their patients over to punitive state authorities.

As the AMA notes: "punishing a person who abuses drugs or alcohol is not generally an effective way of curing their dependency or preventing future abuse" (p. 2667).[55] Furthermore, intimidation and punitive measures are far more likely to deter women from seeking help than from using the drugs upon which they have become dependent.[56,57] On a strictly pragmatic level, by the time a pregnant woman has experienced a stillbirth or a baby is born testing positive for an illicit substance, valuable opportunities have been missed to provide a woman with support and access to good quality health care, including drug treatment.

Support Low-Income Pregnant Women Rather than Infringe Upon Their Civil and Human Rights

Mobilizing the criminal justice system to address a health concern creates a precedent for the supervision and punishment of pregnant women with regard to all aspects of their lives. In Maryland, two women were convicted of reckless endangerment and sentenced to several years in prison for continuing their pregnancies to term and using cocaine during pregnancy, and three other women faced similar charges.[xxv,58,59] The

Maryland Court of Appeals ruled, however, that prosecution of such cases might open the way for pregnant women to be prosecuted for any number of injury-prone activities that might endanger the well-being of an unborn child, such as driving without a seatbelt, skiing, or horseback riding. This ruling, like others before it, is a strong and important recognition of the larger issues of pregnant women's civil and human rights beyond the issue of drug use and addiction. Indeed, the fact that the same legal arguments used to justify the prosecution of pregnant drug and alcohol using women have been used to justify court ordered interventions and arrests of women who do not accede to doctor's advice regarding childbirth makes clear that concerns about the application of fetal homicide laws to drug-dependent pregnant women are not speculative.[60,61]

Court decisions and statutes creating the crime of feticide and unborn victims of violence laws have directly and indirectly become grounds for arresting pregnant drug-using women. In the *Whitner* case mentioned earlier in this article, the state argued that there was precedent for prosecuting Cornelia Whitner for child abuse. That precedent was a case where a man, Horne, brutally stabbed his pregnant wife, causing her to lose the pregnancy. The South Carolina Supreme Court created the crime of feticide in response. *Whitner* argued that experiencing an addiction as a pregnant woman is not the same as a third party attacking a pregnant woman. The court disagreed, stating that if they ruled that way "there would be no basis for prosecuting a mother who kills her viable fetus by stabbing it, by shooting it, or by other such means, yet a third party could be prosecuted for the very same acts. We decline to read *Horne* in a way that insulates the mother from all culpability for harm to her viable child."[xxvi]

The court's reasoning ignores the bald reality that in order to shoot or stab her fetus, the pregnant woman would first have to cut through her own flesh, her own body. The court's rationale requires treating a pregnant woman as if on becoming pregnant she loses her humanity, her capacity to become psychologically and physically addicted like other human beings, her identity as a unique individual whose actions (including stabbing or shooting herself) have obviously different meanings and implications than when another person commits those actions against her.

This distinction has been ignored in states like Texas, where the Prenatal Protection Act (SB 319) was passed in 2003. This law established that for the purposes of murder and aggravated assault, a fetus is considered "an unborn child at every stage of gestation from conception to birth." The bill was ostensibly written to ensure criminal liability in the event of a crime against a pregnant woman that harmed or killed her fetus (e.g., a drunk-driving accident or an incident of domestic violence).[62] The immediate and primary effect of that law, however, was the arrest and prosecution of more than 40 pregnant women and new mothers who were believed to have had drug problems while pregnant.[63] Three weeks after the governor signed the bill into law, 47th District Attorney Rebecca King sent a letter to Potter County physicians informing them that under the Act, "it is now a legal requirement for anyone to report a pregnant woman who is using or has used illegal narcotics during her pregnancy." King reasoned that the new definition of "individual" directly affected the Controlled Substances Act, since the Penal Code provides punishment for "delivery" of narcotics to children, and now to fetuses.[62] Although defense counsel and civil rights organizations were eventually able to overturn the convictions, women were imprisoned for years while a key case worked its way through the court system.[xxvii]

While court decisions overwhelmingly reject the expansion of criminal law as a tool for policing pregnant women and it is still true that, as of this writing, no state legislature has passed a law explicitly criminalizing pregnancy for drug users, many other kinds of laws and policies are being used to police and punish drug-using pregnant women. Take, for example, the Child Abuse Prevention and Treatment Act (CAPTA). In 2003, CAPTA was amended so that states could only receive federal funding under the act if they passed laws to require health care providers involved in the delivery and care of infants to report to child protective services infants "affected" by illegal substance use. The act excludes from consideration fetal alcohol effect or fetal alcohol syndrome.

Neither CAPTA nor any of the civil state reporting laws that pre-dated it mandate universal drug testing. In other words, who gets tested and identified as a drug user, and therefore, who gets reported to authorities is highly discretionary. Nor does CAPTA clearly define what is meant by "drug-affected," leaving states to decide for themselves the criteria health care providers will use to identify infants to be reported to child protective services. Some states require only an unconfirmed positive toxicology screen at birth, others require physical signs of addiction or dependence, and still others mandate an actual assessment of the newborn's imminent risk of harm or need for protection.[64,65]

Although such reporting laws do not mandate that the information be turned over to the police, these laws typically do not prohibit it. As mentioned earlier, hospital workers (including medical staff and social workers) and child welfare workers, who are potentially best situated to provide important care and services to drug-dependent women, are often the very ones who contact law enforcement or who contact child welfare workers, who in turn notify the police.[31,64,65] The result has been that many women who used illicit drugs while they were pregnant are being arrested, interrogated, detained, prosecuted, and punished rather than receiving the services and care they need. Punitive state authorities are willing to mobilize resources to punish and separate families but not to treat and support them.

CONCLUSION

That punitive measures taken under the auspices of protecting the fetus continue to appeal to the public is not surprising. People are genuinely and understandably concerned about the possibility of poor pregnancy outcomes, including sick babies and pregnancy loss. They are sincerely and justifiably interested in ensuring that pregnancies result in healthy babies.[66] Opposing the punishment of pregnant women and the recognition of fetal rights distinct from the rights of pregnant women does not contradict any of these legitimate concerns nor does it deny the value of potential life as matter of religious belief, emotional conviction, or personal experience. Rather, it is to recognize that punitive approaches do not advance either maternal or fetal health, and that on becoming pregnant, women (including those who use drugs and alcohol) do not lose their civil and human rights.

Singling out pregnant women not only for arrest and prosecution, but also for court orders (through family courts and drug treatment courts) and civil commitments, contributes to a climate where pregnant women are increasingly seen as adversaries of the fetuses they carry rather than people who have a stake in a healthy pregnancy and a favorable outcome. There is no question that some people's drug use has become so chaotic and out of control that it can affect their parenting ability. No one is suggesting that such situations be ignored. Too often, however, a single, unconfirmed positive drug test is accepted as incontrovertible evidence of a woman's criminality or unfitness to parent. Rather than a thoughtful evaluation of whether drug use or any other factor has rendered someone incapable of parenting, a single positive drug test result becomes the basis for massive and often highly punitive state intrusions on family life.

Punitive actions against drug-using pregnant women persist even though they remain inconsistent with legal, medical, and public health standards of acceptable practice and even though they do not, in fact, advance maternal, fetal, or child health interests. Our knowledge of existing cases suggests that at some of the points at which a woman is most amenable to help or may benefit most from support (e.g., when she becomes pregnant or gives birth or when she is locked up), our official responses are the harshest and least effective.

This speaks to the need to overcome a national tendency to ignore evidence-based medicine and research and to pursue costly and counterproductive punitive state interventions. The harms to both health and human rights posed by institutionalizing coercive forms of state power are significant. Rather than continue to vilify pregnant women and exaggerate the harms of their drug use, research and experience support the provision of respectful, supportive services to all pregnant women and families who need it as the most effective way to encourage healthy pregnancies and birth outcomes.[1]

NOTES

i. *McFall v. Shimp*, 10 Pa. D. & C.3d 90, 91 (1978) PA Court of Common Pleas, Civil Division (1978) ("For our law to compel the Defendant to submit to an intrusion of his body would change every concept and principle upon which our society is founded. To do so would defeat the sanctity of the individual and would impose a rule which would know no limits and one could not imagine where the line would be drawn.")

ii. *Wisconsin ex. rel. Angela M.W. v. Kruzicki*, 561 N.W.2d 729 (Wis. 1997); *Whitner v. South Carolina*, Pickens County, 382 S.C. 1, 492 S.E.2d 777 (1997), *State v. McKnight*, No. 00-GS-26-432 (S.C. Ct. App. 2002), 352 S.C. 635, 576 S.E.2d 168 (S.C. Jan 27, 2003).

iii. *In re Fetus Brown*, 689 N.E.2d 397, 400 (Ill. App. Ct. 1997) (overturning a court-ordered, forced blood transfusion of a pregnant woman).

iv. See *In re A.C.*, 573 A.2d 1235, 1253 (D.C. 1990) (en banc) (vacating court-ordered cesarean surgery in which the newborn did not survive and that was listed as a contributing factor to the mother's death on her death certificate).

v. Pregnant women also smoke cigarettes and drink alcohol at much lower rates than other women. Less than 1 in 5 pregnant women report smoking cigarettes in the past month (compared to around almost 1 in 3 who were not pregnant). Approximately 1 in 8 pregnant women report drinking alcohol, and less than 4% report binge drinking. By contrast, over half of non-pregnant women report currently drinking alcohol and nearly 1 in 4 report binge drinking.

vi. S.C. CODE ANN. §20-7-50 (Law. Co-op. 1985) ("Any person having the legal custody of any child or helpless person, who shall, without lawful excuse, refuse or neglect to provide...the proper care and attention for such child or helpless person, so that the life, health or comfort of such child or helpless person is endangered or is likely to be endangered, shall be guilty of a misdemeanor and shall be punished within the discretion of the circuit court.").

vii. Affidavit in Support of Arrest Warrant D-038033 (Feb. 5, 1992), *State v. Whitner*, No. 92-GS-39-670 (S.C. Ct. Gen. Sess. Pickens County 1992).

viii. Record at 9, 14-15, *Whitner v. State*, No. 93-CP-39-347 (S.C. Ct. C.P. Pickens County Nov. 1, 1993).

ix. Affidavit of Louise Haynes at 5, *Ferguson v. State*, No. 92-GS-10-7304 (S.C. Ct. Gen. Sess. Charleston County Apr. 27, 1993) (supporting affidavit for motion to dismiss criminal child abuse charges brought against Crystal Ferguson).

x. Record at 2, *State v. Whitner*, No. 92-GS-39-670 (S.C. Ct. Gen. Sess. Pickens County Apr. 20, 1992).

xi. In South Carolina, an activist state Supreme Court with a bare majority twice re-wrote state law to make the word "child" in the state child abuse and homicide statutes include viable fetuses. The court devised a new construction of the word "child" to include viable fetuses, and purported to rely on decisions in the completely different context of civil wrongful death and common law feticide. *Whitner v. South Carolina* reinterpreted these decisions in a new manner, declaring that they "rested on the concept of the viable fetus as a *person* vested with legal rights." The court concluded, "South Carolina has long recognized that viable fetuses are *persons* holding certain legal rights and privileges." Thus the decision was not based on a state interest in fetal protection, but on the flat assertion that "viable fetuses are persons." *Whitner v. South Carolina*, 492 S.E. 2d 777 (S.C. 1997), *cert. denied*, 523 U.S. 1145 (1998).

xii. *United States v. Smith*, 359 F. Supp. 2d 771, 780 n.6 (E.D. Wis. 2005).

xiii. Substance dependence is highest among American Indians and Alaskan Natives and lowest among Asians. Native Hawaiians or other Pacific Islander, Whites, and Hispanics all report slightly higher rates of substance dependence than blacks.

xiv. Methamphetamine, also known as speed, crystal, or crank, is a synthetic stimulant that can be dissolved in liquid, ingested orally, snorted, or injected. Some people have used the drug recreationally ever since the 1960s. A researcher at The Sentencing Project reports that methamphetamine is among the least commonly used drugs; the rate of methamphetamine use has remained stable since 1999 and the rate of use by high school students has actually declined between 1999 and 2005. The rate of use is higher in areas such as Los Angeles, San Diego, San Jose, Omaha, and Portland, Oregon.

xv. Jack Shafer has published several articles in Slate documenting the shortcomings of the press corps' drug coverage, for example "Why Does Drug Reporting Suck?" (August 10, 2005, http://www.slate.com/id/2124298); "Pfft Goes the Methedemic" (July 1, 2006, http://www.slate.com/id/2146303); "Methamphetamine Propaganda" (March 3, 2006, http://www.slate.com/id/2137388). In "How Not To Report About Meth (March 21, 2006, http://www.slate.com/id/2138398)," he offers the following advice: Start your article with an anecdote, preferably one about a user who testifies about how methamphetamine destroyed his life. Toss out some statistics to indicate that meth use is growing, even if the squishy numbers don't prove anything. Avoid statistics that cut against your case. Use and reuse the words "problem" and "epidemic" without defining them. Quote law enforcement officers extensively, whether they know what they're talking about or not. Avoid drug history except to make inflammatory comparisons between meth and other drugs. Gather grave comments from public-health authorities but never talk to critics of the drug war who might add an unwanted layer of complexity to your story.

xvi. *McKnight v. South Carolina*, 2008 WL 2019141 (S.C. May 12, 2008)

xvii. *United States v. Vaughan*, No. F-2172-88B (D.C. Sup. Ct. Aug. 23, 1988).

xviii. *Whitner v. South Carolina* 492 S.E.2d 777 (S.C. 1997). Many charges and convictions of child abuse and neglect, drug distribution, and manslaughter that are leveled against pregnant women have been dropped on the grounds that the legislation was never written with the intent that it be applied to the context of pregnancy. For example, the court in *Ward v. State* held that it is impossible for a fetus to "possess" the drugs since a fetus would not be capable of handling, manipulating or using drugs. *Ward v. State* 184 S.W.3d 874, 876 (Tex. App. 2006). See also *Reinesto v. Arizona*, 894 P.2d 733 (Ariz. Ct. App. 1995); and other cases cited in *State v. Martinez*. Brief for Sutin, Thayer & Browne, P.C. et al. as Amici Curiae Supporting Respondent, *State v. Martinez*, 137 P.3d 1195 (N.M. Ct. App. 2006) (No. 29,775) (National Advocates for Pregnant Women was a signatory to the brief).

xix. *Johnson v. State*, 602 So. 2d 1288, 1297 (Fla. 1992)

xx. See *Ferguson v. City of Charleston*, 532 U.S. 67, 84 n.23 (2001) (noting, in the course of rejecting a Fourth Amendment exception for prosecutorial drug-testing of pregnant women, amicus submissions "claiming a near consensus in the medical community that programs of the sort at issue, by discouraging women who use drugs from seeking prenatal care, harm, rather than advance, the cause of prenatal health").

xxi. *Ferguson v. City of Charleston*, 532 U.S. 67, 83 n.23 (2001).

xxii. Some people experience remission or recover from substance dependence without formal treatment (a phenomenon referred to in the literature as "maturing out," "spontaneous remission" or "spontaneous recovery").

xxiii. See also David Carr's Memoir, The Night of the Gun, describing fatherhood as the primary motivation for one man's recovery. David Carr, The Night of the Gun: A Reporter Investigates the Darkest Story of His Life, His Own (Simon & Schuster 2008).

xxiv. Methadone treatment programs can accommodate fewer than 15% of those whom methadone treatment might help.

xxv. *Kilmon v. State of Maryland*, 905A.2d 306 (Md. App. 2006).

xxvi. *Whitner v. South Carolina*, 492 S.E.2d 783.

xxvii. Tracy Yolanda Ward, a 30-year-old African American woman, gave birth on November 3, 2003, to a baby boy. On October 31, 2003, Ms. Ward experienced pregnancy complications and called an ambulance. According to press reports, Ms. Ward told the ambulance personnel that she smoked cocaine within the previous hour. Following a written directive from the Potter County district attorney, hospital staff notified the Amarillo Police Department. Ms. Ward was charged with delivery of a controlled substance to a minor, a second-degree felony. Ms. Ward filed a motion to dismiss on statutory and constitutional grounds. The motion was denied. Ms. Ward pled guilty to the offense in August 2004, reserving the right to appeal the applicability of the law to her. She was sentenced to 5 years probation. Ms. Ward immediately filed an appeal challenging the legality of her conviction. Ruling on narrow statutory interpretation and evidentiary grounds, the court of appeals held that the delivery of a controlled substance statute requires "an actual" transfer of drugs and that neither possession of drugs nor an actual transfer could be established as having occurred in the context of pregnancy and birth. *Ward v. State*, 188 S.W.3d 874 (Tex. App. 2006).

REFERENCES

1. Daniels CR. At women's expense. Cambridge, MA: Harvard University Press, 1993.

2. Murphy S, Sales P. Pregnant drug user: scapegoats of Reagan/Bush and Clinton era economics. Social Justice 2001; 28:72–95.

3. Arria AM, Derauf C, LaGasse LL, Grant P, Shah R, Smith L, Haning W, Huestis M, Strauss A, Grotta SD, Liu J, Lester B. Methamphetamine and other substance use during pregnancy: Preliminary estimates from the infant development, environment, and lifestyle (IDEAL) study. Maternal Child & Health J 2006; 10:293–302.

4. Substance Abuse and Mental Health Services Administration. Results from the 2005 national survey on drug use and health: National findings Rockville, MD: Office of Applied Studies, NSDUH Series H-30, DHHS Pub. No. SMA 06-4194), 2006:22.

5. U.S. Department of Health and Human Services. Drug use among racial/ethnic minorities. Bethesda, MD: National Institute on Drug Abuse, 2003.

6. Humphries D. Crack mothers: pregnancy, drugs, and the media. Columbus, OH: Ohio State University Press, 1999.

7. Reeves JL and Campbell R. Cracked coverage: Television news, the anti-cocaine crusade, and the Reagan legacy. Durham, NC: Duke University Press, 1994.

8. Center on Addiction and Substance Abuse at Columbia University. Annual report. New York: CASA, 1994.

9. Record at 21, 24, 32-33, *Whitner v. State*, No. 93-CP-39-347 (S.C. Ct. C.P. Pickens County Nov. 1, 1993).

10. U.S. Department of Health and Human Services, Cocaine: Abuse and Addiction, NIH Pub. No. 09-4166 at 6 (May 1999, rev. May 2009) (emphasis added). Available at: http://www.drugabuse.gov/PDF/RRCocaine.pdf.

11. Report to the Congress: cocaine and Federal sentencing policy, May 2002 at 21-21, available at http://www.ussc.gov/r_congress/02crack/ch3.pdf (emphasis added).

12. National Advocates for Pregnant Women. Data file compiled by the authors, 2009.

13. King RS. The next big thing? Methamphetamine in the United States. Washington, DC: The Sentencing Project, 2006.

14. Cnattingius S, Stephansson O. The epidemiology of stillbirth. Seminars Perinatology 2002; 26:25–30.

15. Silver RM, Varner MW, Reddy U, Goldenberg R, Pinar H, Conway D, Bukowski R, Carpenter M, Hogue C, Willinger M, Dudley D, Saade G, Stoll B. Workup of stillbirth: a review of the evidence. Am J Obstet Gyncol 2007; 196:433–44.

16. Evans M. Woman enters plea in death of baby. Associated Press Wire Service. September 21, 2007.

17. Marks JF. For meth mom, a tough road ahead. The Oklahoman. December 22, 2007.

18. U.S. Department of Health and Human Services. Drug use among racial/ethnic minorities. Bethesda, MD: National Institute on Drug Abuse, 2003.

19. Substance Abuse and Mental Health Services Administration. Results from the 2005 National Survey on Drug Use and Health: National Findings. Rockville, MD: Office of Applied Studies, 2006.

20. Lewis DC. Meth Science Not Stigma: Open Letter to the Media, Join Together, http://jointogether.org/news/yourturn/commentary/2005/meth-science-not-stigma-open.html (retrieved July 12, 2005).

21. Oke S. The epidemic that wasn't. NY Times. January 26, 2009.

22. Friedman HJ, Lester D. A critical review of progress toward an animal model of alcoholism. In: Blum K, ed. Alcohol and opiates: neurochemical and behavioral mechanisms. New York: Academic Press, 1977:1–19.

23. Lester B. One hit of meth enough to cause news defects. JoinTogether.org. (retrieved August 17, 2005).

24. King R. The next big thing? Methamphetamine use in the United States. Washington, DC: The Sentencing Project, 2006.

25. Shafer J. 2007. About that methedemic. Slate. (January 31, 2007). http://www.slate.com/toolbar.aspx?action=read&id=2158739

26. Zernike K. 2005. A drug scourge creates its own form of orphan. NY Times. July 11, 2005.

27. Doyle JJ. Child protection and child outcomes: measuring the effects of foster care. Amer Econ Rev 2007; 97:1583–610.

28. Poland M, Ager J, Olson J. Barriers to receiving adequate prenatal care. Am J Obstet Gyncol, 1987; 157:297–303.

29. Lester B, Veer S. A measure of justice for Regina McKnight. State. July 1, 2008.

30. Churchville V. D.C. judge jails woman as protection for fetus: Convicted thief allegedly uses cocaine. Washington Post. July 23, 1988, A1.

31. Weber EM. Child welfare interventions for drug-dependent pregnant women: limitations of a non-public health response. UMKC Law Rev 2007; 75:789–845.

32. Armstrong EM. Conceiving risk, bearing responsibility: fetal alcohol syndrome and the diagnosis of moral disorder. The Johns Hopkins University Press, 2003.

33. Campbell TA, Collins KA. Pediatric toxicologic deaths: a 10 year retrospective study. Am J Forensic Med Pathology 2001; 22:184.

34. Sims MA, Collins KA. Fetal death: a 10-year retrospective study. Am J Forensic Med Pathology 2001; 22:261–5.

35. Silver et al. Workup of stillbirth: a review of the evidence. Am J Obstet Gyncol 2007; 196: 433–44.

36. Termorshuizen, F, Krol A, Prins M, van Ameijden EJC. Long-term outcome of chronic drug use: the Amsterdam cohort study among drug users. Amer J of Epidemiology 2005; 161:271–9.

37. Bischof G, Rumpf HJ, Meyer C, Hapke U, John U. Influence of psychiatric comorbidity in alcohol-dependent subjects in a representative population survey on treatment utilization and natural recovery. Addiction 2005; 100:405–13.

38. Steensma C, Boivin, JF, Blais L, Roy E. Cessation of injecting drug use among street-based youth. J Urban Health 2005; 82:622–37.

39. National Institute on Drug Abuse, Drugs, Brains, and Behavior: The Science of Addiction, NIH Pub. No. 07-5605 at 5 (Apr. 2007), available at http://www.nida.nih.gov/scienceofaddiction/sciofaddiction.pdf

40. American Psychiatric Association. Diagnostic and statistical manual of mental disorders, 4th ed., text revision. Washington, DC: American Psychiatric Association, 2000.

41. Murphy S, Rosenbaum M. Pregnant women on drugs. New Brunswick, NJ: Rutgers University Press, 1999.

42. Sterk CE. Fast lives: women who use crack cocaine. Philadelphia: Temple University Press, 1999.

43. Mallory C, Noerager Stern P. Awakening as a change process among women at risk for HIV who engage in survival sex. Qualitative Health Research 2000; 10:581–94.

44. Newman, RG. Addiction and methadone: one American's view. In: Malinowska-Sempruch K, Gallagher S, eds. War on Drugs, HIV/AIDS and Human Rights. New York: The International Debate Education Association, 2004:271–283.

45. Breitbart V, Chavkin W, Wise P. The accessibility of drug treatment for pregnant women: a survey of programs in five cities. Am J Public Health 1994; 84:1658–61.

46. Pursley-Crotteau S, Noerager Stern P. Creating a new life: dimensions of temperance in prenatal cocaine crack users. Qualitative Health Research 1996; 6:350–67.

47. Guttmacher Institute. Substance abuse during pregnancy: State policies in brief August 1st. Available at: http://www.guttmacher.org/statecenter/spibs/spib_SADP.pdf.

48. O'Brien CP, McLellan TA. Myths about addiction. Lancet 1996; 3471:237–40.

49. Marwick C. Physician leadership on national drug policy finds addiction treatment works. JAMA 1998; 279:1149–50.

50. Davison D. Policy on drug-using moms nets first arrest. The Herald Rock Hill, SC. June 27, 1997.

51. Flavin J. Our bodies, our crimes: the policing of women's reproduction in America. New York: NYU Press, 2009.

52. Stoller N. Improving access to health care for California's women prisoners. Santa Cruz, CA: California Policy Research Center. Available at: http://prisonerswithchildren.org/pubs/stoller.pdf, 2001.

53. Abel EL and Kruger M. Physician attitudes concerning legal coercion of pregnant alcohol and drug users. Am J Obstet Gyncol 2001; 186:768–772.

54. National Center on Addiction and Substance Abuse at Columbia University (CASA). No safe haven: children of substance-abusing parents. New York: CASA, 1999.

55. AMA Board of Trustees report. Legal interventions during pregnancy. JAMA 1990; 264:2663–2670.

56. American College of Obstetricians and Gynecologists. Substance use: obstetric and gynecologic implications in Special issues in women's health. Washington DC: ACOG, 2005.

57. Poland M, Ager J, Olson J. Barriers to receiving adequate prenatal care. Am J Obstet Gyncol, 1987; 157: 297–303.

58. Kinzie S. Charges rejected for moms who bear babies exposed to illegal drugs. Wash Post. August 4, 2006, B6.

59. Harris L. Drugs while pregnant: dangerous vs. 'endangerment'? Salon. September 6, 2006. Available at:salon.com/mwt/broadsheet/2006/09/06/drugs_as_endangerment/index.html.

60. Berkowitz RL. Should refusal to undergo a cesarean delivery be a criminal offense? Obstet Gynecol 2004; 104:1220–1.

61. Minkoff H, Paltrow LM. Melissa Rowland and the rights of pregnant women. Obstet Gynecol 2004; 104:1234–6.

62. Smith J. Naked city, save the fetus: from mom? The Austin Chronicle. September 10, 2004. Available at: http://www.austinchronicle.com/gyrobase/Issue/story?oid=oid%3A228254.

63. Thomas S. Courts: Drugs through birth not a crime. Lubbock Online. October 31, 2006. Available at: http://lubbockonline.com/stories/103106/sta_103106064.shtml.

64. National Clearinghouse on Child Abuse and Neglect Information (NCCANI). Current Trends in Child Maltreatment Reporting Laws. Child Abuse and Neglect State Statutes Series. Washington, DC: NCCANI, 2002.

65. National Clearinghouse on Child Abuse and Neglect Information (NCCANI). Reporting child maltreatment in cases involving parental substance abuse. Washington, DC: NCCANI, 2003. Available at: http://www.calib.com/nccanch/pubs/usermanuals/subabuse/report.cfm.

66. Layne LL. Motherhood lost: a feminist account of pregnancy loss in America. New York: Routledge, 2003.

Prenatal Drug Exposure: Infant and Toddler Outcomes

Emmalee S. Bandstra, MD
Connie E. Morrow, PhD
Elana Mansoor, PsyD
Veronica H. Accornero, PhD

ABSTRACT. This manuscript provides an overview of the current scientific literature on the impact of maternal drug use, specifically opioids and cocaine, during pregnancy on the acute and long-term outcomes of infants and toddlers from birth through age 3 years. Emphasis with regard to opioids is placed on heroin and opioid substitutes used to treat opioid addiction, including methadone, which has long been regarded as the standard of care in pregnancy, and buprenorphine, which is increasingly being investigated and prescribed as an alternative to methadone. Controlled studies comparing methadone at high and low doses, as well as those comparing methadone with buprenorphine, are highlighted and the diagnosis and management of neonatal abstinence syndrome is discussed. Over the past two decades, attention of the scientific and lay communities has also been focused on the potential adverse effects of cocaine and crack cocaine, especially during the height of the cocaine epidemic in the United States. Herein, the findings are summarized from prospective studies comparing cocaine-exposed with non-cocaine-exposed infants and toddlers with respect to anthropometric growth, infant neurobehavior, visual and auditory function, and cognitive, motor, and language development. The potentially stigmatizing label of the so-called "crack baby" preceded the evidence now accumulating from well-designed prospective investigations that have revealed less severe sequelae in the majority of prenatally exposed infants than originally anticipated. In contrast to opioids, which may produce neonatal abstinence syndrome and infant neurobehavioral deficits, prenatal cocaine exposure appears to be associated with what has been described as statistically significant but subtle decrements in neurobehavioral, cognitive, and language function, especially when viewed in the context of other exposures and the caregiving environment which may mediate or moderate the effects. Whether these early findings may herald more significant learning and behavioral problems during school-age and adolescence when the child is inevitably confronted with increasing social and academic challenges is the subject of ongoing longitudinal research.

INTRODUCTION

Substance abuse among women of child-bearing age remains a significant concern in the United States and internationally. According to the 2006-2007 combined National Survey of Drug Use and Health (NSDUH), 5.2% of pregnant and 9.7% of nonpregnant women

Supported by NIH (Grants R01 DA 006556; P50 DA 025484; K01 DA 16720); State of Florida Healthy Start Program; Health Foundation of South Florida; Maribel Lauber, Ed.S., for her editorial assistance between 15 and 44 years reported past-month illicit drug use.[1] The current report focuses on the infancy and toddler outcomes of in utero exposure to two major illicit drugs of abuse: cocaine and opioids. Because mothers who abuse these and other illicit drugs also frequently use varying combinations of alcohol, tobacco, and other drugs, polysubstance use is a salient part of any discussion of the scientific evidence for adverse effects of in utero exposure to drugs of abuse.

Large percentages of both pregnant and nonpregnant women report past-month alcohol consumption and tobacco smoking, despite ubiquitous health warnings. An estimated 11.6% of pregnant women and 53.2% of nonpregnant women aged 15 to 44 years reported current alcohol comsumption.[1] In utero exposure to alcohol, although legal, is extremely hazardous.[2] Fetal alcohol syndrome (FAS) is the leading identifiable, nonhereditary cause of mental retardation in the Western world.[3] The hallmarks are growth retardation, distinctive mid-facial anomalies, and mental retardation associated with central nervous system (CNS) deficits.[4] Fetal alcohol spectrum disorder (FASD) is the umbrella term for FAS, partial FAS, alcohol-related birth defects, and alcohol-related neurodevelopmental disorders.[5] Among women aged 15 to 44 years, 16.4% of pregnant and 28.4% of nonpregnant women reported past month cigarette use.[1] Tobacco smoking by pregnant women has also been implicated in animal and human studies in the pathophysiology of fetal growth restriction and newborn neurobehavioral deficits.[6,7] Furthermore, passive exposure of pregnant women to second-hand tobacco smoke is potentially deleterious to fetal and infant development.[8–10]

OPIOIDS (HEROIN, METHADONE, AND BUPRENORPHINE)

There is no substantive evidence from either preclinical or clinical studies that maternal opioid abuse during pregnancy causes congenital malformations. However, detrimental fetal effects of heroin exposure in terms of prematurity and intrauterine growth restriction have long been recognized.[11,12] Infants exposed to heroin have decreased birth weight, length, and head circumference compared to non-exposed infants; infants born to methadone-maintained mothers have higher birth weights than those born to heroin-dependent mothers not maintained on methadone.[13] Kandall observed that methadone maintenance improves neonatal growth parameters compared to heroin-exposed infants, but this may be partially explained by improved prenatal care and other medical and psychosocial factors.[14]

The National Institutes of Health Consensus Panel considers methadone the standard of care for pregnant opioid-addicted women, but the most desirable dosing schedule continues to be debated. In the early 1990s, the Center for Substance Abuse Treatment Consensus Panel recommended that methadone dosing be individually determined to prevent withdrawal in the mother.[15] Some investigators advocate a low methadone dosing regimen to reduce or eliminate neonatal abstinence syndrome (NAS), whereas others argue that lower doses may lead to maternal withdrawal, craving, and supplemental use of illicit drugs, thus increasing fetal risk. Dashe et al. reported a significant relationship between maternal methadone dose and neonatal abstinence scores, need for pharmacologic intervention, and duration of hospital stay in affected infants.[16] In contrast, Berghalla et al. retrospectively reviewed 21 published investigations on maternal methadone dosage and concluded that maternal methadone dose, comparing <80 mg with ≥ 80 mg daily, does not correlate with neonatal withdrawal.[17]

In 1996, buprenorphine was introduced in France as an opioid substitute and, as discussed in this supplement's accompanying article on the topic, maternal buprenorphine therapy is being prescribed and investigated internationally in the hopes of improving treatment and decreasing maternal and neonatal side effects of methadone maintenance. The logic behind this assumption is that buprenorphine has mixed agonist and antagonist properties with high receptor affinity and low intrinsic activity, resulting in fewer or no autonomic signs and symptoms of opioid withdrawal following abrupt discontinuation in adults. In a review by Johnson et al. of 21 published studies, including 309 infants from 15 cohorts exposed in utero to buprenorphine, 62% of the infants had NAS and 48% of those required therapy.[18] The investigators concluded that buprenorphine-associated NAS is "similar to or less than" that resulting from methadone. Regardless of treatment regimen, pregnant women and their fetuses undergoing opioid substitution therapy should be closely monitored by an addiction specialist and an obstetrician experienced in such care and supported by a multidisciplinary team. Furthermore, because NAS is so common among infants born to mothers using either illicit opiates or prescribed opioid substitutes, physicians and nurses should be well-trained to recognize and adequately treat withdrawal signs. NAS usually relates to withdrawal from opioids such as heroin or methadone, but other narcotics, benzodiazepines, barbiturates, and even alcohol can induce similar signs. The onset of NAS is generally within 2 to 3 days of birth, but may occur as late as 1 month postnatal age. Clinically, NAS presents in 60% to 80% of infants exposed to heroin or methadone and includes varying combinations of CNS, gastrointestinal, metabolic, and autonomic system disturbances. Seizures due to NAS are easily controlled with anticonvulsants and subsequent follow-up of affected infants at 1 year has been shown to be comparable to that of opioid-exposed infants with no seizures.[19] Neurobehavioral effects among infants with prenatal opiate exposure include excessive sucking, hypertonia, high pitched cry, difficulty being consoled, irritability, and jitteriness.[20,21] Central and autonomic nervous system effects were of greater magnitude among opiate-exposed infants compared to those with cocaine exposure[21] and infants exposed to both appear to exhibit the loudest and highest pitched cries.[20]

Supportive care for NAS, regardless of severity, includes provision of a quiet, dimly lit environment and avoidance of noxious stimuli.[22] Loose swaddling may also be an effective adjunct in the supportive care of NAS, but it should be accomplished with appropriate adherence to supine positioning as recommended in the latest American Academy of Pediatrics Task Force on Sudden Infant Death Syndrome's Policy Statement.[23] Treatment of NAS depends on the severity of withdrawal signs as noted clinically or more appropriately as recommended by standardized assessments administered serially at 3 to 4 hour intervals following first appearance of NAS signs to guide initiation and titration of pharmacologic substitutes. There are two popular scoring tools for NAS, the Lipsitz Scale (11 signs each rated from 0 to 3)[24] and the more detailed Finnegan Neonatal Abstinence Score (9 CNS signs, 8 metabolic/vasomotor/respiratory signs, and 4 gastrointestinal signs with variable sign-dependent rating scales),[25] which requires a trained observer. Both scales are more appropriate for full-term infants because the clinical presentation of opioid-exposed premature infants may be influenced by CNS immaturity.

The American Academy of Pediatrics has published guidelines for treating NAS when indicated using opioid substitution therapy. Morphine in the form of diluted tincture of opium (DTO) is preferred over paregoric due to concerns about additives.[26] Practices vary widely and some clinicians advocate morphine or methadone instead of DTO as pharmacotherapy for opiate-induced NAS, thereby avoiding unwanted alcoholic extracts of various alkaloids in the opium tincture.

Phenobarbital is recommended as an adjunctive therapy, usually for anticonvulsant activity, in NAS due to opiates and as a primary treatment for NAS due to sedatives or hypnotics. Although further studies are needed, a preliminary prospective controlled trial of DTO plus phenobarbital compared to DTO alone in a small number of opiate-exposed infants with NAS showed promise in terms of decreased severity of withdrawal accompanied by shorter and less costly hospital stays.[27]

Limited reports on the long-term effects of prenatal opioid exposure on postnatal growth and neurodevelopment are available. Methodological limitations in study design, including small sample sizes, poorly defined comparison groups, and difficulty controlling for important environmental variables, make available results difficult to interpret. Moreover, difficulties associated with the studied population, namely high attrition rates and the lifestyle variability that characterizes the drug abuse culture, have further contributed to the paucity of the literature.[28] Nevertheless, available information suggests that infants prenatally exposed to opiates are at an increased risk for neurodevelopmental impairment.[28,29] Furthermore, the home environment plays a significant modulating role in the developmental outcomes of exposed children,[28–30] although the magnitude of this effect remains unclear.

COCAINE

Many published prenatal cocaine studies from the 1980s and early 1990s included case reports and relatively small series. These methodologically limited studies evoked considerable media attention toward the plight of so-called "cocaine" or "crack" babies with devastating conditions such as congenital anomalies of the brain and other organs, CNS hemorrhage and infarction, and sudden infant death syndrome. Subsequently, several large well-designed prospective studies and meta-analyses have not confirmed these associations.[31–33]

Anthropometric Growth

Maternal cocaine abuse has been shown to be associated with significantly decreased infant birth weight, length, and head circumference, even in covariate-adjusted models accounting for prenatal exposure to other substances.[32,34] The mechanism whereby cocaine diminishes fetal growth is hypothesized to be through vasoconstriction of uterine and placental blood flow as well as direct adverse effects on fetal metabolism and fat deposition. Controlling for gestational age, nutritional indicators such as maternal weight gain, and prenatal exposure to other drugs, cocaine-associated effects on birth growth parameters[34] and lean body mass[34,35] prevail. In both animal and human studies, the magnitude of in utero cocaine-associated fetal growth decrements appear to depend on dose and gestational timing.[36–38]

Studies have yielded mixed results regarding the long-term effects of prenatal cocaine exposure on postnatal growth. These inconsistencies could be partly attributed to differences in cohort size and characteristics, differences in measurement of exposure, and the degree of statistical control for potential confounders and moderating characteristics.[39] A systematic review conducted by Frank et al. concluded that after controlling for level of exposure to other drugs, there is no consistent effect on physical growth, including weight, length, or head circumference, among children 6 years or younger.[40] Shankaran et al. evaluated neonatal size at birth and subsequent growth in prenatally exposed children and found that significant differences in weight, length, and head circumference at birth disappeared for weight and head circumference by age 2 years and for height by age 3 years.[41] Conversely, Covington et al. found that even after controlling for potential covariates, prenatal cocaine exposure was associated with height and weight deficits at age 7 years, particularly for children born to mothers older than 30 years.[42] Similarly, a recent study by Richardson et al. using a longitudinal growth-curve analysis found that children exposed to cocaine during the first trimester grew at a slower rate through 10 years of age compared to unexposed children.[43]

Infant Neurobehavior, Visual and Auditory Function

Numerous studies have documented subtle neonatal neurobehavioral effects associated with prenatal cocaine exposure, although findings have lacked coherence. The most frequently used assessment has been the Brazelton Neonatal Behavioral Assessment Scale (BNBAS), which includes the domains of orientation, habituation, state regulation, autonomic stability, reflexes, tone, motor performance, irritability, alertness, and excitability. Eyler et al. concluded that although subtle cocaine-associated deficits in neurobehavioral functioning were evident across a range of neonatal studies published between 1991 and 1998, there was no consistent pattern of domain-specific findings.[44] Subsequently, larger cohort studies of in utero cocaine exposure have reported subtle impairments in one or more BNBAS neurobehavioral clusters,[45–47] but with considerable variation regarding timing and level of exposure, severity of dysfunction, and specific domains affected.[44,46,47] Morrow et al. found a modest cocaine-associated adverse impact across all neurobehavioral domains except for the reflex cluster score.[46] These findings were partially mediated by fetal growth and appeared dose-dependent. In another large study, Behnke et al. revealed a significant direct effect of prenatal cocaine exposure on the BNBAS qualifier items, but not on the cluster scores.[47] Several investigators reported no significant cocaine-associated findings on the BNBAS at birth[48–51] but did show cocaine-associated greater autonomic instability and abnormal reflexes,[50] impaired motor functions,[48] and dose-dependent difficulties with state regulation and excitability[51] at 2 to 4 weeks postpartum.

Controlled studies have found neurobehavioral deficits among infants exposed to cocaine or opiates using other neurological and physiological assessments.[20,21,32,52,53] For example, cocaine-exposed infants exhibited less arousal, poorer behavior regulation, and higher excitability at 1 month of age than non-exposed infants on the NICU Network Neurobehavioral Scale.[20] Studies have also reported mild cocaine-associated central and autonomic system dysfunction as evidenced by increased irritability, jitteriness, tremors, and hypertonia.[21,32] Using a modified still-face paradigm, Bendersky and Lewis demonstrated significant deficits in arousal modulation among 4-month-old infants with heavy in utero cocaine exposure.[52] Cocaine-exposed infants have also been shown to display abnormal cry characteristics, including high pitched cries and fewer cry utterances, excessive sucking, and sleep alterations.[21,44,54,55] A dose-dependent effect was found, with heavy cocaine exposure resulting in an increased number of cry utterances and short cries, suggestive of an over-aroused (excitable) pattern of neurobehavioral functioning.[20,54]

Studies evaluating the impact of prenatal cocaine exposure on infant cardiac and respiratory systems have shown dose-related alterations in infant regulation. Heavy exposure was associated with the highest increase in heart rate and the greatest decrease in respiratory sinus arrhythmia.[53] In another study, infants with cocaine exposure were found to have lower vagal tone and less heart rate variability at birth, suggestive of decreased autonomic control of the heart.[56] In utero exposure to cocaine may result in ocular/visual problems such as impaired visual attention and tracking,[44] optic nerve hypoplasia, delayed visual maturation, eyelid edema, nystagmus, and strabismus.[36] Research on auditory brainstem responses has evidenced abnormalities in the peripheral auditory system including varying degrees of hearing impairment and slowed brainstem transmission of sensory information among infants prenatally exposed to cocaine[36,57,58] and/or opiates.[57,58]

As may be seen in an emergent field of study, early reports are often characterized by small sample sizes and other methodological issues, resulting in inconsistent findings and lack of generalizability. Later studies addressing methodological issues of concern have begun to document modest cocaine-associated decrements in overall neurobehavioral function rather than a specific pattern of neurobehavioral deficits. In addition, factors such as polydrug use, demographic and environmental influences, caregiving and family issues, and physical and psychological disorders all have the potential to result in inconsistent findings if inadequately controlled.[59] It is also possible that variations across studies are a reflection of cohort-specific differences in neurobehavioral outcomes among infants with prenatal cocaine exposure. To date, a preponderance of the evidence shows subtle impairments in neurobehavioral outcomes due to prenatal cocaine or opiate exposure. The impact of these deficits on later functioning is unclear. Therefore, it is imperative that future studies consider the influence of mediating and moderating variables on the neurodevelopmental trajectories of children with prenatal cocaine, opiate, or polysubstance exposure.

Cognitive and Motor Development

Numerous published studies varying in methodological rigor have evaluated the effects of prenatal cocaine exposure on infant cognitive and motor development. A review of published studies between 1992 and 2000, including only peer-reviewed reports of prospectively enrolled birth cohorts that used examiners blind to exposure status, found that five of the nine studies reviewed reported no cocaine-related effect on mental or physical development, most often assessed by the Bayley Scales of Infant Development (BSID).[40] The remaining four studies reported only subtle cocaine-related effects that did not maintain significance with multivariate statistical control or were evident only within subgroup or cross-sectional analyses. The review concluded that the effects of prenatal cocaine exposure on cognitive development during infancy were not readily discernable from effects due to other contextual factors including prematurity, assessment age, and other prenatal drug exposures.[40] Subsequently, larger prospective cohort studies have suggested a more complex picture in which the teratogenic effects of prenatal cocaine exposure are subtle and most evident when considering factors such as mediating pathways and severity of exposure. Five recent studies have documented cocaine-related effects on the BSID Mental Development Index (MDI) (Table 1). Two studies documented cocaine-related lower MDI scores as well as dose-dependent effects on development, findings not attenuated with statistical control of covariates.[60,61] Very low birth weight ($<$1,500 g) has also been linked to increased risk for cognitive impairment in prenatally cocaine-exposed infants, with one study reporting a 10-point difference in mean MDI scores at age 3 for preterm cocaine-exposed children.[62] Other studies have shown more subtle cocaine-related adverse effects on MDI in longitudinal models including mediating influences, such as birth weight and gestational age, head circumference, and other prenatal drug exposures.[47,63] An almost equal number of recent prospective studies have reported no cocaine-related effects on MDI after covariate adjustment,[64–67] suggesting that prenatal cocaine exposure is a marker for subtle performance decrements in MDI that attenuate with control for other variables such as low birth weight, HIV exposure, disruptions in maternal care, lower socioeconomic status, and maternal vocabulary scores.[67]

Typical motor development, assessed by the BSID Psychomotor Development Index (PDI), has shown little teratogenic sensitivity to prenatal cocaine exposure. In the above-cited 2001 review, only two studies found significant cocaine-related effects on PDI.[40] Our current review of more recent studies reveals a similar picture, with only one study showing a direct cocaine-related effect on PDI scores in longitudinal analyses spanning 12 through 36 months.[61] However, several studies have reported PDI findings specific to timing and degree of exposure. In one study, lower PDI scores were predicted by second trimester self-reported cocaine use,[66] and in another, there was a significant relationship between low birth weight and lower PDI scores in children with heavier cocaine exposure.[64] In a recent longitudinal analysis of global motor development from 1 to 18 months, motor skills for infants with cocaine exposure were lower on average overall, but this finding was most evident at the 1 and 4 month age points with recovery to normal motor function by 18 months.[68]

LANGUAGE DEVELOPMENT

A growing body of research suggests that prenatal cocaine exposure may impact early language development, increasing the risk for language delays in early childhood. In a longitudinal analysis through age 3 years, Morrow et al. reported that children with prenatal cocaine exposure had lower total language scores than non-cocaine-exposed children, with results partially mediated through fetal growth.[69] In the same cohort, increasing level of prenatal cocaine exposure was associated with increased decrements in expressive language functioning at age 3 years.[70] Singer et al. also noted that expressive language skills were more adversely affected in very low birth weight prenatally cocaine-exposed toddlers at age 3 years[62] and reported that heavily cocaine-exposed infants showed lower auditory comprehension and total language on the Preschool Language Scale-3 (PLS-3) than those with lighter or no cocaine exposure.[71] Prenatally cocaine-exposed children aged 14 to 50 months scored lower on the Sequenced Inventory of Communicative Development-Revised (SICD-R) total score but were not different from non-cocaine-exposed children on the Peabody Picture Vocabulary Test, primarily a measure of receptive vocabulary.[72] In a contrasting study, no group differences on the SICD-R were found at age 30

TABLE 1. Infant and Toddler Studies Reporting on Prenatal Cocaine Exposure (PCE) and Child Mental and Motor Development (2001 to Present)

Study	Sample Size and Exposure Groups	Measures[a]	Child Age	Controlled for Other Drug Use	Cocaine-Related Mental and Motor Development Findings
Richardson et al. (2008)[66]	61 PCE 1st trimester; 28 PCE all trimesters; 144 non-PCE	BSID	1 year	Yes; when significant, retained in regression models	PCE was not a significant predictor of MDI scores; 2nd trimester PCE was associated with significantly lower PDI.
Brown et al. (2004)[65]	83 PCE; 63 non-drug; (234 birth cohort; 62% retention)	BSID	2 years	N/A due to negative findings in uncontrolled models	No PCE-related group differences on MDI or PDI. PCE children had higher MDI when in nonparental vs. parental care.
Lewis et al. (2004)[61]	147 PCE; 89 non-PCE; (361 birth cohort; 65% retention)	BSID	12, 18, 24, and 36 months	Yes	Direct cocaine-related effects on MDI and PDI in longitudinal models, and at 12 and 24 months for MDI and 24 months for PDI in cross-sectional models; dose-response PCE-associated effects on MDI and PDI.
Messinger et al. (2004)[67]	522 PCE; 705 non-PCE; 98 opiate; 1,129 non-opiate	BSID-II	1, 2, and 3 years	Yes	MDI scores were lower by 1.6 points in PCE vs. non-PCE groups in uncontrolled models, but were not significantly different after covariate adjustment. Group differences in birth weight did not mediate the effect. No PCE-related group differences were noted for PDI.
Mayes et al. (2003)[63]	265 PCE; 66 non-PCE; 129 non-drug (460 birth cohort; retention across visits 69% to 87%)	BSID-II	3, 6, 12, 18, 24, and 36 months	Not as covariates but in the context of grouping	MDI scores were lower in PCE vs. nonPCE groups across all assessment ages; the PCE-related effect was entirely mediated through birth weight and gestational age. PDI declined in all 3 groups over time; PCE children showed a nonsignificant trend toward a greater decrease than children in the other groups.

Continued on next page

TABLE 1 (Continued)

Study	Sample Size and Exposure Groups	Measures[a]	Child Age	Controlled for Other Drug Use	Cocaine-Related Mental and Motor Development Findings
Behnke et al. (2002)[47]	Birth cohort: 154 PCE; 154 non-PCE	BNBAS; BSID	Birth, 1 and 6 months	Yes	Direct PCE-related effects at birth and 6 months on a "Development" latent construct which included the MDI and PDI in SEM longitudinal modeling; indirect effects at birth, 1 month and 6 months mediated by prenatal alcohol and tobacco exposure and birth head circumference.
Frank et al. (2002)[64]	75 PCE/light; 38 PCE/heavy; 90 non-PCE; (252 birth cohort; 81% retention)	BSID	6, 12, and 24 months	Yes	No PCE-related main effect for level of cocaine exposure on MDI or PDI scores; heavily PCE children who received early intervention had higher MDI scores than all other groups; for children with heavier cocaine exposure, low birth weight was related to lower PDI scores.
Singer et al. (2002)[60]	Birth cohort: 218 PCE; 197 non-PCE; retention: 6 months = 339 (84%); 12 months = 364 (90%); 2 years = 379 (94%)	BSID	6 and 12 months, 2 years (corrected age)	Yes	Direct PCE-related effect on MDI (6-point mean group difference at 2 years); PCE children were twice as likely to have significant developmental delay. MDI was related to higher cocaine metabolites in meconium and higher maternal self-report of amount and frequency of cocaine use during pregnancy. PDI scores were unrelated to PCE.
Singer et al. (2001)[62]	31 PCE VLBW[b]; 38 non-PCE VLBW; 76% of 41 PCE and 93% of 41 non-PCE had BSID data at age 3	BSID	3 years	Not reported	Direct PCE-related effect on MDI (10-point mean difference) and PDI scores (13-point mean difference). A higher percentage of PCE children (46%) vs. non-PCE (16%) scored in the delayed range.

PCE = prenatally cocaine-exposed with other drugs; non-PCE = no cocaine exposure but possible exposure to other drugs (usually alcohol, tobacco, and/or marijuana); BSID = Bayley Scales of Infant Development; PDI = Psychomotor Development Index; non-drug = no known drug exposure; MDI = Mental Development Index; BSID-II = Bayley Scales of Infant Development, 2nd edition; BNBAS = Brazelton Neonatal Behavioral Assessment Scale.

[a]All included studies used measures administered by trained examiners blinded to exposure status.

[b]VLBW = very low birth weight (less than 1500 gm).

months, but prenatally cocaine-exposed children were more restricted and delayed in semantic representations in language samples.[73] In studies using coding of language samples during play, qualitative cocaine-associated deficits in the use of complex language[74] and discourse pragmatics and syntax structure[75] were discerned in children with prenatal cocaine exposure.

Potential mechanisms for prenatal cocaine exposure's effect on language function include disruptions in attention processing due to direct impact on the monoaminergic neurotransmitter systems during fetal development, impaired parent-child dyadic interchanges critical to language development, and impoverished caregiving environments often associated with parental drug use and poverty.[74] Because language development during early childhood is clearly determined by many interacting genetic and environmental influences, from a clinical perspective, viewing prenatal cocaine exposure through the lens of cumulative risk may help to identify affected children in need of remediation. In addition, the study of language development in prenatally cocaine-exposed children into later school age and adolescence will be necessary to elucidate pathways linking language functioning to other critical childhood outcomes, including social, academic, and behavioral outcomes.[76]

Behavioral Teratology: Interpreting Prenatal Drug Effects in Infants and Toddlers

Traditional behavioral teratology models espoused by Vorhees and others incorporate the gradient of effects a toxin may have, extending from morphological abnormalities to functional and behavioral impairments, and acknowledge the role of genetics and the environment in the expression of a teratologic effect.[77,78] Much of the research studying the effects of prenatal substance exposure has been conceptualized from a teratologic approach that acknowledges that the effects of a toxin may not be evident at birth, but may arise later in development as functional and behavioral capacities develop. As noted by Fried, traditional models of behavioral teratology are based primarily on animal research in which control of the postnatal environment is optimized.[79] However, infants and children develop within the context of complex social and environmental conditions that also influence functional and behavioral capacities, making it difficult to ascertain a drug-specific teratogenic effect on developmental processes.[79] In addition, the environment may directly impact the expression or degree of a toxin's effect. For example, the influence of prenatal cocaine exposure on behavioral regulation in children may be exacerbated by stressful environmental conditions or disruptive caregiving environments that have been associated with ongoing parental drug use.[80,81]

Research in the area of developmental psychopathology has long established the importance of responsive parenting to optimal development during infancy and the toddler years. Children with prenatal substance exposure are at increased risk for premature birth, low birth weight, impairments in state regulation and arousal modulation and, especially with opioid exposure, withdrawal symptoms.[82] Infants exposed prenatally to drugs have often been described as irritable, lethargic, unresponsive, and/or easily overstimulated; these characteristics may impede healthy dyadic interchanges and have the potential to impair the quality of mother-child interactions.[83–85] In the case of prenatal cocaine exposure, deficits in infant attention may result in maternal difficulty sustaining interactions with their infant.[84,86,87] In addition, infants exposed to both opiates and cocaine have been found to exhibit higher levels of arousal, and their mothers have been found to be less sensitive and stimulating and more likely to disengage and terminate feeding sessions.[82] Continued cocaine use following delivery among mothers with comorbid depression or anxiety has also been related to greater maternal insensitivity and negative parenting behaviors during feeding interactions.[88] Similarly, mother-child interactions during play sessions were most impaired among children with both prenatal cocaine exposure and ongoing maternal cocaine use.[89] It is important to recognize that multiple factors may moderate or mediate the effects of prenatal substance exposure on the caregiving attachment relationship and, ultimately,

FIGURE 1. Comprehensive prevention and intervention services for substance-abusing mothers and their infants.

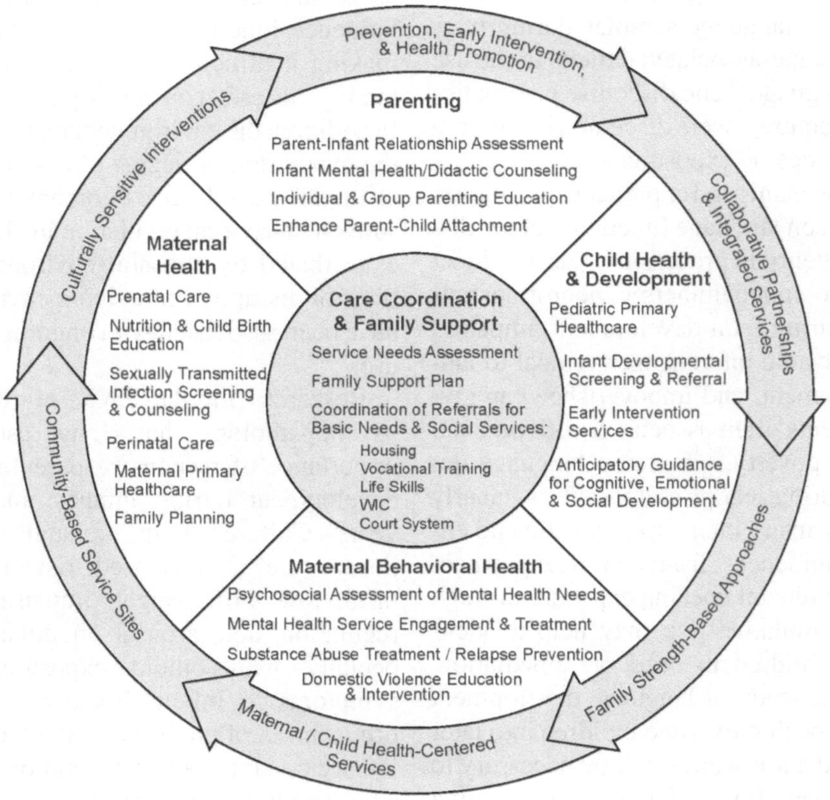

infant development. For example, mothers who use cocaine during pregnancy often abuse other substances, such as alcohol, marijuana, and nicotine, and typically reside in high-risk environments characterized by low-income neighborhoods, poverty, poor nutrition, ongoing caregiver substance use, family instability and homelessness, and limited social support.[83,85,88,90] Illicit substance use during pregnancy combined with these contextual risk factors may exacerbate maternal stress, compromise parenting quality, and negatively impact the caregiving relationship and infant development.

The current manuscript provides an overview of the scientific literature regarding the effects of prenatal opioids and cocaine use on infant and toddler growth and development. Both drugs have the potential to cause significant growth deficits at birth and through the toddler years. In contrast to opioids, which may produce severe NAS and infant neurobehavioral deficits, prenatal cocaine exposure appears to be associated with what has been described as subtle decrements in neurobehavioral, cognitive, and language function. However, even subtle deficits can be extremely costly when they result in significantly higher proportions of children ultimately requiring services for language delays or learning disabilities.[91] Furthermore, these early findings may herald even more significant learning and behavioral problems as the academic and social challenges of the school and community environment create additional stress during early school-age and adolescence. The next article by Lester et al. describes the post-toddler age outcomes of prenatally drug-exposed children. These children, their families, and society in general would be well-served by providing appropriate prevention and intervention services to address the unique needs of substance-abusing pregnant women and their developing offspring. Figure 1 depicts a prevention and intervention model for substance-using mothers and their infants that has inspired the development of various initiatives supported by multiple streams of federal, state, county, and private foundation funding over the past two decades in our Perinatal Chemical Addiction Research and Education Program at the University of Miami Miller School of Medicine. Given the complexities of the environmental context of maternal drug use and the myriad of factors that affect risk and resiliency of their infants and toddlers, we and others[92] are convinced that prevention-intervention programs achieve the most success when maternal and child services are well-integrated and delivered with strong family support, including care coordination to reduce the family's barriers to accessing available services.

REFERENCES

1. Substance Abuse and Mental Health Services Administration. Results from the 2007 National Survey on Drug Use and Health: national findings. NSDUH Series H-34. Rockville, MD: Office of Applied Studies, 2008.

2. Bandstra ES, Accornero VH. Infants of substance-abusing mothers. In: Martin RJ, Fanaroff AA, Walsh MC (eds). Fanaroff and Martin's neonatal-perinatal medicine: diseases of the fetus and newborn. Philadelphia, PA: Mosby Elsevier Press; 2006:733–57.

3. Abel EL, Sokol RJ. Fetal Alcohol Syndrome is now leading cause of mental-retardation. Lancet 1986; 2:1222.

4. Sulik K, Johnston M, Webb M. Fetal alcohol syndrome: embryogenesis in a mouse model. Science 1981; 214:936–938.

5. Committee to Study Fetal Alcohol Syndrome. Fetal Alcohol Syndrome: diagnosis, epidemiology, prevention, and treatment. Washington, DC: National Academy Press, 1996.

6. Slotkin TA. Fetal nicotine or cocaine exposure: which one is worse? J Pharmacol Exp Ther 1998; 285:931–45.

7. Law KL, Stroud LR, LaGasse LL, Niaura R, Liu J, Lester BM. Smoking during pregnancy and newborn neurobehavior. Pediatrics 2003; 111:1318–23.

8. American Academy of Pediatrics Committee on Drugs. Transfer of drugs and other chemicals into human milk. Pediatrics 1989; 84:924–36.

9. Jaddoe V, Troe E, Hofman A, Mackenbach J, Moll H, Steegers E, Witteman J. Active and passive maternal smoking during pregnancy and the risks of low birthweight and preterm birth: the Generation R Study. Paediatr Perinat Epidemiol 2008; 22:162–71.

10. American Academy of Pediatrics Committee on Substance Abuse. Tobacco's toll: implications for the pediatrician. Pediatrics 2001; 107:794–8.

11. Fricker HS, Segal S. Narcotic addiction, pregnancy, and the newborn. Am J Dis Child 1978; 132:360–6.

12. Zelson C, Rubio E, Wasserman E. Neonatal narcotic addiction: 10 year observation. Pediatrics 1971; 48:178–89.

13. Kaltenbach K. Effects of in-utero opiate exposure: new paradigms for old questions. Drug Alcohol Depend 1994; 36:83–7.

14. Kandall SR, Albin S, Lowinson J, Berle B, Eidelman AL, Gartner LM. Differential effects of maternal heroin and methadone use on birth weight. Pediatrics 1976; 58: 681–5.

15. Center for Substance Abuse Treatment Consensus Panel. Pregnant, substance-using women [DHHS Publication No. (SMA) 02–3677]. Treatment Improvement Protocol (TIP) Series #2. Rockville, MD: Substance Abuse and Mental Health Services Administration, 1993.

16. Dashe JS, Sheffield JS, Olscher DA, Todd SJ, Jackson GL, Wendel GD. Relationship between maternal methadone dosage and neonatal withdrawal. Obstet Gynecol 2002; 100:1244–9.

17. Berghella V, Lim PJ, Hill MK, Cherpes J, Chennat J, Kaltenbach K. Maternal methadone dose and neonatal withdrawal. Am J Obstet Gynecol 2003; 189(2):312–7.

18. Johnson RE, Jones HE, Fischer G. Use of buprenorphine in pregnancy: patient management and effects on the neonate. Drug Alcohol Depend 2003; 70:S87–S101.

19. Doberczak TM, Shanzer S, Cutler R, Senie RT, Loucopoulos JA, Kandall SR. One-year follow-up of infants with abstinence-associated seizures. Arch Neurol 1988; 45:649–53.

20. Lester BM, Tronick EZ, LaGasse L, Seifer R, Bauer CR, Shankaran S, Bada HS, Wright LL, Smeriglio VL, Lu J, Finnegan LP, Maza PL. The maternal lifestyle study: effects of substance exposure during pregnancy on neurodevelopmental outcome in 1-month-old infants. Pediatrics 2002; 110:1182–92.

21. Das A, Poole WK, Bada HS. A repeated measures approach for simultaneous modeling of multiple neurobehavioral outcomes in newborns exposed to cocaine in utero. Am J Epidemiol 2004; 159:891–9.

22. Kandall SR. Treatment strategies for drug-exposed neonates. Clin Perinatol 1999; 26:231–43.

23. The American Academy of Pediatrics Task Force on Sudden Infant Death Syndrome. The changing concept of sudden infant death syndrome: diagnostic coding shifts, controversies regarding the sleeping environment, and new variables to consider in reducing risk. Pediatrics 2005; 116:1245–55.

24. Lipsitz PJ. Proposed narcotic withdrawal score for use with newborn-infants: pragmatic evaluation of its efficacy. Clin Pediatr 1975; 14:592–4.

25. Finnegan LP, Kaltenbach K. The assessment and management of neonatal abstinence syndrome. In: Hoekelman N, eds. Primary pediatric care. St. Louis, MO: C.V. Mosby Company, 1992:1367–78.

26. American Academy of Pediatrics Committee on Drugs. Neonatal drug withdrawal. Pediatrics 1998; 101:1079–88.

27. Coyle MG, Ferguson A, LaGasse L, Oh W, Lester B. Diluted tincture of opium (DTO) and phenobarbital versus DTO alone for neonatal opiate withdrawal in term infants. J Pediatr 2002; 140:561–4.

28. Hunt RW, Tzioumi D, Collins E, Jeffery HE. Adverse neurodevelopmental outcome of infants exposed to opiate in-utero. Early Hum Dev 2008; 84:29–35.

29. Ornoy A, Segal J, Bar-Hamburger R, Greenbaum C. Developmental outcome of school-age children born to mothers with heroin dependency: importance of environmental factors. Dev Med Child Neurol 2001; 43: 668–75.

30. Ornoy A, Michailevskaya V, Lukashov I, BarHamburger R, Harel S. The developmental outcome of children born to heroin-dependent mothers, raised at home or adopted. Child Abuse Negl 1996; 20:385–96.

31. Behnke M, Eyler FD, Garvan CW, Wobie K. The search for congenital malformations in newborns with fetal cocaine exposure. Pediatrics 2001; 107:E74.

32. Bauer CR, Langer JC, Shankaran S, Bada HS, Lester B, Wright LL, Krause-Steinrauf H, Smeriglio VL, Finnegan LP, Maza PL, Verter J. Acute neonatal effects of cocaine exposure during pregnancy. Arch Pediatr Adolesc Med 2005; 159:824–34.

33. Behnke M, Davis EF, Conlon M, Wobie K, Stewart WN, Cumming W. Incidence and description of structural brain abnormalities in newborns exposed to cocaine. J Pediatr 1998; 132:291–4.

34. Bandstra ES, Morrow CE, Anthony JC, Churchill SS, Chitwood DD, Steele BM, Ofir AY, Xue L. Intrauterine growth of full-term infants: impact of prenatal cocaine exposure. Pediatrics 2001; 108:1309–19.

35. Frank DA, Bauchner H, Parker S, Huber AM, Kyei-Aboagye K, Cabral H, Zuckerman BS. Neonatal body proportionality and body composition after *in utero* exposure to cocaine and marijuana. J Pediatr 1990; 117:622–6.

36. Church MW, Crossland WJ, Holmes PA, Overbeck GW, Tilak JP. Effects of prenatal cocaine on hearing, vision, growth, and behavior. Ann N Y Acad Sci 1998; 846:12–28.

37. Eyler FD, Behnke M, Conlon M, Woods NS, Wobie K. Birth outcome from a prospective, matched study of prenatal crack/cocaine use: I. Interactive and dose effects on health and growth. Pediatrics 1998; 101:229–37.

38. Bateman DA, Chiriboga CA. Dose-response effect of cocaine on newborn head circumference. Pediatrics 2000; 106:e33.

39. Nordstrom-Klee B, Delaney-Black V, Covington C, Ager J, Sokol R. Growth from birth onwards of children prenatally exposed to drugs: a literature review. Neurotoxicol Teratol 2002; 24:481–8.

40. Frank DA, Augustyn M, Knight WG, Pell T, Zuckerman B. Growth, development, and behavior in early childhood following prenatal cocaine exposure: a systematic review. JAMA 2001; 285:1613–25.

41. Shankaran S, Lester B, Das A, Bauer CR, Bada H, LaGasse L, Higgins R. Impact of maternal substance use during pregnancy on childhood outcome. Semin Fetal Neonatal Med 2007; 12:143–50.

42. Covington CY, Nordstrom-Klee B, Ager J, Sokol R, Delaney-Black V. Birth to age 7 growth of children prenatally exposed to drugs: a prospective cohort study. Neurotoxicol Teratol 2002; 24:489–96.

43. Richardson GA, Goldschmidt L, Larkby C. Effects of prenatal cocaine exposure on growth: a longitudinal analysis. Pediatrics 2007; 120:1017–27.

44. Eyler FD, Behnke M. Early development of infants exposed to drugs prenatally. Clin Perinatol 1999; 26:107–50.

45. Singer LT, Arendt R, Minnes S, Farkas K, Salvator A. Neurobehavioral outcomes of cocaine-exposed infants. Neurotoxicol Teratol 2000; 22:653–66.

46. Morrow CE, Bandstra ES, Anthony JC, Ofir AY, Xue L, Reyes M. Influence of prenatal cocaine exposure on full-term infant neurobehavioral functioning. Neurotoxicol Teratol 2001; 23:533–44.

47. Behnke M, Eyler FD, Garvan CW, Wobie K, Hou W. Cocaine exposure and developmental outcome from birth to 6 months. Neurotoxicol Teratol 2002; 24:283–95.

48. Neuspiel DR, Hamel SC, Hochberg E, Greene J, Campbell D. Maternal cocaine use and infant behavior. Neurotoxicol Teratol 1991; 13:229–33.

49. Myers BJ, Dawson KS, Britt GC, Lodder DE, Meloy LD, Saunders MK, Meadows SL, Elswick RK. Prenatal cocaine exposure and infant performance on the Brazelton Neonatal Behavioral Assessment Scale. Subst Use Misuse 2003; 38:2065–96.

50. Coles CD, Platzman KA, Smith IE, James ME, Falek A. Effects of cocaine and alcohol use in pregnancy on neonatal growth and neurobehavioral status. Neurotoxicol Teratol 1992; 14:23–33.

51. Tronick EZ, Frank DA, Cabral H, Mirochnick M, Zuckerman BS. Late dose-response effects of prenatal cocaine exposure on newborn neurobehavioral performance. Pediatrics 1996; 98:76–83.

52. Bendersky M, Lewis M. Arousal modulation in cocaine-exposed infants. Dev Psychol 1998; 34:555–64.

53. Schuetze P, Eiden RD. The association between maternal cocaine use during pregnancy and physiological regulation in 4–to 8–week-old infants: an examination of possible mediators and moderators. J Pediatr Psychol 2006; 31:15–26.

54. Corwin MJ, Lester BM, Sepkoski C, McLaughlin S, Kayne H, Golub HL. Effects of in utero cocaine exposure on newborn acoustical cry characteristics. Pediatrics 1992; 89:1199–203.

55. Rotta NT, Cunha GB. [Prenatal exposure to cocaine: review of the neurobehavioral effects]. J Pediatr (Rio J) 2000; 76:179–84.

56. Mehta SK, Super DM, Connuck D, Kirchner HL, Salvator A, Singer L, Fradley LG, Kaufman ES. Autonomic

alterations in cocaine-exposed infants. Am Heart J 2002; 144:1109–15.

57. Lester BM, LaGasse L, Seifer R, Tronick EZ, Bauer CR, Shankaran S, Bada HS, Wright LW, Smeriglio VL, Liu J, Finnegan LP, Maza PL. The Maternal Lifestyle Study (MLS): effects of prenatal cocaine and/or opiate exposure on auditory brain response at one month. J Pediatr 2003; 142:279–85.

58. Tan-Laxa MA, Sison-Switala C, Rintelman W, Ostrea EM. Abnormal auditory brainstem response among infants with prenatal cocaine exposure. Pediatrics 2004; 113:357–60.

59. Lester BM, LaGasse LL, Freier K, Brunner SM. Studies of cocaine-exposed human infants. NIDA Res Monogr 1996; 164:175–210.

60. Singer LT, Arendt R, Minnes S, Farkas K, Salvator A, Kirchner HL, Kliegman R. Cognitive and motor outcomes of cocaine-exposed infants. JAMA 2002; 287:1952–60.

61. Lewis MW, Misra S, Johnson HL, Rosen TS. Neurological and developmental outcomes of prenatally cocaine-exposed offspring from 12 to 36 months. Am J Drug Alcohol Abuse 2004; 30:299–320.

62. Singer LT, Hawkins S, Huang J, Davillier M, Baley J. Developmental outcomes and environmental correlates of very low birthweight, cocaine-exposed infants. Early Hum Dev 2001; 64:91–103.

63. Mayes LC, Cicchetti D, Acharyya S, Zhang H. Developmental trajectories of cocaine-and-other-drug-exposed and non-cocaine-exposed children. J Dev Behav Pediatr 2003; 24:323–35.

64. Frank DA, Jacobs RR, Beeghly M, Augustyn M, Bellinger D, Cabral H, Heeren T. Level of prenatal cocaine exposure and scores on the Bayley Scales of Infant Development: modifying effects of caregiver, early intervention, and birth weight. Pediatrics 2002; 110:1143–52.

65. Brown JV, Bakeman R, Coles CD, Platzman KA, Lynch ME. Prenatal cocaine exposure: a comparison of 2-year-old children in parental and nonparental care. Child Dev 2004; 75:1282–95.

66. Richardson GA, Goldschmidt L, Willford J. The effects of prenatal cocaine use on infant development. Neurotoxicol Teratol 2008; 30:96–106.

67. Messinger DS, Bauer CR, Das A, Seifer R, Lester BM, LaGasse LL, Wright LL, Shankaran S, Bada HS, Smeriglio VL, Langer JC, Beeghly M, Poole WK. The maternal lifestyle study: cognitive, motor, and behavioral outcomes of cocaine-exposed and opiate-exposed infants through three years of age. Pediatrics 2004; 113: 1677–85.

68. Miller-Loncar C, Lester BM, Seifer R, LaGasse LL, Bauer CR, Shankaran S, Bada HS, Wright LL, Smeriglio VL, Bigsby R, Liu J. Predictors of motor development in children prenatally exposed to cocaine. Neurotoxicol Teratol 2005; 27:213–20.

69. Morrow CE, Bandstra ES, Anthony JC, Ofir AY, Xue LH, Reyes MB. Influence of prenatal cocaine exposure on early language development: longitudinal findings from four months to three years of age. J Dev Behav Pediatr 2003; 24:39–50.

70. Morrow CE, Vogel AL, Anthony JC, Ofir AY, Dausa AT, Bandstra ES. Expressive and receptive language functioning in preschool children with prenatal cocaine exposure. J Pediatr Psychol 2004; 29:543–54.

71. Singer LT, Arendt R, Minnes S, Salvator A, Siegel AC, Lewis BA. Developing language skills of cocaine-exposed infants. Pediatrics 2001; 107:1057–64.

72. Johnson JM, Seikel JA, Madison CL, Foose SM, Rinard KD. Standardized test performance of children with a history of prenatal exposure to multiple drugs/cocaine. J Commun Disord 1997; 30:45–72.

73. Bland-Stewart LM, Seymour HN, Beeghly M, Frank DA. Semantic development of African-American children prenatally exposed to cocaine. Semin Speech Lang 1998; 19:167–86.

74. Malakoff ME, Mayes LC, Schottenfeld R, Howell S. Language production in 24-month-old inner-city children of cocaine-and-other-drug-using mothers. J Appl Dev Psychol 1999; 20:159-80.

75. Mentis M, Lundgren K. Effects of prenatal exposure to cocaine and associated risk factors on language development. J Speech Hear Res 1995; 38:1303–18.

76. Bandstra ES, Morrow CE, Vogel AL, Accornero VH, Ofir AY, Anthony JC. Language development in children exposed to cocaine *in utero*: a longitudinal perspective. Ital J Pediatr 2003; 29:31–8.

77. Vorhees CV, Butcher RE. Behavioral teratology. In: Snell K, ed. Developmental toxicology. New York: Praeger Press, 1982:249–98.

78. Vorhees CV. Concepts in teratology and developmental toxicology derived from animal research. Ann N Y Acad Sci 1989; 562:31–41.

79. Fried PA. Conceptual issues in behavioral teratology and their application in determining long-term sequelae of prenatal marihuana exposure. J Child Psychol Psychiatry 2002; 43:81–102.

80. Mayes LC. A behavioral teratogenic model of the impact of prenatal cocaine exposure on arousal regulatory systems. Neurotoxicol Teratol 2002; 24:385–95.

81. Mayes LC, Grillon C, Granger R, Schottenfeld RS. Regulation of arousal and attention in preschool children exposed to cocaine prenatally. Ann N Y Acad Sci 1998; 846:126–43.

82. LaGasse LL, Messinger D, Lester BM, Seifer R, Tronick EZ, Bauer CR, Shankaran S, Bada HS, Wright LL, Smeriglio VL, Finnegan LP, Maza PL, Liu J. Prenatal drug exposure and maternal and infant feeding behaviour. Arch Dis Child 2003; 88:F391–9.

83. Johnson MO. Mother-infant interaction and maternal substance use/abuse: an integrative review of research

literature in the 1990s. Online J Knowl Synth Nurs 2001; 8.

84. Mayes LC, Feldman R, Granger RH, Haynes OM, Bornstein MH, Schottenfeld R. The effects of polydrug use with and without cocaine on mother–infant interaction at 3 and 6 months. Infant Behav Dev 1997; 20:489–502.

85. Freier K. In utero drug exposure and maternal-infant interaction: the complexities of the dyad and their environment. Infant Ment Health J 1994; 15:176–88.

86. Bandstra ES, Morrow CE, Anthony JC, Accornero VH, Fried PA. Longitudinal investigation of task persistence and sustained attention in children with prenatal cocaine exposure. Neurotoxicol Teratol 2001; 23:545–59.

87. Accornero VH, Amado AJ, Morrow CE, Xue LH, Anthony JC, Bandstra ES. Impact of prenatal cocaine exposure on attention and response inhibition as assessed by continuous performance tests. J Dev Behav Pediatr 2007; 28:195–205.

88. Eiden RD, Stevens A, Schuetze P, Dombkowski LE. A conceptual model for maternal behavior among polydrug cocaine-using mothers: the role of postnatal cocaine use and maternal depression. Psychol Addict Behav 2006; 20:1–10.

89. Johnson AL, Bandstra ES, Morrow CE, Accornero VH, Xue L, Anthony JC. Maternal cocaine use: estimated effects on mother-child play interactions in the preschool period. J Dev Behav Pediatr 2002; 23:191–202.

90. Espinosa M, Beckwith L, Howard J, Tyler R, Swanson K. Maternal psychopathology and attachment in toddlers of heavy cocaine-using mothers. Inf Men Health J 2001; 22:316–33.

91. Lester BM, LaGasse LL, Seifer R. Cocaine exposure and children: the meaning of subtle effects. Science 1998; 282:633–4.

92. Finnegan LP, Hagan T, Kaltenbach K. Opiod dependence: scientific foundations for clinical practice, pregnancy and substance abuse: perspectives and directions. Proceedings of the New York Academy of Medicine 1991; 67:223–9.

Children of Addicted Women

Barry M. Lester, PhD
Linda L. Lagasse, PhD

ABSTRACT. The purpose of this article was to review follow up studies of children with prenatal drug exposure from preschool through adolescence. Specifically, the authors focus on the effects of prenatal exposure to cocaine, methamphetamine, and opiates on behavior and development. The largest number of studies have examined cocaine-exposed children. The authors identified 42 studies that suggest that there are unique effects of prenatal cocaine exposure on 4- to 13-year-old children, particularly in the areas of behavior problems, attention, language, and cognition. In addition, studies make reasonable attempts to control for possible confounding factors. Systematic research on the long-term effects of prenatal methamphetamine exposure is just beginning but seems to be showing similar effects to that of cocaine. The literature on the on the long-term effects of children with prenatal opiate exposure is more substantial than the methamphetamine literature but it is still relatively sparse and surprising in that there is little recent work. Thus, there are no studies on the current concerns with opiates used for prescription mediation. There is a growing literature using neuroimaging techniques to study the effects of prenatal drug exposure that holds promise for understanding brain/behavior relationships. In addition to pharmacological and teratogenic effects, drugs can also be viewed from a prenatal stressor model. The author discuss this "fetal origins" approach that involves fetal programming and the neuroendocrine system and the potential implications for adolescent brain and behavioral development.

INTRODUCTION

In the previous article, Bandstra et al. reviewed the effects of prenatal drug exposure through infancy and early childhood. Our review will consider prenatal drug exposure effects from preschool through adolescence, specifically the outcomes of exposure to cocaine, methamphetamine, and opiates related to behavior and development. We first provide a review of the published findings of exposure to each drug. We then describe how the effects of these drugs can be viewed from a prenatal stressor model involving fetal programming and the neuroendocrine system and the implications for adolescent brain development.

PRENATAL COCAINE EXPOSURE

Unlike the rather sparse prenatal methamphetamine and opiate literatures, our knowledge about the long-term effects of prenatal cocaine exposure is based on a reasonably large and growing corpus of studies. We were able to identify 42 published, empirical studies of the behavior and development of children with prenatal cocaine exposure between the ages of

4 and 13. These studies were published between 1996 and 2008, most (n = 34) between 2004 and 2008, many of which were longitudinal follow-up reports of the cohorts in the previous Bandstra review. We grouped the studies into categories based on the following outcomes: behavior problems, psychopathology, substance use, IQ, language, cognition (including attention), motor function, school and achievement, quality of relationships, and psychophysiology. In addition, there are 10 neuroimaging studies in this population. We will summarize the findings by category with effects for cocaine considered positive when adjusted for covariates (if applied) and then review covariate and related methodological issues.

Behavior Problems

Behavior problems formed the largest category and included 18 studies,[1–18] 10 of which showed negative effects of prenatal cocaine exposure.[2–4,6–8,10,13,16–18] Of the 18 studies, 8 used the parent report Child Behavior Checklist,[1,2,5,11,12,16–18] 4 used the teacher version (Teacher Report Form),[9,13–15] 4 used other tests (1 child report [Youth Risk Behavior Survey][4] and 3 teacher report [PROBES-14][6–8]), and 2 used behavioral observations (frustration; aggression elicitation).[3,10] For the 12 studies that used the comparable measures (Child Behavior Checklist or Teacher Report Form), only four showed adverse cocaine effects on major subscales (e.g., externalizing) or minor subscales,[2,13,16] with two studies reporting interaction of cocaine exposure, gender, and alcohol exposure (girls exposed to cocaine but not alcohol were more aggressive, whereas boys exposed to both cocaine and alcohol were more delinquent).[13,16]

Psychopathology

Only two studies have examined psychopathology in these children,[12,19] probably because the age of most of the cohorts limited these examinations. One study showed an association between cocaine exposure and ADHD and oppositional defiance disorder[12] and the other studied showed no effects on suicide ideation.[19]

Substance Use

Only 1 study included substance use as an outcome in children. In this study of preadolescents at 10.5 years of age, cocaine-exposed children were more likely to have smoked cigarettes.[4]

IQ

IQ was reported in 14 studies[5,11,14,15,20–29] and, perhaps surprisingly, negative effects of prenatal cocaine exposure were only observed in five of those.[5,21,22,24,28] Of the five studies, gender effects were observed in two studies with lower IQ in boys.[5,22] Among the seven studies reporting analysis of summary IQs and subtests,[5,14,21–23,27,28] six reported significant cocaine effects on Perceptual Reasoning,[28] Verbal Comprehension,[21] Verbal Reasoning (boys only),[5] Short Term Memory,[5] Picture Completion,[23] Object Assembly,[23] Abstract/Visual Reasoning (boys only),[22] Visual-Spatial Skills,[27] General Knowledge,[27] and Arithmetic Skills.[27] In only two cases, summary and subtests scores were reduced by prenatal cocaine exposure but the full IQ score was not.[23,27]

Language

There were eight studies of language in cocaine exposed children.[5,11,24,26,30–34] Only one study did not find negative exposure effects,[11] and one study reported adverse effects for boys only.[5] In a study that examined the trajectory of overall language function from 3 to 7 years, language deficits associated with cocaine exposure were stable across all age points with no increase or decrease over time.[31]

Cognition

Cognition is a somewhat heterogeneous category. The largest single category among cocaine exposure studies is sustained attention, which was examined in seven studies,[14,15,26,35–38] with all but one study[14] reporting adverse exposure effects. Six studies used a continuous performance or vigilance task[14,15,26,35,36,38] that yields scores for omission (poor sustained attention) and commission errors (impulsivity); of these 6 studies, 2 reported exposure effects on omission errors,[35,36] 2 reported both omission and commission errors,[15,26] and 1 reported the effects on both outcomes.[38] Other attention tests (contrary tapping/delay task efficiency) also reported poor attention in exposed children.[37]

Nine studies examined the relationship of cocaine exposure to other cognitive processes, including visual motor integration,[20,26] task persistence observation during a mastery paradigm,[36] central processing (PROBES) for all subjects.[6] or for boys only,[7] visual-spatial short term memory (Gordon Maze),[39,40] maintaining set with interference (Stroop Task),[41] visual attention span and sequencing (Knox Cube),[26] and set switching (Trail Making).[15] Of the nine studies, all but two studies reported harmful exposure effects, both on visual motor integration.[15,20] The diversity of findings is similar to the subscales on IQ tests in that no specific ability emerges across the relevant studies that relate to cocaine exposure. However, in this case, the study-specific selection of paradigms makes replication less likely.

Motor

Of three studies assessing motor abilities, one showed more motor problems in cocaine exposed boys[7] and two showed no cocaine effects on fine motor behavior.[20,26] Unlike the infancy studies described by Bandstra et al. in the previous article in this supplement, relatively few studies examined motor function in older exposed children.

School Performance and Academic Achievement

Of the seven studies of school performance and academic achievement,[14,17,18,24,25,28,42] three showed negative effects of prenatal cocaine exposure.[24,25,42] Two effects were on achievement tests...;[24,25] the other showed an increase in referrals for special education and academic support services.[42] In addition, the one study that anticipated school success by examining school readiness reported negative prenatal cocaine exposure effects.[26]

Relationships

No effects of prenatal cocaine exposure were found in the study of the mother-child relationship using observation of play.[11] No other relationships, such as relationships to peers or teachers, were examined in any study.

Psychophysiology

Only two physiological studies have been reported, and both showed cocaine effects. One showed changes on event-related potentials during the Stroop executive function test of working memory.[41] In the other study, skin conductance, which measures electrodermal activity and reflects autonomic arousal, was altered during stress in children with prenatal cocaine exposure.[18]

Covariates

As has been well documented, early studies of the effects of prenatal cocaine exposure were difficult to interpret because of methodological problems, including small sample size and poor control for confounding factors (e.g., prenatal exposure to other substances and measures of the postnatal caregiving environment) that could also explain what has been ascribed to cocaine exposure. The 42 studies reported above were based on reasonably large sample sizes, with 20 studies based on samples of over 300 participants with the maximum over 1,000 participants. Of course, some studies are based on the same cohorts. There are 14 different cohorts for a total of 4,419 children. Large population studies also allow statistical control for many prenatal and postnatal confounding variables. Studies vary in the criteria used to determine what potentially confounding variables are, such as variables on which the exposed group and the comparison group show statistical differences or variables that have a predetermined relationship (e.g., $P < .10$) with both the predictor variable (prenatal cocaine exposure) and the outcome variable (e.g., IQ). Thus, in the description below, the fact that a variable was not controlled could simply mean that it did not need to be controlled. For example, a study of full-term infants would not control for gestational age. Lack of control could also mean that a factor was not measured.

Prenatal Confounding Variables

Use of legal or illegal substances other than cocaine during pregnancy (tobacco, alcohol, marijuana, or opiates) was controlled in 33 of the 42 studies. Measures of fetal growth, including birthweight, prematurity, head circumference, birth length, and neonatal medical problems, were controlled in 20 studies, and 12 studies controlled for prenatal care.

Postnatal Confounding Variables

Poverty or socioeconomic status was controlled in 27 of the 42 studies. A variety of measures have been used to control for specific aspects of the home environment. The Home Observation Measure of the Environment (Home scale) was used as a covariate in 15.[43] Placement in foster care was used in 23 studies. Related measures of the household included the number of children in the home,the number of regular caregivers, chaos, social support, and early case management. Measures of the caretaker included age, education, marital status, parity, employment, IQ, and self-esteem. Parental psychological problems or symptoms were controlled in 15 studies, and maternal IQ was controlled in 16 studies. Parent's postnatal use of drugs was controlled in 22 studies. Measures of the child included daycare, head start, enrichment programs, services, and blood lead level. Child measures that could be outcomes were also included as covariates, including IQ, physical growth, and depressive symptoms. Two studies controlled for child abuse, one for domestic violence, and six for community violence. Race was used as a covariate in 10 studies and gender was used in 28 studies.

Dose-Response Relationships

One question that is often asked is whether the effects of prenatal cocaine exposure are related to the level of cocaine use. There are no studies in this group in which results of toxicology analysis (e.g., urine or meconium) were reported in relation to prenatal cocaine exposure. However, studies have used maternal interviews to derive measures of cocaine use patterns, such as the frequency of use per week. Of the 42 studies, 10 found effects of heavy cocaine use related to worse outcome: six on behavior problems, two on language, and two on IQ.

Summary

The review of these 42 studies suggests that there are unique effects of prenatal cocaine exposure on 4- to 13-year-old children across a range of domains, including behavior problems, attention, language, and cognition. The evidence is weaker that IQ, school performance, and achievement are affected. In the domains of psychopathology, physiology, and motor performance, only a few studies have been reported. It is important to note that, in general, the effects that have been observed have been conducted on reasonably large samples with adjustment for confounding variables, suggesting that these are "true" cocaine effects. There is also evidence for dose response relationships, especially with behavior problems.

It is also interesting to note dimensions that have not been well studied. Substance use by the children and more studies of psychopathology will undoubtedly be undertaken as the age of children in longitudinal cohorts increases. It is somewhat surprising that there is only one study of parent-child relationships because this was an important focus in the infancy research, and that there are only two psychophysiological studies. There are also few studies using direct observation of behavior. Maternal report, paper and pencil forms, or computerized tests were used in 39 of the 42 studies.

In addition to determining the unique effects of cocaine, it is also important to determine how cocaine interacts with other factors in predicting child outcome. There are no studies on the interaction between genetic markers and prenatal cocaine exposure. The field of genetics provides an interesting metaphor in that we now know that most diseases do not obey the laws of classical Mendelian genetics and this is likely even more the case for behavioral phenotypes. For most outcomes, the genetic "main effect" is relatively small, allowing the study of gene-environment interactions to take center stage. This approach is starting to appear in the prenatal cocaine exposure literature. For example, studies have examined mediators or moderators of prenatal cocaine exposure effects, including gender, alcohol, head circumference, and foster care. The impact of puberty on this complex matrix has yet to be studied. More sophisticated statistical modeling is starting to be used to study more complex relationships between prenatal cocaine exposure and child outcome, including structural equation modeling, generalized estimated equations, and hierarchical linear modeling.

Neuroimaging

Quantitative neuroimaging studies represent another way in which the field of prenatal cocaine exposure has matured. We chose to review these 10 studies separately because this is a new area for this field and many are preliminary with relatively small sample sizes and were not able to control for confounding variables as in the 42 studies reviewed above. Quantitative neuroimaging studies in children with prenatal cocaineinclude anatomical magnetic resonance imaging (MRI), diffusion tensor imaging, functional MRI, and magnetic resonance spectroscopy (MRS).

In anatomicor structural MRI, the volumes of cortical gray matter, white matter, subcortical structures, corpus callosum, and cerebellum have been studied. In a study of 41 11-year-old children, Behnke et al. reported a decrease in the volume of the right anterior cerebellum in cocaine-exposed children.[44] Singer et al. reported a decrease in gray matter volume in the right parietal and left occipital lobes, as well as a decrease in corpus callosum volume in 35 cocaine-exposed children aged 7 to 8.[44] They also found a decrease in the corpus callosum, which contains the largest fiber tract in the brain. A mean decrease in the caudate volumes in 49 cocaine-exposed children at 13 to 15 years of age has also been reported.[45] We[46] reported a volumetric decrease in cortical gray matter, thalamus, and putamen in a sample of 22 cocaine-exposed and comparison children between 9 and 11 years of age. We also found an inverse "dose response" relationship between prenatal exposure level and these volumes. The caudate and putamen findings in these last two studies[45,46] are noteworthy because these are major dopaminergic areas. Finally, although lower mean cortical gray matter and total parenchymal volumes were reported by Rivkinin in a study of 35 children aged 10 to 14, cocaine effects did not remain[47] when adjusted for prenatal exposure to other drugs.

In a study using diffusion tensor imaging, cocaine-exposed children (age: 10.6 years, N = 53) had increased average diffusion in left frontal callosal and right frontal projection fibers.[48] They found no differences in fractional anisotropic values. A brain MRS study of children exposed to cocaine in utero showed increased Creatine in the frontal white matter, with normal N-acetyl aspartate in the absence of any visible volumetric brain abnormalities on MRI.[49] It was suggested that the increased Creatine could be due to glial proliferation or an abnormal energy metabolism. Using perfusion fMRI, Rao et al. reported a 10% decrease in global cerebral blood flow in 49 adolescents with prenatal cocaine exposure.[50] They found an increase in cerebral blood flow in the anterior and superior brain regions and suggested that this may be due to development of compensatory mechanisms for reduced global cerebral blood flow during neural ontogeny. In an fMRI study of 34 adolescents, both fMRI activation patterns during task and performance on a separate executive function test were similar between cocaine exposed and comparison groups.[51] We[52] measured fMRI activation during a response inhibition task in 24 children aged 8 and 9 years. Groups did not differ in task performance by design. Cocaine-exposed children showed greater activation in the right inferior frontal cortex and the caudate during response inhibition, suggesting that prenatal cocaine may affect the development of brain systems involved in the regulation of attention and response inhibition.

Recent advances in MRI quality have greatly contributed to our understanding of prenatal cocaine exposure effects on the developing human brain. Longitudinal studies with careful control of other factors (exposure to other drugs and postnatal environmental factors) will add to the excitement of these findings. It will be important to determine whether these imaging findings are related to the child's behavior and performance on psychological tests outside of the scanner. It is also important to be mindful of the fact that imaging findings do not denote causal mechanisms, but rather associations between a condition and brain involvement, not that the condition was caused by said brain findings. For example, we might speculate that the increases in fMRI,[52] Creatine,[53] diffusion,[48] and cerebral blood flow[50] could represent compensatory mechanisms related to other (as yet unknown) areas of brain involvement. Nor do we know the developmental course of these findings, their presence or absence at birth, the effects of prenatal cocaine exposure on normative processes of brain development and maturation, or the role of the postnatal environment in shaping brain architecture, structure, and function.

PRENATAL METHAMPHETAMINE EXPOSURE

Systematic research on the long-term effects of prenatal methamphetamine exposure is limited.[54] As mentioned in the previous Bandstra review in this supplement, the only published findings from the NIH longitudinal Infant Development Environment and Lifestyle (IDEAL) study are from the infancy period. IDEAL is a multisite (Iowa, Oklahoma, California, and Hawaii) longitudinal study of children with prenatal exposure to methamphetamines. Preliminary findings from approximately half of that sample at age 3 show (Figure 1) no differences between methamphetamine-exposed and comparison children on the Bayley Scales (MDI shown here) at ages 1, 2, or 3 years of age.

On the Child Behavior Checklist at age 3, the number of children with total problem behavior scores above the clinical cutoff was similar for the methamphetamine exposed (28 of 133; 21%) and comparison group (25 of 138; 18%). This finding should be considered in light of our study of cocaine exposed children. Differences in IQ between cocaine exposed and controls did not emerge until 4.5 years of age and increased from ages 4.5 to 7.[55] Adverse cocaine effects on the Child Behavior Checklist were not observed

FIGURE 1. Mean Bayley MDI scores in methamphetamine exposed and comparison children at ages 1, 2, 3.

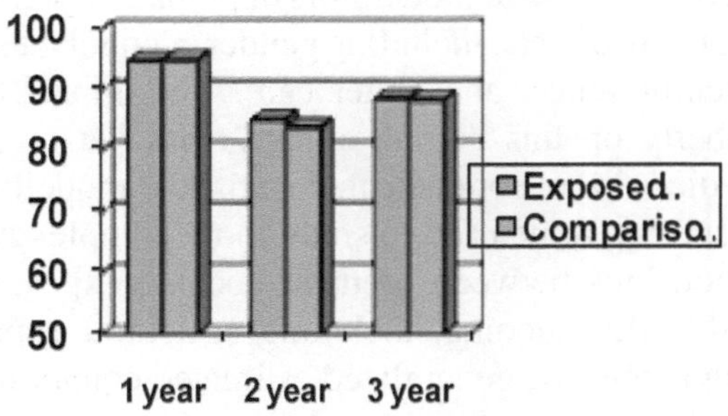

until age 5 but remained stable from ages 5 to 7.[2] It is possible that stimulant drugs, such as cocaine and methamphetamine, affect areas of the brain whose functions become more easily tested as children are forced to deal with settings that place more demands on executive function abilities and require higher cortical functioning, such as school. Continued follow-up is critical to determine whether the methamphetamine effects continue to parallel the cocaine effects.

The only published work on prenatal methamphetamine exposure in school-age children draws from a series of studies from Sweden examining 66 amphetamine-exposed children who have been studied to the age of 14.[56] At age 4,[57] there were no differences in physical growth or health. Mean IQ was lower than a separately selected control group from the population. The amphetamine group had more disturbed or problem children if the mother was still addicted. Also at age 4,[58] child adjustment correlated with maternal alcohol and drug use, maternal stress, and paternal criminal convictions. At age 8,[59] the extent of prenatal exposure could be related to psychometric outcome, aggression, peer problems, adjustment, and general assessment, as well as alcohol exposure and pregnancy attitudes. Maternal psychiatric treatment, alcohol abuse, and the number of custodians correlated with aggressive behavior and general assessment. The children had problems with advancement in school due to delays in math and language, and at age 14 they had difficulties with physical fitness activities.[56] The limitations of this work include lack of a control group, small sample size, and prenatal polydrug use (30% of the mothers used heroin, 81% used alcohol with 1/3 meeting criteria for alcohol abuse, and 80% smoked more than 10 cigarettes a day). The study is also based on self-report and the route of administration of amphetamine was injection, which is less common today in the United States.

Neuroimaging

Two MRI studies of children exposed prenatally to methamphetamine have been reported.[53,60] Smith et al.[53] used proton magnetic resonance spectroscopy (^{1}H MRS) to evaluate neurochemical alterations in 12 children between 7 and 8 years old who were exposed prenatally to methamphematine and other substances (alcohol and tobacco) and 14 controls. Increases were found in total creatine in the basal ganglia of the methamphetamine exposed group, suggesting possible alterations in cellular energy metabolism; however, no differences were found in N-acetyl-containing compounds that would indicate neuronal damage or loss. In the second study,[60] volumetric MRI differences in brain regions were found between 13 methamphetamine-exposed (and other drug) children and a group of 15 non-drug exposed controls at 7 and 8 years of age. Methamphetamine was associated with reduced volumes of the globus pallidus, putamen, and hippocampus. However, the reductions in the methamphetamine-exposed group were not related to performance on attention and verbal memory tests.

PRENATAL EXPOSURE TO OPIATES

The literature on the long-term effects of children with prenatal opiate exposure is more substantial than the methamphetamine literature but it is still relatively sparse[61] and surprising in that little work has been done since the thorough reviews published ten years ago.[61,62] The opiates studied include heroin and methadone. Currently, there is concern about the abuse of opiate-based prescription medication (e.g., Vicodin or hydrocodone and OxyContin or oxycodone) by pregnant women, as well as the recently approved drug, buprenorphine. No studies have yet been published on the effects of these drugs on the post-infancy child. Methodological similarities and differences exist between the literature studying prenatal cocaine (and to some extent methamphetamine) and opiate exposure. Both literatures face the problem of how to control for virtually the same set of confounding factors when trying to isolate the effects of the target drug. Most pregnant women who use cocaine or opiates are polydrug users and most of their children are raised in high-risk social environments. One major difference between the prenatal cocaine/methamphetamine and opiate studies is that the opiates studies tend to have small sample sizes (20 subjects per group is typical), which precludes statistical adjustment for confounding variables, whereas cocaine studies deal with larger population samples, allowing more valid adjustment for confounding variables.

Some studies were cross-sectional rather than longitudinal. In one such study,[63] 3 to 6 year old children exposed to heroin performed more poorly than the comparison groups on the general cognitive index and on the perceptual, quantitative, and memory subscales of the McCarthy Scales. There were three comparison groups—drug-nave subjects in drug-using households, a group with multiple high risk factors, and a socioeconomic comparison group—but there were only 15 to 22 children in each group, including the heroin exposed group. No effects of heroin exposure on measures of speech and language, activity level, mental maturity, or developmental status were found. In a study of 126 offspring of heroin addicts between 8 and 17 years old,[64] school absence, school failure, and behavior problems in school were more common than in comparison group from the same neighborhoods. Cubas and Field[65] compared 20 children aged 6 to 13 with prenatal exposure to methadone and a control group of 20 non-exposed children. No differences were found on cognitive tests, although methadone exposure was associated with lower IQ scores. Methadone-exposed children exhibited greater anxiety, aggression, and rejection than did those in the control group, and their mothers reported more behavior problems.

looseness-1In three longitudinal studies, no differences were found on the McCarthy scales related to prenatal opiate exposure. These include: a study comparing methadone-exposed (N = 26), heroin-exposed (N = 25), and a drug-free comparison group (N = 41) in 3 to 6 year old children;[66] a study of 27 methadone-exposed and 17 non-drug exposed children at age 4 years;[67] and a study of methadone-exposed (N = 33) and non-drug exposed comparison children (N = 30) at age 5 years.[68] In the latter study, during the testing session, the drug-exposed children were more active, energetic, immature, and showed more task irrelevant activity during the testing session.[68] In a longitudinal follow-up of the previously reported sample,[63] 32 prenatally exposed 6- to 11-year-old children were compared with 12 controls.[69] Behavior problems in school and psychiatric referrals were related to maternal opiate use, although the number of cases was small (7 psychiatric referrals in the exposed group and 1 in the comparison group). In a 10-year follow-up of 36 methadone-exposed children and a similar group of comparison children, Hans[62] found that drug-exposed children were somewhat more likely to receive ADHD and disruptive behavior diagnoses and made more errors on an attentional (continuous performance) task.

As mentioned above, it is known that many of these children grow up in high-risk environments.[62] Similar learning and behavioral problems have been reported in school-age children either exposed to drugs in utero[70] or living with drug-dependent parents who were not exposured in utero.[71,72] Some studies have attempted to isolate the effects of in utero opiate exposure by using different types of comparison groups. An early study compared 6- to 15-year-old, opiate-exposed children to a narcotic-environment group (no in utero exposure but caregivers used opiates) using measures of neurological and behavioral functioning.[73] Opiate-exposed children had impairments in perceptual, motor, and attentional functioning, whereas the narcotic environmental group did not. In more recent work, lower scores were found on the McCarthy scales at age 4.5 in a Norwegian study of 64 exposed and 52 comparison children under conditions of minimal postnatal social risk.[74] Social risk was "controlled" by studying children of heroin users (and other drugs) placed in the care of foster or adoptive parents who were specially selected to provide care for infants at risk. In an Israeli study attempting to control the postnatal environment, the development of children aged 5 to 12 years born to mothers with heroin dependency who were raised at home or adopted was studied in comparison with children with environmental deprivation alone (i.e., low parental socioeconomic status and evidence of neglect), children born to fathers with heroin dependency,[75] and control individuals of average socioeconomic status.[76] Children born to parents with heroin dependency who were raised at home showed impaired verbal, performance, and reading and arithmetic skills. Children born to mothers with heroin dependency but who were adopted at a young age had normal intellectual and learning abilities, but some had reduced function on performance IQ. Children born to parents with heroin dependency had a high rate of ADHD, including those who were adopted; the highest rate of ADHD was seen in children born to mothers with heroin dependency who were raised at home.

One physiological study attempted to control for opiate-related environmental factors, comparing a group of children born to mothers who began drug use after the child was born to a group of children with intrauterine opiate exposure for environmental influences associated with parental drug use.[77] Heart rate variability (vagal tone) was measured during an attention task. When distracters were added to the attention task, opiate-exposed boys failed to suppress vagal tone compared to both control groups. However, both the opiate-exposed boys and the environmental controls made fewer correct responses than non-drug-exposed controls on this task. Thus, physiological responses to increased attention demands may be affected by prenatal opiate exposure as well as environmental influences.

In a neuroimaging study of this population,[78] morphometric cerebral characteristics were studied in 9- to 11-year-old children with prenatal exposure to opiates and other drugs (n = 14) compared to unexposed controls (n = 14).

Compared to controls, the drug-exposed children had smaller intracranial and brain volumes, including smaller cerebral cortex, amygdala, accumbens area, putamen, pallidum, brainstem, cerebellar cortex, cerebellar white matter, and inferior lateral ventricles, as well as a thinner cortex of the right anterior cingulate and lateral orbitofrontal cortex. There was some association between volumes of the right anterior cingulate, the right lateral orbitofrontal cortex, and the accumbens area and cognitive ability and behavior problems.

UNDERSTANDING THE EFFECTS OF PRENATAL DRUG EXPOSURE

One determinant of the long-term effects of prenatal drug exposure is the pathophysiology of the drug itself. Typically, we think of drugs as teratogens that cause malformations or defects depending on the drugs' mechanisms of action. For example, the effects of cocaine on blocking the reuptake of neurotransmitters, especially dopamine, have been well documented. However, in addition to teratogenic effects, there may also be non-teratogenic effects of drugs. We[79] have described a model in which cocaine, as well as other substances, acts as an intrauterine stressor that disrupts the neuroendocrine environment and the genetic programming of fetal-placental development.

Increasing evidence from preclinical, prospective clinical and epidemiological studies suggest that, at least in the case of disease, early development does echo throughout life.[80–82] The literature on the influence of prenatal stress on the offspring suggests that many biological factors acting during prenatal life are associated not only with the development of common adult cardiovascular and metabolic disorders but also with neurobehavioral abnormalities[83–93] and behavioral disorders.[94–97] These findings have given rise to the concept of "*fetal origins of adult disease*" or the "*developmental origins of health and disease.*" Although original studies related low birthweight to adult disease, it is generally accepted that low birth weight per se is not at the heart of these disorders, but that there are common factors that influence intrauterine growth, as well as adult physiological systems.[82] The "fetal origins" observations are due, in part, to environmental factors acting early in life that "program" developing systems, altering structure and function and probably behavioral expression. Prenatal drug exposure may be one of those factors that alter the set-points or "hard-wire" physiological systems. Stress hormones such as catecholamines and glucocorticoids can alter regulation of the neuroendocrine environment by acting on the hypothalamic-pituitary-adrenal (HPA) axis, which results in an altered set point for physiologic, metabolic, and behavioral outcomes.[98] Because they are an important feature of the stress response, glucocorticoids have become prominent candidates as mediators of the effects of "programming."

Fetal Programming and Brain

The brain is particularly sensitive to prenatal programming including effects on the HPA axis. Pregnant dams exposed to stress show increased adrenocorticotrophic hormone (ACTH) and corticosterone (CORT).[82,99,100] Prenatal stress also increases CORT and ACTH levels in adult offspring.[80–82,96,98] The effect of prenatal stress on adult hippocampal corticosteroid receptor density[95,101–104] may have implications for emotional reactivity. Prenatally, stressed rats have a high degree of "emotionality,"[105] indicated by decreased locomotion and increased defecation.[105–108] They also show less play,[109] more defensive freezing,[110] less movement in an activity wheel,[111] and increased vocalizations.[100] Prenatal stress affects cognitive abilities including operant discrimination,[112] reversal task in a water maze,[113,114] and memory.[115] In other animal studies, maternal stress during pregnancy results in offspring that are more irritable, anxious, and difficult to control.[82,116–119]

Brain neurotransmitter systems and glucocorticoids interact to modulate both behavior and HPA activity.[120] Disturbances in HPA regulation and brain monoamine levels have been associated with affective and anxiety disorders in humans.[121–124] Also, in human studies, poor health outcomes, such as low birthweight, preterm birth, and intrauterine growth retardation, have been related to prenatal stress.[125,126] Moderate to severe stressful life events during midgestation was related to birth weight and small head circumference, suggesting effects on the brain.[127] Maternal first-trimester exposure to the stress of war has also been associated with an increased risk of the offspring developing schizophrenia in adult life.[128] Similar to the "emotionality" reported in animal studies, human infants exposed to stress in utero show high reactivity, activity, and irritability.[129–131] Psychological and behavioral abnormalities, including learning and behavior problems, have also been reported in children exposed to prenatal stress.[132–135] The effects of prolonged exposure to chronic stress, called allostatic load,[136] and, concomitantly, prolonged activation of the neuroendocrine stress axes has also been related to physical disease and behavioral disorders.[137]

Drugs and Gene Expression

Our model[79] argues for the effects of an adverse intrauterine environment, created by maternal use of cocaine and other substances, on catecholamines and glucocorticoids. As a stressor, a drug such as cocaine programs the HPA axis as well as behavior, due in part to plasticity of brain monoamine systems. Specifically, a drug as a stressor alters the expression of key candidate genes and gene networks important to placental function in late gestation. We focus on the norepinephrine transporter (NET) and a steroid metabolic enzyme, 11β-HSD-2 and placental gene networks.

Placental NET and 11ß-HSD-2 are pivotal placental genes that program the intrauterine neuroendocrine environment during development by protecting the fetus from excess catecholamines and glucocorticoids, which have harmful effects on the fetus.[138] Lower placental 11ß-HSD-2 activity is associated with smaller fetuses in rats[139] and humans.[140–143] Mutations of 11ß-HSD-2 are also associated with low birth weight in human infants[144] and increased fetal cortisol levels are associated with IUGR[145] 11ß-HSD-2 modulates the programming effects of prenatal glucocorticoid exposure.[146,147] The HPA axis is highly sensitive to the effects of glucocorticoids on perinatal programming.[82,148–150] High levels of maternal glucocorticoids have been shown to disrupt intrauterine growth, postnatal HPA axis function, and neurobehavioral outcome in offspring. Placental expression of this key enzyme is potently downregulated at the RNA, protein, and functional level by norepinephrine, which is in turn regulated by NET. Downreguàltion of NET is associated with adverse intrauterine events, including maternal/placental disorders such as preeclampsia and exposure to drugs such as cocaine and nicotine.[151,152] Reduced placental NET expression from drug exposure may lead to increased circulating catecholamines, downregulation of 11β-HSD-2 and chronic fetal hypercortisolism, leading to altered neuroendocrine (HPA axis) activity and dysregulated neurobehavioral functioning. Because catecholamines are released during stress, this may be a mechanism linking prenatal stress with altered fetal development mediated by effects on 11β-HSD-2.

The altered expression of these two key candidate genes is likely associated with changes in networks of genes involved in critical placental functions that maintain physiological homeostasis in utero and otherwise promote intrauterine growth, development, and preparation for postnatal life. Epigenetic mechanisms (i.e., environmentally induced changes in gene expression without altering DNA sequences) are thought to be involved. Our preliminary findings[79] showed that these changes in placental gene expression are associated with altered methylation of placental genomic DNA, particularly in promoter regions. We found that dysregulation of 11β HSD2 related to cocaine or nicotine use during pregnancy was associated with hypermethylation, suggesting DNA silencing. Significant interest exists in the concept that modifications of DNA mechanistically affect "adaptation to the environment." Complex processes such as the development of memory are now being attributed to chromatin remodeling, epigenetic modifications of DNA, and lasting alterations in gene expression.[153] Drugs of abuse induce "adaptations" in brain regions. This may occur through alterations in gene expression, altered chromatin remodeling, and alterations in the number and projections of neurons in specific regions. Recently, cocaine was shown to induce neuroadaptations through altered gene expression.[154] It is becoming widely accepted that chromatin remodeling is an important regulatory mechanism underlying gene environment interactions, learning, and drug-induced neural and behavioral plasticity. Similar alterations in DNA methylation and histone acetylation are seen following intrauterine growth restriction.[155] It is thus likely that altered expression of these key candidate genes and associated changes in networks of genes involved in placental function follows intrauterine exposure to stress, cocaine, and other substances. Some of these changes may lead to permanent "epigenetic" alterations in placental gene expression through DNA methylation and chromatin remodeling. Because of the unique nature of intrauterine development, these observations suggest mechanisms whereby an altered placental environment can have effects on neurodevelopmental outcome.

Behavioral Dysregulation

In our model,[79] these disruptions in the placental environment alter HPA set points, resulting in neuroendocrine and behavioral dysregulation in the newborn that can lead to the type of childhood behavioral, emotional, and neurocognitive deficits related to prenatal drug exposure described earlier. These deficits may, in turn, have implications for adolescent psychopathology, including early onset of substance use in adolescence. Behavioral dysregulation can begin in utero and is proposed to be a dynamic developmental process as alterations in the quality of the environment (prenatal and postnatal) modify behavioral expression. Behavioral dysregulation is evidenced during infancy as neurobehavioral and neuroendocrine disorganization. During childhood, indicators of behavioral dysregulation reflect a deficient capacity to control behavior and regulate emotion. These phenotypes are important because they appear to be prognostic indicators for substance use.[156] The earlier a drug is used, the greater the likelihood of its abuse during adolescence and adulthood.[157,158] These phenotypes reflect major domains of psychological function, cognition, affect, and behavior and include impulsivity, reactive aggression, sensation seeking, excessive risk taking,[159,160] irritability, negative affect, difficult temperament,[161–163] conduct disorder, attention deficit hyperactivity disorder, oppositional defiant disorder, anxiety, depression,[164]and impaired executive function.[165–167] This collection of disturbances in emotion regulation and behavior control is included in the construct of neurobehavioral disinhibition and is thought to reflect disturbances in the prefrontal cortex.[168] Some of these disturbances have already been reported in the prenatal cocaine exposure studies reported above and may become more visible as these youths enter adolescence. Disruption of neuroendocrine homeostasis in utero by prenatal drug exposure can be observed at birth and may lead to lasting behavioral dysregulation that increases vulnerability to substance use, resulting in early onset substance use in adolescents.

Adolescent Brain Development

The understanding that addiction is a developmental disease means that it is critical to consider the influence of specific developmental periods.[169] In addition to fetal development, we know that brain development continues well beyond childhood and adolescence.[170,171] The "immaturity" or abnormal development of the adolescent brain may be related to risk taking behavior, including substance use.

Extensive maturational changes that occur in brain development in adolescence may confer vulnerability to substance use through disruption of the HPA system.[172–174] Maturation of high-order association cortices, including changes in prefrontal cortex, occurs later than low-order sensory cortices during late adolescence.[75] Neurophysiologic,[175,176] and fMRI[177] studies have shown disruption of the frontal cortex in youths at high risk for substance use onset. These youths show deficits related to substance use onset, including poor affect modulation, behavior control, and executive function processes thought to reflect a neuromaturational disturbance subserved by neural systems in the anterior cerebral cortex.[160,178–180] Stress reactivity is related to pubertal development and brain regions, such as the hippocampus, prefrontal cortex, and amygdale, and anatomic areas that are highly sensitive to stress hormones and regulate emotionality and continue to mature during the peripubertal period.[181] Glucocorticoid receptors are present in both subcortical (paraventricular nucleus and other hypothalamic nuclei, the hippocampus and parahippocampal gyrus) and cortical structures, with a preferential distribution in the prefrontal cortex.[120,182–184] The distribution of glucocorticoid receptors in the primate brain are more closely related to the human brain in terms of neocortex development.[185,186] Non-human primate studies suggest that the behavioral effects of prenatal cocaine exposure may not be manifested until later in development.[187,188] Chronic exposure to stress or allostatic load leads to atrophy and impaired neuronal function in the hippocampus and medial prefrontal cortex,[189–191] regions that are responsible for executive function and adaptation to stress. Cocaine and other substance related to "fetal programming" could have long-term effects on HPA axis activity, resulting in a physiological endophenotype of cortisol reactivity that could be a harbinger of substance use. Although there are studies of cortisol reactivity related to prenatal drug exposure in infancy, as described in the previous article by Bandstra et al., we did not find any studies relating prenatal cocaine, methamphetamine, or opiate exposure to cortisol in older children.

The advent of the "Genome Era" has dissolved disciplinary boundaries and transformed the research landscape. The sequencing of the human genome has lead to advances in our understanding of the cellular, molecular, and biochemical mechanisms that regulate development, learning, behavior, and the molecular pathways that could be altered due to prenatal substance exposure. These are exciting times as advances in neurobiology, including genetics, epigenetics, fetal programming, and neural plasticity, will provide a better understanding of the pathophysiology and long-term implications of prenatal drug exposure that should have implications for public policy, preventive intervention and treatment.

REFERENCES

1. Accornero VH, Morrow CE, Banstra ES, Johnson AL, Anthony JC. Behavioral outcome of preschoolers exposed to cocaine: role of maternal behavioral health. J Ped Psych 2002; 27:259–69.

2. Bada HS, Das A, Bauer CR, Shankaran S, Lester B, LaGasse L, Hammond J, Wright LL, Higgins R. Impact of prenatal cocaine exposure on child behavior problems through school age. Pediatrics 2007; 119:e348–59.

3. Bendersky M, Bennett D, Lewis M. Aggression at age 5 as a function of prenatal exposure to cocaine, gender, and environmental risk. J Pediatr Psychol 2006; 31: 71–84.

4. Bennett D, Bendersky M, Lewis M. Preadolescent health risk behavior as a function of prenatal cocaine exposure and gender. J Dev Behav Pediatr 2007; 28: 467–72.

5. Bennett DS, Bendersky M, Lewis M. Children's intellectual and emotional–behavioral adjustment at 4 years as a function of cocaine exposure, maternal characteristics, and environmental risk. Dev Psych 2002; 38:648–58.

6. Covington C, Nordstrom–Klee B, Delaney–Black V, Templin T, Ager J, Sokol RJ. Development of an instrument to assess problem behavior in first grade students prenatally exposed to cocaine. Part II: validation. Subst Abus 2001; 22:217–33.

7. Delaney–Black V, Covington C, Nordstrom B, Ager J, Janisse J, Hannigan JH, Chiodo L, Sokol RJ. Prenatal cocaine: quantity of exposure and gender moderation. J Dev Behav Pediatr 2004; 25:254–63.

8. Delaney–Black V, Covington C, Templin T, Ager J, Martier S, Sokol R. Prenatal cocaine exposure and child behavior. Pediatrics 1998; 102:945–50.

9. Delaney–Black V, Covington C, Templin T, Ager J, Nordstrom-Klee B, Martier S, Leddick L, Czerwinski RH, Sokol RJ. Teacher–assessed behavior of children prenatally exposed to cocaine. Pediatrics 2000; 106:783–91.

10. Dennis T, Bendersky M, Ramsay D, Lewis M. Reactivity and regulation in children prenatally exposed to cocaine. Dev Psychol 2006; 42:688–97.

11. Kilbride HW, Castor CA, Fuger KL. School–age outcome of children with prenatal cocaine exposure following early case management. J Dev Behav Pediatr 2006; 27:181–7.

12. Linares TJ, Singer LT, Kirchner HL, Short EJ, Min MO, Hussey P, Minnes S. Mental health outcomes of cocaine–exposed children at 6 years of age. J Pediatr Psychol 2006; 31:85–97.

13. Nordstrom Bailey B, Sood BG, Sokol RJ, Ager J, Janisse J, Hannigan JH, et al. Gender and alcohol moderate prenatal cocaine effects on teacher–report of child behavior. Neurotoxicol Teratol 2005; 27:181–9.

14. Richardson GA, Conroy ML, Day NL. Prenatal cocaine exposure: effects on the development of school–age children. Neurotoxicol Teratol 1996; 18:627–34.

15. Savage J, Brodsky NL, Malmud E, Giannetta JM, Hurt H. Attentional functioning and impulse control in cocaine–exposed and control children at age ten years. J Dev Behav Pediatr 2005; 26:42–7.

16. Sood BG, Nordstrom Bailey B, Covington C, Sokol RJ, Ager J, Janisse J, Hannigan JH, Delaney-Black V. Gender and alcohol moderate caregiver reported child behavior after prenatal cocaine. Neurotoxicol Teratol 2005; 27:191–201.

17. Hurt H, Brodsky NL, Roth H, Malmud E, Giannetta JM. School performance of children with gestational cocaine exposure. Neurotoxicol Teratol 2005; 27:203–11.

18. Kable JA, Coles CD, Lynch ME, Platzman K. Physiological responses to social and cognitive challenges in 8–year olds with a history of prenatal cocaine exposure. Dev Psychobiol 2008; 50:251–65.

19. O'Leary CC, Frank DA, Grant–Knight W, Beeghly M, Augustyn M, Rose–Jacobs R, Cabral HJ, Gannon K. Suicidal ideation among urban nine and ten year olds. J Dev Behav Pediatr 2006; 27:33–9.

20. Arendt RE, Short EJ, Singer LT, Minnes S, Hewitt J, Flynn S, et al. Children prenatally exposed to cocaine: developmental outcomes and environmental risks at seven years of age. J Dev Behav Ped 2004; 25:83–90.

21. Asanbe CB, Lockert E. Cognitive abilities of African American children with prenatal cocaine/polydrug exposure. J Health Care Poor Underserved 2006; 17: 400–12.

22. Bennett DS, Bendersky M, Lewis M. Children's cognitive ability from 4 to 9 years old as a function of prenatal cocaine exposure, environmental risk, and maternal verbal intelligence. Dev Psychol 2008; 44:919–28.

23. Frank DA, Rose–Jacobs R, Beeghly M, Wilbur M, Bellinger D, Cabral H. Level of prenatal cocaine exposure and 48–month IQ: importance of preschool enrichment. Neurotoxicol Teratol 2005; 27:15–28.

24. Marques PR, Pokorni JL, Long T, Teti LO. Maternal depression and cognitive features of 9–year–old children prenatally–exposed to cocaine. Am J Drug Alcohol Abuse 2007; 33:45–61.

25. Morrow CE, Culbertson JL, Accornero VH, Xue L, Anthony JC, Bandstra ES. Learning disabilities and intellectual functioning in school–aged children with prenatal cocaine exposure. Dev Neuropsychol 2006; 30:905–31.

26. Pulsifer MB, Radonovich K, Belcher HME, Butz AM. Intelligence and school readiness in preschool children with prenatal drug exposure. Child Neuropsychology 2004; 10:89–101.

27. Singer LT, Minnes S, Short E, Arendt R, Farkas K, Lewis B, Klein N, Russ S, Min MO, Kirchner HL. Cognitive outcomes of preschool children with prenatal cocaine exposure. JAMA 2004; 291:2448–56.

28. Singer LT, Nelson S, Short E, Min MO, Lewis B, Russ S, Minnes S. Prenatal cocaine exposure: drug and environmental effects at 9 years. J Pediatr 2008; 153: 105–11.

29. Wasserman GA, Kline JK, Bateman DA, Chiriboga C, Lumey LH, Friedlander H, Melton L, Heagarty MC. Prenatal cocaine exposure and school–age intelligence. Drug Alcohol Depend 1998; 50:203–10.

30. Bandstra ES, Morrow CE, Vogel AL, Fifer RC, Ofir AY, Dausa AT, Xue L, Anthony JC. Longitudinal influence of prenatal cocaine exposure on child language functioning. Neurotox Teratol 2002; 24:297–308.

31. Bandstra ES, Vogel AL, Morrow CE, Xue L, Anthony JC. Severity of prenatal cocaine exposure and child language functioning through age seven years: a longitudinal latent growth curve analysis. Substance Use and Misuse 2004; 39:25–59.

32. Beeghly M, Martin B, Rose–Jacobs R, Cabral H, Augustyn M, Bellinger D, Frank DA. Prenatal cocaine exposure and children's language functioning at 6 and 9.5 years: moderating effects of child age, birthweight, and gender. J Pediatr Psychol 2006; 31:98–115.

33. Lewis BA, Kirchner HL, Short EJ, Minnes S, Weishampel P, Satayathum S, Singer LT. Prenatal cocaine and tobacco effects on children's language trajectories. Pediatrics 2007; 120:e78–85.

34. Lewis BA, Singer Lt SEJ, Minnes S, Arendt R, Weshampel P, Klein N, Min MO. Four year language outcomes of children exposed to cocaine in utero. Neurotoxicol.Teratol. 2004; 26:617–27.

35. Accornero VH, Amado AJ, Morrow CE, Xue L, Anthony JC, Bandstra ES. Impact of prenatal cocaine exposure on attention and response inhibition as assessed by continuous performance tests. J Dev Behav Pediatr 2007; 28:195–205.

36. Bandstra ES, Morrow CE, Anthony JC, Accornero VH, Fried PA. Longitudinal investigation of task persistence and sustained attention in children with prenatal cocaine exposure. Neurotoxicol Teratol. 2001; 23: 545–59.

37. Bendersky M, Gambini LS, Lastella A, Bennett DS, Lewis M. Inhibitory motor control at five years as a function of prenatal cocaine exposure. J Dev Behav Ped 2003; 24:345–51.

38. Noland JS, Singer LT, Short EJ, Minnes S, Arendt RE, Kirchner HL, Bearer C. Prenatal drug exposure and selective attention in preschoolers. Neurotoxicol Teratol 2005; 27:429–38.

39. Mayes L, Snyder PJ, Langlois E, Hunter N. Visuospatial working memory in school–aged children exposed in utero to cocaine. Child Neuropsychol 2007; 13:205–18.

40. Schroder MD, Snyder PJ, Sielski I, Mayes L. Impaired performance of children exposed in utero to cocaine on a novel test of visuospatial working memory. Brain Cog 2004; 55:409–12.

41. Mayes LC, Molfese DL, Key AP, Hunter NC. Event–related potentials in cocaine–exposed children during a Stroop task. Neurotoxicol Teratol 2005; 27:797–813.

42. Levine TP, Liu J, Das A, Lester B, Lagasse L, Shankaran S, Bada HS, Bauer CR, Higgins R. Effects of

prenatal cocaine exposure on special education in school–aged children. Pediatrics 2008; 122:e83–91.

43. Caldwell B, Bradley R. HOME inventory and administration manual. Littlerock: University of Arkansas for Medical Sciences and University of Arkansas at Littlerock, 2001.

44. Dow–Edwards DL, Benveniste H, Behnke M, Bandstra ES, Singer LT, Hurd YL, et al. Neuroimaging of prenatal drug exposure. Neurotoxicol Teratol 2006; 28:386–402.

45. Avants BB, Hurt H, Giannetta JM, Epstein CL, Shera DM, Rao H, et al. Effects of heavy in utero cocaine exposure on adolescent caudate morphology. Pediatr Neurol 2007; 37:275–9.

46. Neyzi N, Quinn B, Kekatpure D, Kennedy S, Sheinkopf B, Lester B, et al. Automated segmentation of brain structures in a pediatric population with prenatal cocaine exposure. In: 2007 meeting of the Society for Neuroscience. San Diego, CA; 2007.

47. Rivkin MJ, Davis PE, Lemaster JL, Cabral HJ, Warfield SK, Mulkern RV, Robson CD, Rose-Jacobs R, Frank DA. Volumetric MRI study of brain in children with intrauterine exposure to cocaine, alcohol, tobacco, and marijuana. Pediatrics 2008; 121:741–50.

48. Warner TD, Behnke M, Eyler FD, Padgett K, Leonard C, Hou W, Garvan CW, Schmalfuss IM, Blackband SJ. Diffusion tensor imaging of frontal white matter and executive functioning in cocaine–exposed children. Pediatrics 2006; 118:2014–24.

49. Smith LM, Chang L, Yonekura ML, Grob C, Osborn D, Ernst T. Brain proton magnetic resonance spectroscopy and imaging in children exposed to cocaine in utero. Pediatrics 2001; 107:227–31.

50. Rao H, Wang J, Giannetta J, Korczykowski M, Shera D, Avants BB, Gee J, Detre JA, Hurt H. Altered resting cerebral blood flow in adolescents with in utero cocaine exposure revealed by perfusion functional MRI. Pediatrics 2007; 120:e1245–54.

51. Hurt H, Giannetta JM, Korczykowski M, Hoang A, Tang KZ, Betancourt L, Brodsky NL, Shera DM, Farah MJ, Detre JA. Functional magnetic resonance imaging and working memory in adolescents with gestational cocaine exposure. J Pediatr 2008; 152:371–7.

52. Sheinkopf SJ, Lester BM, Sanes JN, Eliassen JC, Hutchison ER, Seifer R, Lagasse LL, Durston S, Casey BJ. Functional MRI and response inhibition in children exposed to cocaine in utero. Dev Neurosci 2009; 31(1–2):159–66.

53. Smith LM, Chang L, Yonekura ML, Grob C, Osborn D, Ernst T. Brain proton magnetic resonance spectroscopy in children exposed to methamphetamine in utero. Neurology 2001; 57:255–60.

54. Wouldes T, LaGasse L, Sheridan J, Lester B. Maternal methamphetamine use during pregnancy and child outcome: what do we know? NZ Med J 2004; 117(1206):1–10.

55. Lester B, Das A, LaGasse L, Seifer R, Bauer C, Shankaran S, Bada H, Messinger D, Wright L, Smeriglio V, Poole K. Prenatal cocaine exposure and 7–year outcome: IQ and special education. Ped Res 2004; 53:534A.

56. Cernerud L, Eriksson M, Jonsson B, Steneroth G, Zetterstrom R. Amphetamine addiction during pregnancy: 14–year follow–up of growth and school performance. Acta Paediatr 1996; 85:204–8.

57. Billing L, Eriksson M, Steneroth G, Zetterstrom R. Pre–school children of amphetamine–addicted mothers. I. Somatic and psychomotor development. Acta Paediatr Scand 1985; 74:179–84.

58. Billing L, Eriksson M, Steneroth G, Zetterstrom R. Predictive indicators for adjustment in 4–year–old children whose mothers used amphetamine during pregnancy. Child Abuse Negl 1988; 12:503–7.

59. Billing L, Eriksson M, Jonsson B, Steneroth G, Zetterstrom R. The influence of environmental factors on behavioral problems in 8–year–old children exposed to amphetamine during fetal life. Child Abuse Negl 1994; 18: 3–9.

60. Chang L, Smith LM, LoPresti C, Yonekura ML, Kuo J, Walot I, Ertist T. Smaller subcortical volumes and cognitive deficits in children with prenatal methamphetamine exposure. Psychiatry Res 2004; 132:95–106.

61. Kaltenbach KA. Exposure to opiates: behavioral outcomes in preschool and school– age children. NIDA.Res.Monogr. 1996; 164:230–41.

62. Hans SL. Prenatal drug exposure: behavioral functioning in late childhood and adolescence. NIDA Res Monogr 1996; 164:261–76.

63. Wilson GS, McCreary R, Kean J, Baxter JC. The development of preschool children of heroin–addicted mothers: a controlled study. Pediatrics 1979; 63:135–41.

64. Sowder B, Burt M. Children of Heroin addicts: an assessment of health, learning, behavioral, and adjustment problems. New York, NY: Praeger, 1980.

65. de Cubas MM, Field T. Children of methadone–dependent women: developmental outcomes. Am J Orthopsychiatry 1993; 63:266–76.

66. Lifschitz MH, Wilson GS, Smith EO, Desmond MM. Factors affecting head growth and intellectual function in children of drug addicts. Pediatrics 1985; 75: 269–74.

67. Kaltenbach K, Finnegan L. Children exposed to methadone in–utero: Assessment of developmental and cognitive ability. Ann N Y Acad Sci 1989; 562:360–362.

68. Strauss ME, Lessen–Firestone JK, Chavez CJ, Stryker JC. Children of methadone–treated women at five years of age. Pharmacol Biochem Behav 1979; 11(Suppl): 3–6.

69. Wilson GS. Clinical studies of infants and children exposed prenatally to heroin. Ann N Y Acad Sci 1989; 562:183–94.

70. Olofsson M, Buckley W, Andersen GE, Friis–Hansen B. Investigation of 89 children born by

drug–dependent mothers. II. Follow–up 1–10 years after birth. Acta Paediatr Scand 1983; 72:407–10.

71. Hejanic B, Barredo V, Hejanic M, Tomelleri C. Children of heroin addicts. Inter J Addict 1979; 14:919–31.

72. Nichtem S. The children of drug users. J Amer Acad Child Adolesc Psych 1973; 12:24–31.

73. Davis DD, Templer DI. Neurobehavioral functioning in children exposed to narcotics in utero. Addict Behav 1988; 13:275–83.

74. Moe V. Foster–placed and adopted children exposed in utero to opiates and other substances: prediction and outcome at four and a half years. J Dev Behav Pediatr 2002; 23:330–9.

75. Gogtay N, Giedd JN, Lusk L, Hayashi KM, Greenstein D, Vaituzis AC, Nugent TF, 3rd, Herman DH, Clasen LS, Toga AW, Rapoport JL, Thompson PM. Dynamic mapping of human cortical development during childhood through early adulthood. Proc Natl Acad Sci USA 2004; 101:8174–9.

76. Ornoy A, Segal J, Bar–Hamburger R, Greenbaum C. Developmental outcome of school–age children born to mothers with heroin dependency: importance of environmental factors. Dev Med Child Neurol 2001; 43:668–75.

77. Hickey JE, Suess PE, Newlin DB, Spurgeon L, Porges SW. Vagal tone regulation during sustained attention in boys exposed to opiates in utero. Addict Behav 1995; 20:43–59.

78. Walhovd KB, Moe V, Slinning K, Due-Tonnessen P, Bjornerud A, Dale AM, van der Kouwe A, Quinn BT, Kosofsky B, Greve D, Fischl B. Volumetric cerebral characteristics of children exposed to opiates and other substances in utero. Neuroimage 2007; 36:1331–44.

79. Lester B, Padbury J. The Third Pathophysiology of Prenatal Cocaine Exposure. Dev Neurosci 2009; 31(1–2):23–35.

80. Barker DJ, Osmond C, Rodin I, Fall CH, Winter PD. Low weight gain in infancy and suicide in adult life. BMJ 1995; 311:1203.

81. Gluckman PD, Hanson MA. Living with the past: evolution, development, and patterns of disease. Science 2004; 305:1733–6.

82. Welberg LA, Seckl JR. Prenatal stress, glucocorticoids and the programming of the brain. J Neuroendocrinol 2001; 13:113–28.

83. Barker D. Fetal programming of coronary heart disease. Trends Endocrinol Metab 2002; 13:364–8.

84. Barker DJ. The fetal origins of adult hypertension. J Hypertens Suppl 1992; 10:S39–44.

85. Barker DJ, Osmond C, Golding J, Kuh D, Wadsworth ME. Growth in utero, blood pressure in childhood and adult life, and mortality from cardiovascular disease. BMJ 1989; 298:564–7.

86. Falkner B. Birth weight as a predictor of future hypertension. Am J Hypertens 2002; 15(2 Pt 2):43S–5S.

87. Hales CN, Barker DJ, Clark PM, Cox LJ, Fall C, Osmond C, Winter PD. Fetal and infant growth and impaired glucose tolerance at age 64. BMJ 1991; 303(6809):1019–22.

88. McMillen IC, Robinson JS. Developmental origins of the metabolic syndrome: prediction, plasticity, and programming. Physiol Rev 2005; 85:571–633.

89. Ong KK, Dunger DB. Birth weight, infant growth and insulin resistance. Eur J Endocrinol 2004; 151(Suppl 3):U131–9.

90. Phillips D, Barker D, Hales C, Hirst S, Osmond C. Thinness at birth and insulin resistance in adult life. Diabetologia 1994; 37:150–4.

91. Rich-Edwards JW, Colditz GA, Stampfer MJ, Willett WC, Gillman MW, Hennekens CH, Speizer FE, Manson JE. Birthweight and the risk for type 2 diabetes mellitus in adult women. Ann Intern Med 1999; 130(4 Pt 1):278–84.

92. Sallout B, Walker M. The fetal origin of adult diseases. J Obstet Gynaecol 2003; 23:555–60.

93. Stein CE, Fall CH, Kumaran K, Osmond C, Cox V, Barker DJ. Fetal growth and coronary heart disease in south India. Lancet 1996; 348:1269–73.

94. Allin M, Rooney M, Cuddy M, Wyatt J, Walshe M, Rifkin L, Murray R. Personality in young adults who are born preterm. Pediatrics 2006; 117:309–16.

95. Gale CR, Martyn CN. Birth weight and later risk of depression in a national birth cohort. Br J Psychiatry 2004; 184:28–33.

96. Thompson C, Syddall H, Rodin I, Osmond C, Barker DJ. Birth weight and the risk of depressive disorder in late life. Br J Psychiatry 2001; 179:450–5.

97. Wals M, Reichart CG, Hillegers MH, Van Os J, Verhulst FC, Nolen WA, Ormel J. Impact of birth weight and genetic liability on psychopathology in children of bipolar parents. J Am Acad Child Adolesc Psychiatry 2003; 42:1116–21.

98. Matthews SG. Antenatal glucocorticoids and the developing brain: mechanisms of action. Semin Neonatol 2001; 6:309–17.

99. Slotkin TA, Orband–Miller L, Queen KL, Whitmore WL, Seidler FJ. Effects of prenatal nicotine exposure on biochemical development of rat brain regions: maternal drug infusions via osmotic minipumps. J Pharmacol Exp Ther 1987; 240:602–11.

100. Williams MT, Hennessy MB, Davis HN. Stress during pregnancy alters rat offspring morphology and ultrasonic vocalizations. Physiol Behav 1998; 63:337–43.

101. Barbazanges A, Piazza PV, Le Moal M, Maccari S. Maternal glucocorticoid secretion mediates long–term effects of prenatal stress. J Neurosci 1996; 16:3943–9.

102. Henry C, Kabbaj M, Simon H, Le Moal M, Maccari S. Prenatal stress increases the hypothalamo–pituitary–adrenal axis response in young and adult rats. J Neuroendocrinol 1994; 6:341–5.

103. Maccari S, Piazza PV, Kabbaj M, Barbazanges A, Simon H, Le Moal M. Adoption reverses the long–term impairment in glucocorticoid feedback induced by prenatal stress. J Neurosci 1995; 15(1 Pt 1):110–6.

104. Vallee M, Mayo W, Dellu F, Le Moal M, Simon H, Maccari S. Prenatal stress induces high anxiety and postnatal handling induces low anxiety in adult offspring: correlation with stress–induced corticosterone secretion. J Neurosci 1997; 17:2626–36.

105. Fride E, Dan Y, Feldon J, Halevy G, Weinstock M. Effects of prenatal stress on vulnerability to stress in prepubertal and adult rats. Physiol Behav 1986; 37:681–7.

106. Pfister HP, Muir JL. Prenatal exposure to predictable and unpredictable novelty stress and oxytocin treatment affects offspring development and behavior in rats. Int J Neurosci 1992; 62(3–4):227–41.

107. Poltyrev T, Keshet GI, Kay G, Weinstock M. Role of experimental conditions in determining differences in exploratory behavior of prenatally stressed rats. Dev Psychobiol 1996; 29:453–62.

108. Wakshlak A, Weinstock M. Neonatal handling reverses behavioral abnormalities induced in rats by prenatal stress. Physiol Behav 1990; 48:289–92.

109. Takahashi LK, Haglin C, Kalin NH. Prenatal stress potentiates stress–induced behavior and reduces the propensity to play in juvenile rats. Physiol Behav 1992; 51:319–23.

110. Takahashi LK, Turner JG, Kalin NH. Prenatal stress alters brain catecholaminergic activity and potentiates stress–induced behavior in adult rats. Brain Res 1992; 574:131–7.

111. Lambert KG, Kinsley CH, Jones HE, Klein SL, Peretti SN, Stewart KM. Prenatal stress attenuates ulceration in the activity stress paradigm. Physiol Behav 1995; 57:989–94.

112. Weller A, Glaubman H, Yehuda S, Caspy T, Ben–Uria Y. Acute and repeated gestational stress affect offspring learning and activity in rats. Physiol Behav 1988; 43:139–43.

113. Hayashi A, Nagaoka M, Yamada K, Ichitani Y, Miake Y, Okado N. Maternal stress induces synaptic loss and developmental disabilities of offspring. Int J Dev Neurosci 1998; 16:209–16.

114. Szuran T, Zimmermann E, Welzl H. Water maze performance and hippocampal weight of prenatally stressed rats. Behav Brain Res 1994; 65:153–5.

115. Vallee M, MacCari S, Dellu F, Simon H, Le Moal M, Mayo W. Long–term effects of prenatal stress and postnatal handling on age–related glucocorticoid secretion and cognitive performance: a longitudinal study in the rat. Eur J Neurosci 1999; 11:2906–16.

116. Meaney M, Seckl J. Glucocorticoid programming. Ann N Y Acad Sci 2004; 1032:63–84.

117. Roughton EC, Schneider ML, Bromley LJ, Coe CL. Maternal endocrine activation during pregnancy alters neurobehavioral state in primate infants. Am J Occup Ther 1998; 52:90–8.

118. Schneider M, Moore C, Kraemer G. Moderate level alcohol during pregnancy, prenatal stress, or both and limbic–hypothalamic–pituitary–adrenocortical axis response to stress in rhesus monkeys. Child Dev 2004; 75:96–109.

119. Schneider ML. Prenatal stress exposure alters postnatal behavioral expression under conditions of novelty challenge in rhesus monkey infants. Dev Psychobiol 1992; 25:529–40.

120. McEwen BS. Glucocorticoid–biogenic amine interactions in relation to mood and behavior. Biochem Pharmacol 1987; 36:1755–63.

121. Maes M, Meltzer HY, D'Hondt P, Cosyns P, Blockx P. Effects of serotonin precursors on the negative feedback effects of glucocorticoids on hypothalamic–pituitary–adrenal axis function in depression. Psychoneuroendocrinology 1995; 20:149–67.

122. Meador–Woodruff JH, Greden JF, Grunhaus L, Haskett RF. Severity of depression and hypothalamic–pituitary–adrenal axis dysregulation: identification of contributing factors. Acta Psychiatr Scand 1990; 81:364–71.

123. Nemeroff CB, Widerlov E, Bissette G, Walleus H, Karlsson I, Eklund K, Kilts CD, Loosen PT, Vale W. Elevated concentrations of CSF corticotropin–releasing factor–like immunoreactivity in depressed patients. Science 1984; 226(4680):1342–4.

124. van Praag HM. Depression. Lancet 1982; 2:1259–64.

125. Wadhwa PD, Garite TJ, Porto M, Glynn L, Chicz-DeMet A, Dunkel-Schetter C, Sandman CA. Placental corticotropin–releasing hormone (CRH), spontaneous preterm birth, and fetal growth restriction: a prospective investigation. Am J Obstet Gynecol 2004; 191:1063–9.

126. Wadhwa PD, Sandman CA, Garite TJ. The neurobiology of stress in human pregnancy: implications for prematurity and development of the fetal central nervous system. Prog Brain Res 2001; 133:131–42.

127. Lou HC, Hansen D, Nordentoft M, Pryds O, Jensen F, Nim J, Hemmingsen R. Prenatal stressors of human life affect fetal brain development. Dev Med Child Neurol 1994; 36:826–32.

128. van Os J, Selten J. Prenatal exposure to maternal stress and subsequent schizophrenia. Br J Psychiatry 1998; 172:324–6.

129. Field T. Stress and coping from pregnancy through the postnatal period. In: Cummings EG, Greene AL, eds. Life–Span developmental psychology: perspectives on stress and coping. Hillsdale, NJ: Lawrence Erlbaum Associates; 199:45–59.

130. Huizink AC, Robles de Medina PG, Mulder EJ, Visser GH, Buitelaar JK. Stress during pregnancy is associated with developmental outcome in infancy. J Child Psychol Psychiatry 2003; 44:810–8.

131. Levy–Shiff R, Dimitrovsky L, Shulman S, et al. Cognitive appraisals, coping strategies, and support resources as correlates of parenting and infant development. Dev Psychobiol 1998; 34:1417–27.

132. Meijer A. Child psychiatric sequelae of maternal war stress. Acta Psychiatr Scand 1985; 72:505–11.

133. Stott DH. Follow–up study from birth of the effects of prenatal stresses. Dev Med Child Neurol 1973; 15:770–87.

134. Ward AJ. Prenatal stress and childhood psychopathology. Child Psychiatry Hum Dev 1991; 22:97–110.

135. DePietro J. The role of prenatal maternal stress in child development. Current Directions in Psychological Science 2004; 13:71–4.

136. McEwen BS. Protective and damaging effects of stress mediators. N Engl J Med 1998; 338:171–9.

137. McEwen BS. Early life influences on life–long patterns of behavior and health. Ment Retard Dev Disabil Res Rev 2003; 9:149–54.

138. Meyer JS. Biochemical effects of corticosteroids on neural tissues. Physiol Rev 1985; 65:946–1020.

139. Benediktsson R, Lindsay RS, Noble J, Seckl JR, Edwards CR. Glucocorticoid exposure in utero: new model for adult hypertension. Lancet 1993; 341:339–41.

140. McTernan CL, Draper N, Nicholson H, Chalder SM, Driver P, Hewison M, Kilby MD, Stewart PM. Reduced placental 11beta–hydroxysteroid dehydrogenase type 2 mRNA levels in human pregnancies complicated by intrauterine growth restriction: an analysis of possible mechanisms. J Clin Endocrinol Metab 2001; 86:4979–83.

141. Murphy VE, Zakar T, Smith R, Giles WB, Gibson PG, Clifton VL. Reduced 11beta–hydroxysteroid dehydrogenase type 2 activity is associated with decreased birth weight centile in pregnancies complicated by asthma. J Clin Endocrinol Metab 2002; 87:1660–8.

142. Shams M, Kilby MD, Somerset DA, Howie AJ, Gupta A, Wood PJ, et al. 11Beta–hydroxysteroid dehydrogenase type 2 in human pregnancy and reduced expression in intrauterine growth restriction. Hum Reprod 1998; 13:799–804.

143. Stewart P, Roberson F, Mason J. Type 2 11–hydroxysteroid dehydrogenase messenger RNA and activity in human placenta and fetal membranes: its relationship to birth weight and putative role in fetal steroidogenesis. J Clin Endocrinol Metab 1995; 80:885–90.

144. Dave–Sharma S, Wilson R, Harbison M. Extensive personal experience: examination of genotype and phenotype relationships in 14 patients with apparent mineralocorticoid excess. J Clin Endocrinol Metab 1998; 83:2244–54.

145. Seckl JR, Cleasby M, Nyirenda MJ. Glucocorticoids, 11beta–hydroxysteroid dehydrogenase, and fetal programming. Kidney Int. 2000; 57:1412–7.

146. Edwards CR, Benediktsson R, Lindsay RS, Seckl JR. Dysfunction of placental glucocorticoid barrier: link between fetal environment and adult hypertension? Lancet 1993; 341:355–7.

147. Seckl JR. Glucocorticoids, feto–placental 11 beta–hydroxysteroid dehydrogenase type 2, and the early life origins of adult disease. Steroids 1997; 62:89–94.

148. Bohn MC. Granule cell genesis in the hippocampus of rats treated neonatally with hydrocortisone. Neuroscience 1980; 5:2003–12.

149. Gould E, Woolley CS, Cameron HA, Daniels DC, McEwen BS. Adrenal steroids regulate postnatal development of the rat dentate gyrus: II. Effects of glucocorticoids and mineralocorticoids on cell birth. J Comp Neurol 1991; 313:486–93.

150. Gould E, Woolley CS, McEwen BS. Adrenal steroids regulate postnatal development of the rat dentate gyrus: I. Effects of glucocorticoids on cell death. J Comp Neurol 1991; 313:479–85.

151. Bottalico B, Larsson I, Brodszki J, Hernandez-Andrade E, Casslen B, Marsal K, Hansson SR. Norepinephrine transporter (NET), serotonin transporter (SERT), vesicular monoamine transporter (VMAT2) and organic cation transporters (OCT1, 2 and EMT) in human placenta from pre–eclamptic and normotensive pregnancies. Placenta 2004; 25:518–29.

152. Bzoskie L, Yen J, Tseng YT, Blount L, Kashiwai K, Padbury JF. Human placental norepinephrine transporter mRNA: expression and correlation with fetal condition at birth. Placenta 1997; 18:205–10.

153. Jacob S, Moley KH. Gametes and embryo epigenetic reprogramming affect developmental outcome: implication for assisted reproductive technologies. Pediatr Res 2005; 58:437–46.

154. Colvis CM, Pollock JD, Goodman RH, Impey S, Dunn J, Mandel G, Champagne PA, Mayford M, Korzus E, Kumar A, Renthal W, Theobald DE, Nestler EJ. Epigenetic mechanisms and gene networks in the nervous system. J Neurosci 2005; 25:10379–89.

155. Kumar A, Choi KH, Renthal W, Tsankova NM, Theobald DE, Truong HT, Russo SJ, Laplant Q, Sasaki TS, Whistler KN, Neve RL, Self DW, Nestler EJ. Chromatin remodeling is a key mechanism underlying cocaine–induced plasticity in striatum. Neuron 2005; 48:303–14.

156. Loeber R, Burke JD, Lahey BB, Winters A, Zera M. Oppositional defiant and conduct disorder: a review of the past 10 years, part I. J Am Acad Child Adolesc Psychiatry 2000; 39:1468–84.

157. Ellickson PL, Tucker JS, Klein DJ. High–risk behaviors associated with early smoking: results from a 5–year follow–up. J Adolesc Health 2001; 28:465–73.

158. Hawkins JD, Graham JW, Maguin E, Abbott R, Hill KG, Catalano RF. Exploring the effects of age of alcohol use initiation and psychosocial risk factors on subsequent alcohol misuse. J Stud Alcohol 1997; 58: 280–90.

159. Brook JS, Whiteman MM, Finch S. Childhood aggression, adolescent delinquency, and drug use: a longitudinal study. J Genet Psychol 1992; 153:369–83.

160. Tarter R, Vanyukov M, Giancola P, Dawes M, Blackson T, Mezzich A, Clark DB. Etiology of early age onset substance use disorder: a maturational perspective. Dev Psychopathol 1999; 11:657–83.

161. Blackson TC, Butler T, Belsky J, Ammerman RT, Shaw DS, Tarter RE. Individual traits and family contexts predict sons' externalizing behavior and preliminary relative risk ratios for conduct disorder and substance use

disorder outcomes. Drug Alcohol Depend 1999; 56:115–31.

162. Chassin L, Barrera MJ. Substance use escalation and substance use restraint among adolescent children of alcoholics. Psychol Addict Bahav 1993; 7:3–20.

163. Tarter RE, Blackson T, Brigham J, Moss H, Caprara GV. The association between childhood irritability and liability to substance use in early adolescence: a 2–year follow–up study of boys at risk for substance abuse. Drug Alcohol Depend 1995; 39:253–61.

164. Clark DB, Parker AM, Lynch KG. Psychopathology and substance–related problems during early adolescence: a survival analysis. J Clin Child Psychol 1999; 28: 333–41.

165. Aytaclar S, Tarter RE, Kirisci L, Lu S. Association between hyperactivity and executive cognitive functioning in childhood and substance use in early adolescence. J Am Acad Child Adolesc Psychiatry 1999; 38:172–8.

166. Giancola PR, Martin CS, Tarter RE, Pelham WE, Moss HB. Executive cognitive functioning and aggressive behavior in preadolescent boys at high risk for substance abuse. J Stud Alcohol 1996; 57:352–9.

167. Shoal G, Giancola P. Executive cognitive functioning, negative affectivity, and drug use in adolescent boys with and without a family history of a substance use disorder. J Child Adolesc Subst Abuse 2001; 10:111–21.

168. Tarter RE, Kirisci L, Mezzich A, Cornelius JR, Pajer K, Vanyukov M, Gardner W, Blackson T, Clark D. Neurobehavioral disinhibition in childhood predicts early age at onset of substance use disorder. Am J Psychiatry 2003; 160:1078–85.

169. Volkow ND, Li TK. Drugs and alcohol: treating and preventing abuse, addiction and their medical consequences. Pharmacol Ther 2005; 108:3–17.

170. Sowell ER, Thompson PM, Peterson BS, Mattson SN, Welcome SE, Henkenius AL, Riley EP, Jernigan TL, Toga AW. Mapping cortical gray matter asymmetry patterns in adolescents with heavy prenatal alcohol exposure. Neuroimage 2002; 17:1807–19.

171. Sowell ER, Thompson PM, Toga AW. Mapping changes in the human cortex throughout the span of life. Neuroscientist 2004; 10:372–92.

172. Barnea–Goraly N, Eliez S, Menon V, Bammer R, Reiss AL. Arithmetic ability and parietal alterations: a diffusion tensor imaging study in velocardiofacial syndrome. Brain Res Cogn Brain Res 2005; 25:735–40.

173. Giedd J. Brain development, IX: human brain growth. Am J Psychiatry 1999; 156:4.

174. Paus T, Zijdenbos A, Worsley K, Collins DL, Blumenthal J, Giedd JN, et al. Structural maturation of neural pathways in children and adolescents: in vivo study. Science 1999; 283:1908–11.

175. Bauer LO, Hesselbrock VM. P300 decrements in teenagers with conduct problems: implications for substance abuse risk and brain development. Biol Psychiatry 1999; 46:263–72.

176. Giancola P, Tarter R. Executive cognitive functioning and risk for substance abuse. Psychol Sci 1999; 10:203–5.

177. Schweinsburg AD, Paulus MP, Barlett VC, Killeen LA, Caldwell LC, Pulido C, Brown SA, Tapert SF. An FMRI study of response inhibition in youths with a family history of alcoholism. Ann N Y Acad Sci 2004; 1021:391–4.

178. Chambers RA, Taylor JR, Potenza MN. Developmental neurocircuitry of motivation in adolescence: a critical period of addiction vulnerability. Am J Psychiatry 2003; 160:1041–52.

179. Fuster JM. Executive frontal functions. Exp Brain Res 2000; 133:66–70.

180. Spear L. Neurobehavioral changes in adolescence. Curr Dir Psycholog Sci 2000; 9:111–4.

181. Romeo RD, McEwen BS. Stress and the adolescent brain. Ann N Y Acad Sci 2006; 1094:202–14.

182. Diorio D, Viau V, Meaney MJ. The role of the medial prefrontal cortex (cingulate gyrus) in the regulation of hypothalamic–pituitary–adrenal responses to stress. J Neurosci 1993; 13:3839–47.

183. McEwen BS, De Kloet ER, Rostene W. Adrenal steroid receptors and actions in the nervous system. Physiol Rev 1986; 66:1121–88.

184. Meaney MJ, Aitken DH. [3H]Dexamethasone binding in rat frontal cortex. Brain Res 1985; 328:176–80.

185. Patel PD, Lopez JF, Lyons DM, Burke S, Wallace M, Schatzberg AF. Glucocorticoid and mineralocorticoid receptor mRNA expression in squirrel monkey brain. J Psychiatr Res 2000; 34:383–92.

186. Sanchez MM, Young LJ, Plotsky PM, Insel TR. Distribution of corticosteroid receptors in the rhesus brain: relative absence of glucocorticoid receptors in the hippocampal formation. J Neurosci 2000; 20:4657–68.

187. Chelonis JJ, Gillam MP, Paule MG. The effects of prenatal cocaine exposure on reversal learning using a simple visual discrimination task in rhesus monkeys. Neurotoxicol Teratol 2003; 25:437–46.

188. Paule MG, Gillam MP, Allen RR, Chelonis JJ. Effects of chronic in utero exposure to cocaine on behavioral adaptability in rhesus monkey offspring when examined in adulthood. Ann N Y Acad Sci 2000; 914:412–7.

189. Isgor C, Kabbaj M, Akil H, Watson SJ. Delayed effects of chronic variable stress during peripubertal–juvenile period on hippocampal morphology and on cognitive and stress axis functions in rats. Hippocampus 2004; 14:636–48.

190. McEwen BS. Glucocorticoids, depression, and mood disorders: structural remodeling in the brain. Metabolism 2005; 54(5 Suppl 1):20–3.

191. Radley JJ, Rocher AB, Miller M, Janssen WG, Liston C, Hof PR, McEwen BS, Morrison JH. Repeated stress induces dendritic spine loss in the rat medial prefrontal cortex. Cereb Cortex 2006; 16:313–20.

Index

Page numbers in *Italics* represent tables.
Page numbers in **Bold** represent figures.

academic and social challenges 142
acamprosate 95–6
acquired immune deficiency syndrome (AIDS) 1; women 19, *see also* human immunodeficiency virus (HIV)
addiction: health concern 125; treatment 1; women's history 1
addiction groups 21; gender 21
Addiction Survey Index (ASI) 38
adrenocorticotrophic hormone (ACTH) 155
African American women 80
alcohol 17, 29; postpartum 66; preconception 66; pregnancy 66
Alcohol Use Disorder Identification Test (AUDIT) 66
alcohol withdrawal syndrome 75
America: anti-drug legislation 7
American Academy of Pediatrics 66, 92, 125, 135
American Academy of Pediatrics Task Force 135
American College of Obstetricians and Gynecologists 60
American Diabetes Association 31
American Gynecological Society 6
American Heart Association (AHA) 30
American Medical Association (AMA) 125, 126
American Psychiatric Association 125
American Society of Addiction Medicine 125
amphetamines: postpartum 71; preconception 70; pregnancy 71
Anslinger, H. 8
anthropometric growth 136
Anti-Drug Abuse Act 10
Anti-Drug Abuse Amendment 10
anti-drug legislation 7
Attention Deficit Hyperactivity Disorder (ADHD) 3, 154
autonomy 56–7; beneficence 57–9; physician's obligations 57; pregnant women 58

Bandstra, E.S.: *et al* 147
barbiturate 69
Bayley MDI scores **152**
Bayley Scales of Infant Development (BSID) 138; Mental Development Index (MDI) 138; Psychomotor Development Index (PDI) 138
behavior problems 148; Child Behavior Checklist 148
behavioral dysregulation 157
Belcher, L.: *et al* 85
Bendersky, M.: and Lewis, M. 137
beneficence autonomy 57–9
beneficence enforcement 59
benzodiazepine 68
Berghalla, V.: *et al* 134
Beth Israel Medical Center: MMT program 98
Billie's Place 98
biophysical profile: ultrasound 74
body mass index (BMI) 73
Boedicker, A.E.: and Westmeyer, J. 18
Bolivia: cocaine 6
Booth, R.E.: *et al* 82
brain development: adolescents 157
brain function: heroin 39
Brazelton Neonatal Behavioral Assessment Scale (BNBAS) 136
breast cancer 32, 35; cases 27; tobacco 35
buprenorphine 108–9; methadone 109
buprenorphine exposure during pregnancy *111*

caffeine: postpartum 66; preconception 65; pregnancy 65
cardiovascular disease 30, 35; tobacco 35
Carey, M.P.: *et al* 84–5
catechol-O-methyl transferase gene (COMT) 91
Center for Substance Abuse Treatment: Consensus Panel 134
Centers for Disease Control and Prevention (CDC) 66; HIV screening 82
central nervous system (CNS) 65; depression 96
cervical cancer: human papillomavirus (HPV) 36
Child Abuse Prevention and Treatment Act (CAPTA) 127
Child Behavior Checklist 152
childbearing age: substance abuse 63
childcare 20
China: opium dens 7; Opium Wars 5
chronic liver disease 75
Chronic Obstructive Pulmonary Disease (COPD) 34–5; deaths 35; tobacco 34–5
cocaine: Bolivia 6; Peru 6; postpartum 70; preconception 69; pregnancy 69–70
cocaine/crack: passive exposure 60
Columbia University: Center on Addiction and Substance Abuse 120
Comprehensive Crime Control Act 10
contraction stress testing 74
Controlled Substances Act 127
Copeland, A.L.: and Sorenson, J.L. 83
coronary heart disease 30
corticosterone (CORT) 155
covariates 149
Covington, C.Y.: *et al* 136
crime: heroin 5
Cut down, Annoyed, Guilty, Eye-opener (CAGE) 33

cytochrome P-450 (CYP) 107

de Cubas, M.M.: and Field, T. 153
Department of Justice 122
dependence: progression 18
depression 19; women 19
detoxification 9
developed neonatal abstinence signs (NAS) 110
development: cognitive and motor 137–8
developmental delay 72
diabetes mellitus 31
disulfiram 95
Dole, V. 94
Drug Abuse Treatment Outcome Studies (DATOS) 95
drug effects: infants 141–3
Drug Enforcement Agency 98
drug interactions 107; gender 107
drug use 15; costs 27; gender 15; poverty and crime 12; pregnancy 63; research 15; revulsion 56; sexuality 8, 9

Eighth Amendment 59
endometrial cancer 36; tobacco use 36
enforcement: beneficence 59
Epidemiologic Data 16
esophageal cancer: studies 37
ethical principles 56
Exner, T.M.: *et al* 83–4
Eyler, F.D.: *et al* 136

family dysfunction 60
Federal Bureau of Narcotics 8
fetal: health 28; programming 155–6; rights 55; withdrawal symptoms 109
fetal alcohol spectrum disorder (FASD) 66
fetal/neonatal cerebral cavitary lesions 71
field cancerization theory 41
Field, T.: and de Cubas, M.M. 153
Finnegan, L.P.: *et al* 112
Finnegan Neonatal Abstinence Score 135
Fischer, G.: *et al* 110
Flavin, J.: and Paltrow, L.M. 2–3
Food and Drug Administration Fetal Risk Summary 68

gender: biological response 17; cocaine experience 17; medical consequences 18–19; medical problems 18; opioids 106; susceptibility 106
gene expression 156; drugs 156
genital/urinary cancer 33
Genome Era 158
Gordon Maze 149
government: research funding 4
Great Britain: Opium Wars 5
growth restriction: placental insufficiency 73
gynecological complaints 7

Hargreaves, W.A. 94
Harrison Act 11
health care: pregnant women 53
Health and Human Services Department 11
health insurance 20
Healthy Moms Trial 66
hepatitis B 67
hepatitis C 67
Hernandez, T.L. 121–2
heroin: brain function 39
high-risk subpopulations 22
highly active antiretroviral therapy (HAART) 83; regimen 83
Hispanic women 80
Home Observation Measure of the Environment 150
human immunodeficiency virus (HIV) 1, 19; American women 80; intervention 84; risk behavior 83; risk reduction 21; substance abuse 81; women 19, *see also* acquired immune deficiency syndrome (AIDS)
human papillomavirus (HPV): cervical cancer 36
hypothalamic-pituitary-adrenal axis (HPA) 90; neuroendocrine environment 155

in utero exposure 1
incarceration rates 12
infant neurobehavior: deficits 3, 142; visual and auditory function 136–7
infertility 37, 64
Information-Motivation-Behavior model 84
intimate partner violence 42
intrauterine growth restriction (IUGR) 70
intravenous drug users (IVDUs) 92

John Harvey Kellogg clinic 8
Johnson, J. 124
Johnson, R.E.: *et al* 107
Joint Commission on the Accreditation of Healthcare Organizations (JCAHO) 98
Jones, H.E.: *et al* 107
justice 57; pursuit 59–60

Kakko, J.: *et al* 113
Kandall, S.R.: *et al* 134
Keeley institute 8
King, R. 127
Knox Cube 149
Korsten, T.R. 94

labetolol 76
labour: management 75
language 148; development 138
Lee, H. 7
LeJeune, C.: *et al* 110
levomethadyl acetate (LAAM) 106
Lewis, M.: and Bendersky, M. 137
Lim, S. 112
Lipsitz score 113
liver disease 29–30
Long Day's Journey into Night (O'Neill) 7
long QT syndrome (LQTS) 108
lung cancer 32, 34; tobacco 34

McCarthy, J.J.: *et al* 113
McCarthy scales 153
McKnight, R. 123
magnetic resonance imaging (MRI) 151
magnetic resonance spectroscopy (MRS) 151
Manhattan General Hospital 88
marijuana: postpartum 72; preconception 71; pregnancy 71–2
Maryland Court of Appeals 127
maternal drug use: science 124
maternal morbidity **I** 63; illicit use **I** 63
Maternal Opioid Treatment: Human Experimental Research (MOTHER) 111; international study 114; study 2, 113
maternal psychiatric treatment 152

maternal rights 56
Maxwell, S.: and Shinderman, S. 94
medical consequences: gender 18–19
Medical Eligibility Criteria for Contraceptive Use: World Health Organization (WHO) 97
medical treatment: gender 106–7
Medical University of South Carolina 58
Mendelian genetics 150
menopause 20
mental retardation 72
methadone: buprenorphine 109; drug codependency 94–6; maintenance 12; overdose 93; pharmacology 91–3; retention 93–4
methadone maintenance treatment (MMT) 88; medical issues 96; patients 93; safety 89
Michigan Alcoholism Screening Test 33
molecular genetics 90–1
morphine 109
Morrow, C.E.: *et al* 136–7
Mortimer, W.G. 7

N-methyl-D-aspartate (NMDA) 91
Narcotics Unit of the Treasury Department 8
National Advocates for Pregnant Women 120, 126
National Coalition for Child Protection Reform 122
National Council on Alcoholism and Drug Dependence 125
National Institute on Drug Abuse (NIDA) 10, 121
National Institutes of Health (NIH) 28; Consensus Panel 134; Infant Development Environment and Lifestyle (IDEAL) 152
National Osteoporosis Foundation: osteoporosis 32
National Survey of Drug Use and Health (NSDUH) 52, 63–4; pregnant women survey 133–4; Substance Abuse and Mental Health Services Office 16
neonatal: death 53; withdrawal 67
neonatal abstinence syndrome (NAS) 1, 112–13; methadone 114; pilot studies 111–12
neurasthenia 6
neurobiological studies 89–90; gender 89–90
neuroimaging 151–2; resonance spectroscopy 153; study 154
New York State Council on Children 11
New York State Department of Health 98
New York State Office of Substance Abuse Services 98
New York Times 122
nicotine 17; gender 17
NICU Network Neurobehavioral Scale 137
norepinephrine transporter (NET) 156
Norsigian, J. 28

obesity 31; alcohol 31
O'Neill, E. 7
O'Neill, K.: *et al* 85
opiates: children 154; development 147; neurobiological aspects 89; opioids 40; prenatal exposure 153
opioids 38; international treatment 115; neurological consequences 38–9; opiates 40; postpartum 68; preconception 66–7; pregnancy 67–8; telescoping 38
Opium Wars: China 5; Great Britain 5
osteoporosis 31–2; National Osteoporosis Foundation 32
Ostrea, E.M.: *et al* 112
Our Bodies, Ourselves (Norsigian) 28
ovarian cancer 36; tobacco 36

Paltrow, L.M.: and Flavin, J. 2–3
Peabody Picture Vocabulary Test 138
perinatal substance abuse: criminalization 55, 59
perinatal substance exposure *54*
Perkins, C.A. 18; cessation trials 18
Peru: cocaine 6
pharmacokinetic interaction 92
pharmacology: methadone 91
physiological effects: stimulants 40–1
physiology: stimulants 41
Pierce, R.V. 6
placental abruptions 69
placental insufficiency: growth restriction 73
positron-emission tomography (PET) 95
postnatal: confounding variables 150; substance abuse 52
poverty and crime: drug use 12
pregnancy: abuse management 72; civil rights 126–7; drug use 63; treatment 82
pregnant women: autonomy 58; health care 53–4
prenatal cocaine exposure (PCE) *139–40*; mechanisms 141
prenatal confounding variables 150
prenatal drug exposure 3; understanding 155
prenatal glucocorticoid 156
prenatal opiates 153
Prenatal Protection Act 127
prescription painkillers 17; Substance Abuse and Mental Health Services Administration (SAMHSA) 38; women 17
preterm birth 53
prevention services **142**
primate studies 158
prison treatment programmes 21
propofol 76
psychiatric disorders 19
psychological effects: stimulants 41–2
psychopathology 148; developmental 141
psychophysiology 149
psychosocial intervention 64
punishment: problems 122–4
Pure Food and Drug Act 8

race and class bias 121
relationships 149
reproductive system: tobacco 36
Revolutionary War 5
Richardson, G.A.: *et al* 136
Robert Wood Johnson Foundation: Substance Abuse Policy Research Program 55
Rockefeller: General Hospital 88; Institute for Medical Research 88; Institute in New York 9
Rosen, D.: and Tolman, R.M 42
Rubin, D.H. 60

Schindler, S.D.: *et al* 110
Schottenfeld, R.S.: *et al* 107
sedative-hypnotics: postpartum 69; preconception 68–9; pregnancy 69
Self-Administered Screening Test 33
Sequenced Inventory of Communicative Development-Revised (SICD-R) 138
sex risk behavior 81
sexual abuse: children 21
sexuality: drug use 8, 9
Shankaran, S.: *et al* 136
Shinderman, S.: and Maxwell, S. 94
Sorenson, J.L.: and Copeland, A.L. 83

stillbirth 53
stimulants 40; physiology 41; physiological effects 40–1; psychological effects 41–2
stress: reactivity 158
Stroop Task 149
substance abuse: childbearing age 63; epidemic 52
Substance Abuse and Mental Health Services Administration (SAMHSA) 29, 98; prescription drugs 38
Substance Abuse Policy Research Program: Robert Wood Johnson Foundation 55
substance use disorders: screening 29
Sudden Infant Death Syndrome (SIDS) 37; Policy Statement 135
Supreme Court of Florida 124

telescoping 22; cocaine 40; OPIOIDS 38
teratogenic exposure 72
The House of Mirth (Wharton) 7
The Snake Pit (Ward) 9
Thomas, T.G. 6
thrombocytopenia 76
To Kill a Mockingbird (Lee) 7
tobacco: postpartum 65; preconception 64; pregnancy 64–5; reproductive system 36
Tolerance, Annoyed, Cut-down, Eye-opener (T-ACE) 33
Tolerance, Worry, Eye-Opener, Amnesia, Cut-down (TWEAK) 33
Tolman, R.M: and Rosen, D. 42
torsade de pointes ventricular tachycardia (TdP) 108
Toth, A.R.: and Varga, T. 39
Trail Making 149
treatment: funding 27; interventions 22; programs 21

ultrasound: biophysical profile 74
United Nations (UN): Millenium Development Goals 105
United States Preventative Services Task Force 66
U.S. Food and Drug Administration (FDA) 91
U.S. Sentencing Commission 121

Varga, T.: and Toth, A.R. 39
Vaughan, B. 123
A Voice in the Wilderness (Weed) 7

Ward, M.J. 9
Weed, M. 7
Western society: women's role 89
Westmeyer, J.: and Boedicker, A.E. 18
Wharton, E. 7
Whitner, C. 120–1; child abuse 127
withdrawal symptoms: management 76
women: acquired immune deficiency syndrome (AIDS) 19; bodily integrity 119; human immunodeficiency virus (HIV) 19; liberty 119; midlife 19–20; prosecution 11; treatment entry 20
Women's Movement 10
women's social movement 28
World Health Organization (WHO) 42; barrier methods 97; Gender Policy 105; Medical Eligibility Criteria for Contraceptive Use 97
Wright, H. 8

Yu, L. 90

zidovudine (AZT) 11